GW01081094

Parasitology and Microbiology Research

Edited by Gilberto Antonio Bastidas Pacheco
and Asghar Ali Kamboh

Published in London, United Kingdom

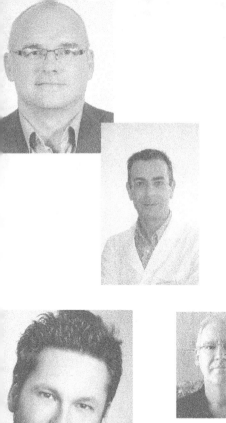
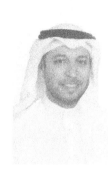
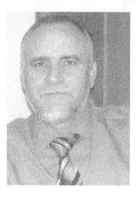
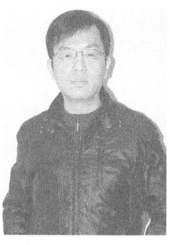
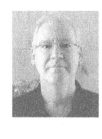
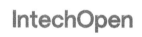
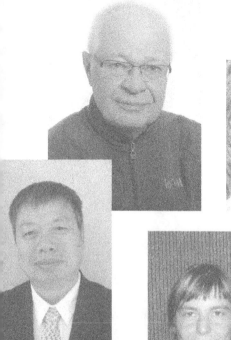
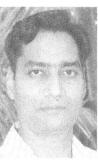
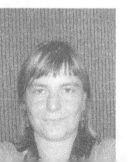
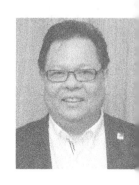
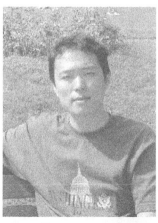

IntechOpen

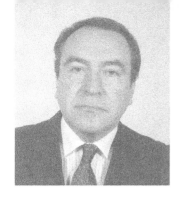
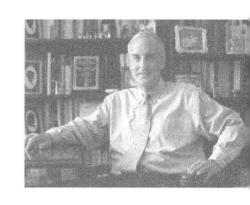
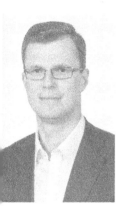
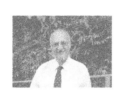
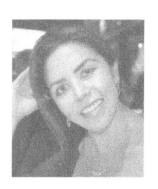

Supporting open minds since 2005

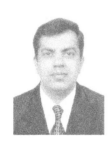
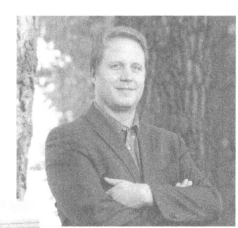
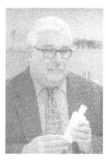
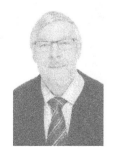
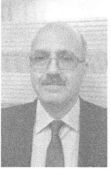
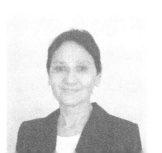
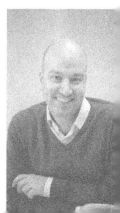

Parasitology and Microbiology Research
http://dx.doi.org/10.5772/intechopen.82990
Edited by Gilberto Antonio Bastidas Pacheco and Asghar Ali Kamboh

Contributors

Carlos Vicente, María-Estrella Legaz, Elena Sánchez-Elordi, Eva Díaz, Rae Robertson-Anderson, Shea Ricketts, Bekele Gurmessa, Nour Mammari, Mohamad Adnan Halabi, Haseeb Anwar, Shahzad Irfan, Ghulam Hussain, Humaira Muzaffar, Imran Mukhtar, Imtiaz Mustafa, Saima Malik, Muhammad Irfan Ullah, Muhammad Naeem Faisal, Helena Lucia Carneiro Santos, Karina Mastropasqua Rebello, Teresa Cristina Bergamo Bomfim, Harris Bernstein, Carol Bernstein, Muhammad Sarwar, Kailash Pandey, Rahul Pasupureddy, Sriram Seshadri, Rajnikant Dixit, Greanious Alfred Alfred Mavondo, Blessing Nkazimulo Mkhwanazi, Mayibongwe Mzingwane, Obadiah Moyo, Joy Mavondo, Francis Farai Chikuse, Blessing Zambuko, Rachael Dangarembizi, Tariroyashe Mpofu, Greanious Alfred Mavondo, Colleen Runyararo Emily Rakabopa, Valeria Regia Franco Sousa, Arleana Almeida, Naiani Gasparetto, Maria Elena Villagrán Herrera, Susanta Ghosh, Pradeep Kumar Srivastava, Alpana Mukhuty, Chandrani Fouzder, Snehasis Das, Dipanjan Chattopadhyay, Salwa S Sheikh, Amaar Amir, Baraa Amir, Abdulrazack Amir, Eduardo Gómez-Conde, Miguel Ángel Vargas Mejía, María Alicia Díaz-Orea, Luis David Gómez-Cortes, Tayde Guerrero Gonzalez, Eduardo França, Jose Nivaldo Da Silva, Adenilda Cristina Honorio-França, José De La Fuente, José Francisco Lima Barbero, Margarita Villar, Ursula Höfle, Adenilda Honorio-Franca, Saulo Pereira Cardoso, Giane Regina Paludo, Ricardo Francisco Mercado-Curiel, José Trinidad López-Vázquez, Maria del Carmen Aburto-Fernández, Nicolás Camacho-Calderón, Javier Ávila-Morales, José Antonio De Diego-Cabrera

© The Editor(s) and the Author(s) 2020
The rights of the editor(s) and the author(s) have been asserted in accordance with the Copyright, Designs and Patents Act 1988. All rights to the book as a whole are reserved by INTECHOPEN LIMITED. The book as a whole (compilation) cannot be reproduced, distributed or used for commercial or non-commercial purposes without INTECHOPEN LIMITED's written permission. Enquiries concerning the use of the book should be directed to INTECHOPEN LIMITED rights and permissions department (permissions@intechopen.com).
Violations are liable to prosecution under the governing Copyright Law.

Individual chapters of this publication are distributed under the terms of the Creative Commons Attribution 3.0 Unported License which permits commercial use, distribution and reproduction of the individual chapters, provided the original author(s) and source publication are appropriately acknowledged. If so indicated, certain images may not be included under the Creative Commons license. In such cases users will need to obtain permission from the license holder to reproduce the material. More details and guidelines concerning content reuse and adaptation can be found at http://www.intechopen.com/copyright-policy.html.

Notice
Statements and opinions expressed in the chapters are these of the individual contributors and not necessarily those of the editors or publisher. No responsibility is accepted for the accuracy of information contained in the published chapters. The publisher assumes no responsibility for any damage or injury to persons or property arising out of the use of any materials, instructions, methods or ideas contained in the book.

First published in London, United Kingdom, 2020 by IntechOpen
IntechOpen is the global imprint of INTECHOPEN LIMITED, registered in England and Wales, registration number: 11086078, 7th floor, 10 Lower Thames Street, London, EC3R 6AF, United Kingdom
Printed in Croatia

British Library Cataloguing-in-Publication Data
A catalogue record for this book is available from the British Library

Additional hard and PDF copies can be obtained from orders@intechopen.com

Parasitology and Microbiology Research
Edited by Gilberto Antonio Bastidas Pacheco and Asghar Ali Kamboh
p. cm.
Print ISBN 978-1-78985-901-0
Online ISBN 978-1-78985-902-7
eBook (PDF) ISBN 978-1-83880-737-5

We are IntechOpen,
the world's leading publisher of
Open Access books
Built by scientists, for scientists

4,900+
Open access books available

123,000+
International authors and editors

140M+
Downloads

Our authors are among the

151
Countries delivered to

Top 1%
most cited scientists

12.2%
Contributors from top 500 universities

WEB OF SCIENCE™

Selection of our books indexed in the Book Citation Index
in Web of Science™ Core Collection (BKCI)

Interested in publishing with us?
Contact book.department@intechopen.com

Numbers displayed above are based on latest data collected.
For more information visit www.intechopen.com

Meet the editors

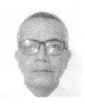 Prof. Bastidas is a physician with degrees in Pre-hospital Emergency Care, Executive Direction for Senior Management in Health, and Occupational Health and Safety. With a Health Management Course equivalent to the Public Health Middle Course; Magister Scientise in Education Management and also in Protozoology, Prof. Bastidas holds a Ph.D. in Parasitology. He is a full professor in the Faculty of Health Sciences, Department of Public Health, University of Carabobo, Valencia, Venezuela. He has authored several articles published in national and international journals. He is also an arbitrator of scientific articles, member of the editorial committees of several journals, and a textbook writer and lecturer.

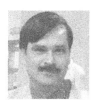 Dr. Asghar Ali Kamboh was born in Mehrabpur, Sindh, Pakistan in 1979. He completed his studies in Veterinary Medicine and Masters in Veterinary Microbiology in 2003 and 2007 respectively, with distinguished grades. In 2009, he was awarded an oversees scholarship by the Government of Pakistan and proceeded to China for doctoral studies. Currently, he is working as an Associate Professor and Chairperson of the Department of Veterinary Microbiology, Sindh Agriculture University, Tandojam. He has published more than 80 research and review articles in national and international peer reviewed journals. He has supervised/co-supervised more than 30 M.Phil students. He is also the author of many books and book chapters. In addition, he is an editor/editorial board member of many scholarly journals in the area of animal health and production.

Contents

Preface

The analysis of ribosomal sequences of parasitic life agents has shown the extreme differentiation of the groups to which they belong, with distances magnitudes greater than those observed between mammals and fish. Hence there is a need for continuous research of the different aspects that determine parasitic life. These include microbial and parasite biology, ecophysiology, genetics, and molecular biology. In addition, knowledge of the pathogenesis, epidemiology, symptomatology, immune reaction, diagnosis, treatment, and prevention of parasitic diseases is of the utmost importance.

It is absolutely clear that systematic research is the only way to unveil the intricate mechanisms involved in parasitic associations. For example, with description of the direct dependence of the parasite on the genetic expressions of the hosts, with the adaptive convergences among which include the successful evasion of the immune system (to the point of not being considered strange), and with the chemical dialogue, so to speak, that occurs between molecules, specifically, in the molecular exchange. Likewise, research has shown parasitism as the basic mechanism that allowed the differentiation of eukaryotes.

It should be understood that variability as a result of genetic and phenotypic adaptation is key in parasitism in order to maintain the species, which ranges from microscopic to macroscopic organisms, with multiple forms of reproduction. The study of the antagonistic association that defines parasitism is fascinating and essential, particularly the physiological aspects, biochemical interdependence, and loss or mutual acquisition of genetic information.

In this sense, this book brings together in three sections current information in the fields of microbiology and parasitology. The first section covers aspects of cytokines and receptors on parasites and microbes. In the second section we dive into the study of the biology of parasites and microbes. Finally, in the third section we discuss the state of the art of parasitic diseases. I would like to acknowledge the extraordinary investigative work carried out by the chapter authors as well as their great commitment to enriching world knowledge on such an interesting subject. Finally, I express my sincere thanks to the IntechOpen publishing team for their advice in all stages of the construction of this book.

Gilberto Bastidas
Department of Public Health and Center for Medical
and Biotechnological Research,
Faculty of Health Sciences,
University of Carabobo,
Venezuela

Asghar Ali Kamboh
Sindh Agriculture University,
Pakistan

Section 1

Cytocises and Receptors on Parasites and Microbes

Chapter 1

Role of the Cytoskeletal Actomyosin Complex in the Motility of Cyanobacteria and Fungal Spores

Elena Sánchez-Elordi, Eva María Díaz, Carlos Vicente and María Estrella Legaz

Abstract

This study demonstrates the involvement of the cytoskeleton in the movement of cyanobacteria and fungal spores to their hosts to establish a state of symbiosis or pathogenicity. The term symbiosis sensu lato is referred not only to commensalism and mutualism but also to the parasitic aberrations. The establishment of association implies that the endohabitant can move on a wet surface until finding an entry point in the exohabitant surface. In aqueous media, the exohabitant secretes glycoproteins that form a chemoattraction gradient for the invading cells. In lichens, the gradient consists of fungal lectins whose function is to recognize a compatible green alga or cyanobacterium. In the case of pathogens, the secreted proteins usually are a mixture that includes false quorum and chemoattractant signals, and cell wall digestive enzymes. The results indicate that fungal lectins and defense proteins bind to specific cell wall receptors for signaling the activation of cytoskeleton, causing successive cycles of cell contraction-relaxation that permits the migration of the endohabitant. In this study, different biochemical and microscopy techniques have been used. The mechanisms through which the cytoskeleton carries out these cycles of cell contractionrelaxation are described, being this a remarkable advance compared to previous results.

Keywords: actin, chemotaxis, cytoskeleton, lichens, motility, myosin, *Nostoc*, pathogens, *Sporisorium*

1. Introduction

The main interactions between plants include epiphytism, mutualism, commensalism, and parasitism, although the frontier between these types of association can be confusing [1]. For example, most epiphytes do not negatively influence their phytophores since they absorb water and nutrients directly from the atmosphere [2]. It is the case of many bromeliads or the crassulaceae *Aeonium arboreum*, growing on the *Phoenix dactylifera* stipe without damaging it (**Figure 1A**), although in some cases, drift toward parasitism is evident, as has been demonstrated by Montaña et al. [3] for epiphytic Bromeliads growing upon *Cercidium praecox*. Many

IntechOpen

lichens are also epiphytic, although they can behave as hemiparasitic if the phytophore is vitally weakened by environmental circumstances, such as drought or severe air pollution (**Figure 1B**). Examples include *Evernia prunastri* growing on *Quercus rotundifolia* [4] or on *Betula pendula* [5]. In other cases, nonlichenized fungi are decidedly parasites (**Figure 1C**).

In this respect, lichens, traditionally considered as an example of mutual symbiosis, exhibit a characteristic that can lead to a decided parasitism: the specificity between symbionts. The fungus selectively chooses individuals from an algal species from its surroundings to form the thallus, while those from other different species will be rejected. This implies that a fungus susceptible to lichenization is able to discriminate between compatible or incompatible algae: the former will form the association while the latter will be eliminated [6]. The argument can be further complicated: if the algae that make up the association split up inside an established thallus, the newly hatched algae may not be recognized as compatible and should therefore be removed (**Figure 1D**), unless they are able to set up the appropriate recognition systems in time.

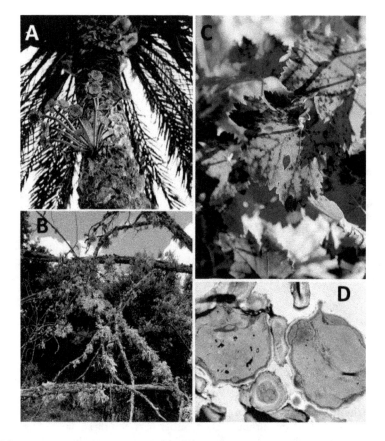

Figure 1.
(A) Aeonium arboreum, *a crassulacean species epiphytically growing on the stipe of* Phoenix canariensis. *(B) Hemiparasitic action of a dense population of epiphytic lichens that defoliated branches of their oak substrate. (C) Red spots on the leaves of* Vitis vinifera, *symptoms of the disease called tinder. The causal agents are fungi from* Stereum hirsutum *and* Phellinus igniarius *species. (D) Parasitic drift of* Xanthoria parietina *mycobiont on its phycobiont,* Trebouxia, *devoid of the receptor for recognition lectin.*

Lichen thalli can be reproduced by propagules containing some compatible algal cells surrounded by fungal hyphae. But there is also the possibility that a free-living fungus may find compatible algal cells in its environment. These algae, living in an aqueous film that covers the substrate (soil, rock, tree trunk), can move toward the fungal mass that would envelop them after being recognized. A similar situation is established when a single-cell organism (bacteria, fungal spore) is deposited on the wet surface of a plant, and the higher organism must discriminate whether it is an epiphytic, potential endosymbiont, or decidedly pathogenic microorganism. In the latter two cases, the cells must move in the water film until a suitable point of penetration is found.

Therefore, two main problems arise to explain the mechanisms used to establish this type of interspecific relationship: how unicellular organisms, potential endobionts, move toward the points of contact or entry and how they are recognized by the potential exohabitant when it reaches this position.

Lichens generally secrete glycoproteins to the environment depending on the availability of water [7]. Since most of these glycoproteins were enzymes, it was long time assumed that secretion was a function of the chemical composition of the substrate. This secretion might be taken as a kind of exocellular digestion of the compounds in the medium in order to be internalized into the thallus as simpler structures. However, using the lichen *Xanthoria parietina* growing on different substrates, rock or tree branches, it was found that the composition of the substrate did not influence the secretion of particular enzymes, which resulted in an exclusive function of the water availability and the degree of hydration of the thalli [8].

The aim of this study is to investigate the mechanism by which both prokaryotic and eukaryotic cells that do not have motile organs can move in liquid media thanks to the properties of their actomyosin cytoskeleton.

2. Secreted proteins

In the early stages of the establishment of lichen symbiosis, parasitic attack of the mycobiont (the fungal partner) against a variable number of photobiont cells (algae or cyanobacteria) can occur, which can be attenuated, according to Ahmadjian [9], by subjecting the neo-association to conditions of deprivation of organic nutrients. In this way, the fungus must keep a vital and active population of green cells, on whose photosynthetic products it depends to maintain its chemoorganic metabolism. This parasitic attack is carried out by invasion of the photosynthetic cells by fungal haustoria or by secretion of proteins that cause changes in genetic expression, structure disorganization, and cell death. These actions require proteins such as arginine methyltransferase, arginase, dioxygenases, or chitinases, according to Joneson et al. [10], secreted by the fungus *Cladonia grayi* in contact with the single-celled green alga *Asterochloris* sp. The appearance of chitinase as a secreted protein during the first stages of recognition has been explained as a defensive reaction of the algal partner against the fungus that attempts parasitism, which means that for the association to be successful, the secretion and production of this enzyme must be avoided [11].

In the case of fungal recognition of an algae considered genetically incompatible, the contact ends with the disorganization of the photosynthetic apparatus and the enzymatic rupture of the cell wall, with the loss of protoplast and death of the cell [12]. When the fungal-secreted arginase does not find a specific receptor in the algal cell wall, the enzyme penetrates the cell wall and activates its own β-1,4-glucanase up to 10 times above its normal physiological level, causing total digestion of specific areas of the cell wall. Such a drastic response contradicts the assertion of Wang et al. [13] when they state that *Endocarpon pusillum* mycobiont interacts with their photobiont, *Diplosphaera chodatii*, by means of secreted small proteins much weaker than those that produce pathogenic fungi.

Another model of interaction between individuals, studied in our laboratory, is the pathosystem *Saccharum officinarum-Sporisorium scitamineum*. Plant invasion by the pathogen causes the production of at least 5–6 defense proteins, among which a dirigent protein [14], secreted arginase, β-1,3- and β-1,4-glucanases, chitinase as well as a sixth protein that acts as a positive chemotactic factor have been identified [15]. The actions that these secreted proteins carry out on the spores of the pathogen are varied. On one hand, arginase secreted by the plant causes a false quorum effect on the fungal teliospore population. The quorum effect exists by itself. The teliospores themselves secrete authentic quorum signals to increase the population of cells at the points of invasion in such a way as to ensure the survival of a sufficient number of them in the event that the plant emits effective defense factors. The false quorum signal causes the teliospores to form large aggregates over which the hydrolytic enzymes of the plant, chitinase, and glucanases would act [16].

Therefore, the behavior of the former inhabitant against a process of recognition of compatibility in the symbiosis or defense against a pathogen presents molecular similarities, but a very different characteristic in each case. For lichens, the mycobiont secretes a protein (a lectin) able to discriminate between compatible and

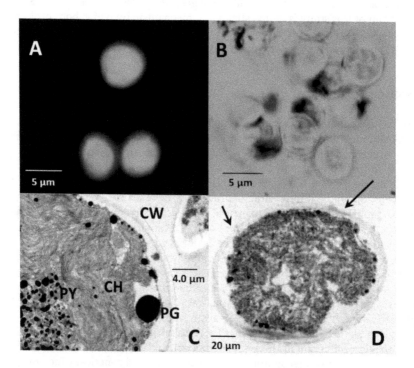

Figure 2.
(A) Trebouxia cells isolated from X. parietina after the binding of the fluorescent lectin isolated from the compatible mycobiont. Fluorescence is superficially located on the algal cell wall. (B) The same algal cells lacking the specific lectin receptor. (C) Transmission electron micrograph of Trebouxia cells corresponding to (A). The integrity of the cells permits to distinguish the intact cell wall (CW), the chloroplast (CH) showing the complex lamellae system, the pyrenoid (PY), and one plastoglobuli (PG). (D) Transmission electron micrograph of Trebouxia cells corresponding to (B). The chloroplast has been disorganized, pyrenoid disappears, and the cell wall shows zones partially digested (black arrows).

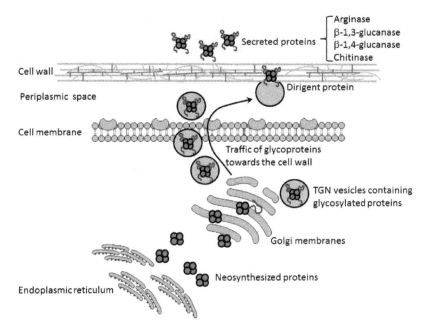

Figure 3.
Defense proteins produced by sugarcane cells are synthesized in the endoplasmic reticulum, glycosylated in the Golgi cisternae, and internalized in the trans-*Golgi network (TGN) vesicles to be transported to periplasmic space, crossing the cell membrane, to deposit them on the inner surface of the cell wall or to be secreted outside the cells.*

incompatible algae [17]. Only in the latter case, the secreted protein behaves as an aggressive factor (**Figure 2**). In the case of host-pathogen interactions, the proteins secreted by the host are always defense proteins (**Figure 3**). To carry out these actions, the potential endohabitant, symbiont or pathogen, must possess receptors for the secreted proteins that transmit the signal of compatibility or resistance to the cell machinery when they receive the recognition protein.

3. Receptors

The nature of these receptors, both in lichen photobionts as well as in some sugarcane pathogens, has been investigated in our laboratory. The occurrence of a glycosylated urease located in the phycobiont cell wall of *X. parietina* has been identified as an arginase-lectin receptor [18]. This identity has also been extended to other lichen species, such as *E. prunastri* [6], *Leptogium corniculatum* [19], and *Peltigera canina* [20]. *X. parietina* and *E. prunastri* contain a green algae from the *Trebouxia* genus as chlorobiont, while *L. corniculatum* and *P. canina* are associated with *Nostoc* sp. (a cyanobacterium). Recently isolated photobionts from thalli of these four lichen species contained an active urease associated with the cell wall. However, this activity was completely inhibited when cell wall fractions isolated from phycobiont or cyanobiont cells were incubated for 2 h at 37°C with the corresponding, previously purified lectin. In addition, hydrolysis of the galactoside moiety of urease in intact algae with α-1,4-galactosidase releases high amounts of D-galactose and impedes the binding of the lectin to the algal cell wall. However, the use of β-1,4-galactosidase releases low amounts of D-β-galactose from the algal cell wall and does not change the pattern of binding of the lectin to its ligand [21]. The production of glycosylated urease is restricted to the season in which algal cells divide, and this assures the recognition of new phycobiont produced after cell division by its fungal partner [22]. This should be interpreted as meaning that the polypeptide sequence of arginase (the lectin produced by the mycobiont) possesses an amino acid domain capable of stereochemically recognizing the remains of D-β-galactose in β-1,3 bonds of the glycosylated, algal urease.

This mode of binding a lectin to the polysaccharide moiety of its ligand by an affinity reaction equals, at the level of action mechanism, the secreted lichen argi-nases with other, well-known lectins from higher plants, such as concanavalin A (ConA) from *Canavalia ensiformis*, and ricin A (RCA) from *Ricinus communis*. Studies carried out by using α-methyl-mannose as a ligand suggest that the sugar forms seven hydrogen bonds with the peptide of ConA, four with –NH groups of Lys99, Tyr100, Arg228 and Lys229, and three with amino acids interacting with Ca^{2+}, Asn 14 and Asp208 [23]. On the other hand, Fontaniella et al. [24] showed that a commercial ConA was able to develop arginase activity that increased more than 40 times in the presence of 1.7 mM Mn^{2+}. Another similarity between ConA and fungal arginases lies in the fact that their activity as enzymes requires Mn^{2+}, while their activity as lectin is dependent on Ca^{2+} and both cations, at the level of biological activity, are mutually excluding. The comparison between crystalline structures of ConA-containing or not Ca^{2+} suggests that the cation pulls from Tyr12, Asp208, and Arg228 to conform the site to bind the specific sugar [25]. It is probable that the binding of Ca^{2+} to the specific domain for the cation changes the tertiary structure of the domain defined as site for the sugar binding and, for the same reason, the structure of the catalytic site for arginine. The ability to bind both cations together in order to develop their binding capacity to specific galactose ligands has been demon-strated for other lectins, such as that purified and crystallized from *Spatholobus parviflorus* [26].

According to this, Marx and Peveling [27] found that many cultured phycobionts isolated from several lichen species bind to commercial lectins, includ-ing Con A and RCA. In addition, Fontaniella et al. [24] found that ConA is able to bind to the cell wall of algal cells recently isolated from *E. prunastri* and *X. parietina* thalli. This binding involves a ligand, probably a glycoprotein containing mannose, which has been isolated by affinity chromatography. Analysis by SDS-PAGE of the purified ligand revealed that it is a dimeric protein composed by two monomers of 54 and 48 kDa. This ligand shows to be different from the receptor for natural lichen lectins, previously identified as a polygalactosylated urease.

The binding of sugarcane glycoproteins to their cell wall ligands in the bacterial endophyte *Gluconacetobacter diazotrophicus* [28] and in the bacterial pathogen *Xanthomonas albilineans* [29] results in cell recruitment (**Figure 4**) rather than a defense mechanism. Similar results on cytoagglutination were obtained using *Herbaspirillum rubrisubalbicans* treated with sugarcane glycoproteins of

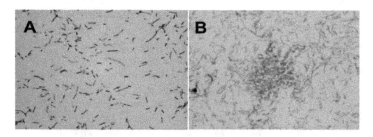

Figure 4.
Effect of secreted sugarcane glycoproteins on the cytoagglutination of Xanthomonas albilineans. *(A) Bacterial cells immediately after the contact with plant defense glycoproteins and (B) 3 h after the contact.*

mid- (MMMG) and high molecular mass (HMMG). MMMG were preferentially desorbed from the bacterial cell wall with sucrose and galactitol, whereas HMMG were mainly desorbed with glucose and mannose [30]. This would indicate that, against this bacterium, MMMG behaves as signal molecules that bind to their receptor, or receptors, using their polysaccharide moiety, whereas, on the contrary, HMMG would use their peptide moiety for binding to different receptors, similar to the action mode of the lectin ConA [24], from *Canavalia ensiformis*.

Surprisingly, receptors for both HMMG and MMMG do not behave as the typical adhesion receptors containing polysaccharides that bind by affinity to a specific peptide domain in the signaling molecule, the recognition of which implies the binding of this to selected carbohydrate moieties in their ligands [31]. In this case, the carbohydrate moiety of the signal molecule seems to be used to recognize a particular amino acid domain on the ligand (receptor) in an inverse way to that described for plant lectins and animal selectins. This fact suggests that HMMG and MMMG, with independence of their possible enzymatic activities [32], behave as true protein of resistance (PR), according to Su et al. [33], that would require ligands similar to toll-like receptors (TLRs), studied in animals [34].

The cytoagglutinating effect of sugarcane glycoproteins on smut teliospores was clearly reduced using invertase-digested glycoproteins. This suggested that the hydrolyzed glycidic moiety, which contains fructose residues polymerized as β-D-fructofuranosyl-1,2-β-D-fructose, could be involved in the process of binding since the extensive hydrolysis of β-$(1 \rightarrow 2)$ bonds impeded cell adhesion. To obtain experimental evidence of the presence of such cell-wall receptor, or receptors, glycoproteins were isolated from the cell wall of the fungal pathogen. These glycoproteins were separated by affinity chromatography through activated agarose columns to which sugarcane glycoproteins from different cultivars had been previously bound. Fungal cell-wall receptors retained by sugarcane glycoproteins were then recovered, desorbed by certain monosaccharides used as eluents [35]. Sugarcane HMMG and MMMG fractions exhibited a high affinity for N-acetyl-D-glucosamine, component of the cell wall of filamentous fungi. Interestingly, this binding mechanism differed, for example, from that described by Blanco et al. [27] for the cell wall receptors of *G. diazotrophicus*. In this case, glycoproteins bound through a domain β-$(1 \rightarrow 2)$-fructofuranosyl fructose from its glycidic moiety to the bacterial cell wall receptors, which exhibited a binding site for this saccharide residue. Therefore, in the cases that HMMG or MMMG bound to their ligands using their polysaccharide moiety, either to bacterial cells or to fungal teliospores, they did not behave as lectins but as recognition factors using monosaccharide units or glycosidic bonds to bind to a particular domain of their ligands [36]. In addition, and as previously explained, HMMG and MMMG fractions behaved differently in their binding mechanisms to cell walls of *H. rubrisubalbicans*. These differences in the recognition mechanism could be interpreted as a discrimination factors between pathogens and endosymbionts.

4. Cytoskeleton as the main responsible for displacement of *Nostoc* and *Sporisorium scitamineum* cells

Directed cell migration is a physical process that involves dramatic modifications in cell shape and, generally, adhesion to the extracellular matrix [37]. Chemoattractive displacement is typically linked to the reorganization of actin filaments in cells, since polarization is the triggering event of cell migration [38]. A ligand on cell surface must activate a signaling pathway that leads to contraction/

relaxation of the cytoskeleton. Then, cell polarizes and as a consequence, it moves to the chemoattractant source.

Moreover, many intracellular signaling molecules are involved in cell motility, such as MAPK cascades, lipid kinases, phospholipases, Ser/Thr and Tyr kinases, and scaffold proteins. Specially, GTP molecules play an essential role in both signal transduction and actin organization through Rho GTPases, which appear as the most important components of signaling cascade related to cell migration [38, 39].

Cell migration is the core to modern cell biology. However, progress has been hindered by experimental limitations and the complexity of the process. This has led to the popularity of *Dictyostelium discoideum*, with its experimentally friendly lifestyle and small, haploid genome, as a tool to dissect the pathways involved in migration. *Dictyostelium* has the potential to unlock many fundamental questions in the cell motility field [37]. Here, the involvement of the cytoskeleton in movement is analyzed in two very different systems, such as the compatible association fungus-alga in the lichen *Peltigera canina* and the plant-pathogen interaction between *Sporisorium scitamineum* and sugarcane plants.

4.1 Cytoskeleton reorganization in *Nostoc* cells in response to the binding of a fungal lectin

For symbiotic interaction, germinating hyphae of the mycobiont needs to meet a compatible photobiont cell, to recognize it, and to make contact [40]. When an isolated fungus and an isolated alga associate, the photobiont migrates toward its potential compatible partner, which implies that the cyanobiont would develop organelles to move toward the fungus. Displacement is particularly relevant in cyanolichens, in which the cyanobiont forms filaments inside the thallus, a segment of which can break off and migrate toward other locations [19]. The recognition process continues during thallus growth, since it is necessary that new generations of photobiont cells become involved in the association [9].

Lectins found in both prokaryotic and eukaryotic cells play an important role in cell interaction processes. Synthesis of fungal lectins with arginase activity and the occurrence of an algal receptor showing urease activity are absolutely required in the formation of lichen associations [41]. Urease on the algae cell wall acts as a ligand for fungal arginase, fixing it on the cell wall and preventing it to penetrate the cell [20]. So, lectins with arginase activity participate as recognizing proteins of compatible alga binding to a specific receptor on the cell wall. However, they penetrate and cause destruction of algae cells if the specific receptor does not exist [41]. This is the case of noncompatible interaction, as it is shown in **Figure 5**.

The search for the chemoattractant attracting photobiont cells leads to the discovery of the attractant properties of fungus lectin. In particular, chemotaxis of *Nostoc* cells from *P. canina* toward the lectin isolated from the same lichen species has been amply studied [42]. Many multicellular filamentous cyanobacteria move on solid surfaces by gliding, in absence of pili or fimbriae. It is the case of filaments and hormogonia of *Nostoc* [43]. This mechanism, which occurs in a parallel direction to the cell long axis, is associated with the production of polysaccharide slime and the attachment of the cell to a surface is needed. On the other hand, blebbing and the release of small vesicles by the cyanobacterial outer membrane have been observed in distantly related symbiotic and nonsymbiotic cyanobacteria such as *Nostoc*, the cyanobiont of *Peltigera* spp. [44]. Blebs are spherical membrane protrusions produced by contractions of the actomyosin cortex often considered to be a hallmark of apoptosis. However, blebs are also frequently observed during cytokinesis and migration in three-dimensional cultures and in vivo conditions [45].

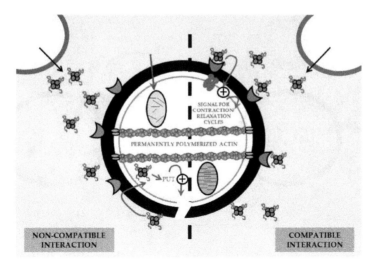

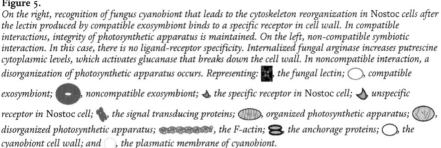

Figure 5.
On the right, recognition of fungus cyanobiont that leads to the cytoskeleton reorganization in Nostoc *cells after the lectin produced by compatible exosymbiont binds to a specific receptor in cell wall. In compatible interactions, integrity of photosynthetic apparatus is maintained. On the left, non-compatible symbiotic interaction. In this case, there is no ligand-receptor specificity. Internalized fungal arginase increases putrescine cytoplasmic levels, which activates glucanase that breaks down the cell wall. In noncompatible interaction, a disorganization of photosynthetic apparatus occurs. Representing:* ▒*, the fungal lectin;* ◯*, compatible exosymbiont;* ⬤*, noncompatible exosymbiont;* ⬧*, the specific receptor in* Nostoc *cell;* ⬧ *unspecific receptor in* Nostoc *cell;* ✎*, the signal transducing proteins;* ▨*, organized photosynthetic apparatus;* ▨*, disorganized photosynthetic apparatus;* ▧*, the F-actin;* ⬨ *the anchorage proteins;* ◯*, the cyanobiont cell wall; and* ◯*, the plasmatic membrane of cyanobiont.*

However, neither gliding nor blebbing can explain the invaginations observed by electron microscopy in one of the poles of *Nostoc* cells during the displacement [42], as can be seen in **Figure 6**. That is why the cytoskeleton has been revealed as responsible of migration of photobionts toward the fungus during a compatible interaction.

Some bacterial actin-like proteins or MreB have been already described in free-living cyanobacteria [46–47] but, contrary to that expected, chemotaxis assays of *Nostoc* displacement in presence of S-(3,4-dichlorobenzyl) isothiourea (A22), an inhibitor of MreB functionality, did not prevent the movement of cells toward the source of the lectin. Conversely, when *Nostoc* cells were incubated with the actin inhibitor phalloidin during chemoattraction assays, the drug inhibited chemotaxis by 50%. Also latrunculin A, which blocks actin polymerization, impedes *Nostoc* migration. The occurrence of F-actin fibers in *Nostoc* have also been found by immunocytochemical techniques associated with transmission electron microscopy.

Interestingly, when phalloidin was combined with blebbistatin, an eukaryotic myosin II inhibitor, the negative effect on displacement increases (78%), suggesting that blebbistatin may target a molecular target related to chemotaxis in cyanobacteria [42].

This means that, in the presence of compatible fungus, the binding of the lectin to its specific cell wall receptor would activate the signaling pathway that involves cytoskeleton reorganization. It must take place probably by means of GTPase activity, since the inhibition of chemotaxis produced by the combined action of phalloidin and blebbistatin is largely reversed by GTP and its analogs, GTP(γ)S and

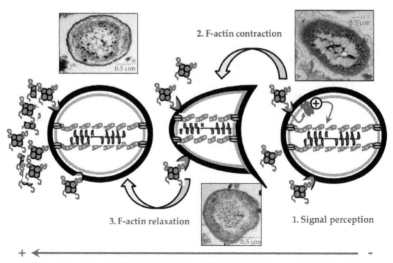

2. F-actin contraction

3. F-actin relaxation

1. Signal perception

+ ← ———————————————————————————————— -

Migration of the cell in the direction of the lectin concentration gradient

Figure 6.
Scheme of movement of Nostoc *cells during symbiotic interaction that explains how motility of lichen cyanobionts is due to contraction-relaxation episodes of the cytoskeleton. (1) Chemoattractant lectins released by fungus bind to specific receptors in photobiont cell walls. As a result, the transduction signal that implies cytoskeleton reorganization is activated. (2) Polar cell invaginations are produced by interaction of an ATPase with contractile ability, sensitive to blebbistatin, with F-actin cytoskeleton. (3) After this, depolymerization of F-actin is achieved at the opposite pole, repolymerization of which produces the cell advancement. Representing: , the fungal lectin; the specific receptor in* Nostoc *cell; the signal transducing proteins; , the actin monomeres; , the F-actin; , the contractile protein; , the anchorage proteins; , the cell wall; and , the plasmatic membrane. Ferritin-labelled F-actin can be seen in micrographs obtained by transmission electron microscopy (TEM).*

GDP(β)S, as well as by cyclic AMP [48]. On the contrary, when it is a noncompatible interaction, lectin penetrates into the cell, promoting putrescine synthesis. The diamine, which causes disorganization of photosynthetic apparatus, activates glucanase that breaks down the cell wall. Compatible and noncompatible interaction effect on cytoskeleton organization is schematized in **Figure 5**.

The absence of superficial elements (fimbriae, pili, or flagellum), related to cell movement, and the appearance of invaginated cells during or after movement, verified by scanning electron microscopy, support the hypothesis that the motility of lichen cyanobionts could be achieved by contraction-relaxation episodes of the cytoskeleton induced by fungal lectin [42]. However, other issues raised included (1) how cytoskeleton is reorganized during migration, (2) how is the mechanism of force generation of movement for cyanobacteria from *P. canina*, and (3) how it can be related to the invaginations previously observed by electron microscopy. The answers to all of these questions have led to elaborate a proposal of migration mechanism in cyanobacteria.

Figure 6 represents F-actin contraction/relaxing cycles in the *Nostoc* photobiont cells during migration following the lectin gradient. Firstly, binding of arginase molecules to cell wall receptors induces F-actin contraction by means of the activation of a signaling cascade where GTPases must play a main role. At the same time, contraction of filaments must be responsible for invagination appearance in one of the poles of the cell, which is followed by the actin depolarization at the opposite pole. This fact releases the tension from the actin-like cable bound to the membrane, and, finally, induces recovery of the spherical cell shape and movement of the cell [42].

4.2 Cytoskeleton reorganization in *S. scitamineum* cells in response to the binding of sugarcane glycoproteins

In the early stages of smut disease, spore germination occurs on the internode surface of host stalks, followed by the formation of appressoria, mainly on the inner scale of young buds and on the bases of emerging leaves [49]. Penetration into the plant meristem takes place between 6 and 36 h after fungal cells are deposited on the surface [50]. Since the pathogens normally use the opened stomata of sugarcane leaves to penetrate, it is easy to think that the teliospores deposited at random on the surface of a leaf, far from stomata, should develop a mechanism of displacement toward the way of entry [51]. For this rationale, it is important to demonstrate the existence of these mechanisms and to study how they can be carried out.

Cytoskeleton reorganization in response to the binding of glycoproteins also occurs during *Sporisorium scitamineum*-sugarcane recognition. Moreover, displacement after recognition also results in cytoagglutination of smut teliospores in the same way that activation and chemotaxis of lichen photobionts induced by fungal lectins cause cell aggregation [15]. Interestingly, if glycoproteins are produced by sugarcane-resistant varieties, chemotaxis initially directed to plant invasion results in a "suicide" mechanism.

It has been proposed that at least three classes of glycoproteins exist in the mixture of sugarcane defensive glycoproteins produced by resistant cultivars: (i) a chemotactic glycoprotein, yet uncharacterized; (ii) a cytoagglutinating factor endowed with arginase activity, which also inhibits germination; and (iii) enzymatic proteins that mediate the breakdown of the teliospore cell wall. It has been demonstrated that agglutination of a lot of smut cells in a small region in contact with sugarcane glycoproteins confers resistance, since degradative activity also contained in these glycoproteins (β-1,3-, β-1,4-glucanase, and chitinase) can hydrolyze cell wall of many teliospores at the same time [15]. In this context, it must be pointed out that defensive agglutination depends necessarily on early chemoattraction of cells. For this reason, it is very interesting to go into some depth about how the teliospores movement is stimulated by sugarcane signals. Currently, it has been found that the early chemoattractive effect is fully relevant to trigger a successful defensive response [52]. Lower levels of chemoattractant power exhibited by glycoproteins released by nonresistant cultivars have been directly related to the minor capacity of these plants to defend themselves.

Brand and Gow [53] summarize the knowledge on spore movement in plant-pathogen interactions. The two most frequently proposed mechanisms are submicroscopical contractions of helically arranged fibrils within the cell walls and the occurrence of motile appendages in zoospores. Other species of pathogenic fungi produce spores that are capable of gliding in the same way that it occurs for many species of cyanobacteria. Gliding is a form of cell movement that differs from crawling or swimming in which it does not rely on any obvious external organ or change in cell shape and it occurs only in the presence of a substrate [54].

Light and electron microscopy images showed the absence of motile external structures in smut teliospores. However, in the same way that it occurs for *Nostoc*, the invaginations observed during the cellular displacement suggested that cytoskeleton could be the responsible of spore displacement after the contact with sugarcane glycoproteins. Indeed, chemotactic movement of teliospores was strongly inhibited by phalloidin, latrunculin A, and blebbistatin, and the presence of actin and myosin in *S. scitamineum* teliospores has been revealed by immunohistochemical techniques [52].

Teliospores do not need to develop lamellipodia in the direction of movement because they do not "crawl" on a substrate, but "swim" in solution because of the rigidity of the cell wall. Therefore, invagination at the opposite pole would be the only mechanical requirement for cell motion [52]. Again as in *Nostoc* migration, a movement model has been proposed for smut teliospores displacement, which is schemed in **Figure** 7. Firstly, glycoprotein binding to its ligand on cell wall generates a signaling cascade that will trigger cytoskeletal remodeling (1). Translocation of actin filaments has been described as a consequence of the interaction of contractile myosin activity with F-actin cytoskeleton. It leads to an increase in the cell volume at the front of advance and the retraction of the opposite pole. At this pole, filaments must be anchored to cell membrane, since invaginations are observed (2). Finally, depolymerization of F-actin is achieved at the opposite pole, the repolymerization of which leads to cell advancement (3) [30, 52].

Also in the case of *S. scitamineum* cells, GTPases seem to be relevant in the activation of the movement. GTP causes an enhancement of the inhibition exerted by blebbistatin during migration. However, a large reversion is achieved by addition of GTPγS, the poorly hydrolysable GTP analogue [30, 55] or GDPβS, a deactivator of Rho [56] GTPases, and a total reversion of inhibition can be observed by combining GTP and GTPγS. GTP slightly reverts latrunculin A effect probably at the Rho pathway. However, when GTP analogues, GTPγS and GDPβS are added to the incubation media in the presence of latrunculin A, no reversion of the chemostatic inhibition is observed. These results indicate that GTPγS behaves as a strong activator of the small Rho-GTPase and its downstream pathways, which results in its final switch-off. Conversely, GDPβS blocks this signaling cascade, likely by inhibiting GTP exchange on Rho. These results, that are *not a priori* easy

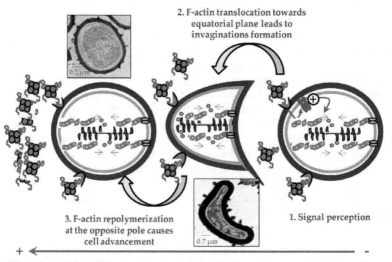

2. F-actin translocation towards equatorial plane leads to invaginations formation

3. F-actin repolymerization at the opposite pole causes cell advancement

1. Signal perception

Migration of the cell in the direction of the glycoprotein concentration gradient

Figure 7.
Scheme of movement of S. scitamineum *cells during sugarcane-pathogen interaction that explain how motility of teliospores is due to contraction-relaxation episodes of the cytoskeleton. (1) chemoattractant glycoprotein released by sugarcane plants binds to specific receptors in fungal cell walls. As a result, the transduction signal that implies cytoskeleton reorganization is activated. (2) Polar cell invaginations are produced by interaction of myosin II with F-actin cytoskeleton. The translation of the actin filaments into the interior of the cell must begin at its less end, located in the equatorial plane of teliospore. This permits an increase of the cell volume in the front of advance and the retraction of the opposite pole, which produces cell invagination. (3) Repolymerization of F-actin in the front of cell produces the cell advancement. Representing:* ▣ *the glycoproteins;* ⬓ *the receptor in fungal cell;* ⬧ *the signal transducing proteins;* ○, *the actin monomeres;* ▰▰▰▰▰, *the F-actin;* ⌐, *the myosin;* ⬮ *the anchorage proteins;* ○, *the cell wall;* ○, *the plasmatic membrane; and* ← *the direction of retrograde flow. F-actin specific labeled ferritin can be seen in micrographs obtained by transmission electron microscopy (TEM).*

to understand, manifest that GTPases should participate in a meticulous regulation of actin organization.

Moreover, microtubules seem to be also involved in migration mechanism since nocodazole inhibits chemotactic displacement. Interestingly, assays revealed that the negative effect that this drug exerts on chemoattraction is related to a blockage of actin polarization. This demonstrates that actin and microtubules interact, participating together in the establishment of cellular polarity during migration (**Figure 8**). Microtubules-actin interactions regulate important processes in which dynamic cellular asymmetries need to be established such as cell motility, neuronal pathfinding, cellular wound healing, cell division, and cortical flow [57]. The presence of tubulin has also been demonstrated by immunohistochemical techniques in *S. scitamineum* cells [58].

It is obvious that cytoskeleton reorganization in fungal cells is also involved in germination, in addition to chemotaxis. This is because hyphae of filamentous fungi are very polarized cells and a continuous migration of vesicles from the teliospore cytoplasm through the hyphal cell body to the growing hyphal tip is necessary for organism development [59, 60]. It is clear that cytoskeleton plays a crucial role in polarity establishment in fungal cells during germination: microtubules support nuclei division and long-distance-transport functions in filamentous fungi, whereas actin microfilaments are required for localized targeting events [61]. Microtubule organization in *S. scitamineum* teliospores seems to be crucial for a successful germination [58]. *S. scitamineum* secretes its own arginase, which activates a signal transduction cascade that accelerates teliospore germination when it binds its cell wall. Moreover, it has been recently suggested that microtubule stabilization during germination of smut teliospores could be triggered by the production of moderate levels of spermidine. *In vitro* microtubule polymerization assays in the presence of spermidine indicate that this polyamine interacts positively with cytoskeleton, probably by means of the positive charges of the molecule. Thus, polyamines are able to bind strongly to existing negative charges in different cellular components, such as nucleic acids, proteins, and phospholipids [62]. Spermidine could act in this way interacting and stabilizing the cytoskeleton.

So, polarization of cytoskeleton occurs during both teliospore movement and germination. Herein lies one of the most surprising discover about *S. scitamineum*-sugarcane interaction: glycoproteins from resistant to smut plants stimulate the

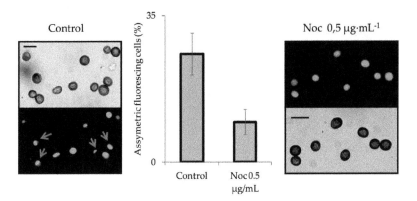

Figure 8.
Micrographs obtained by fluorescence optical microscope that show F-actin distribution in S. scitamineum cells in the absence (on the left) or in the presence (on the right) of nocodazole (Noc) 0.5 µg.mL-1, an inhibitor of microtubule polymerization. F-actin was detected using phalloidin labeled with fluorescein isothiocyanate (FITC). Red arrows indicate polarized cell. In the middle, percentage of cells with an asymmetric distribution of F-actin in the absence (control) or in the presence of Noc 0.5 µg.mL-1.

organization of the actin cytoskeleton to induce the movement of the teliospores toward the cytoagglutination points but stimulate its depolymerization for avoiding germination. Thus, after displacement as a consequence of cytoskeleton reorganization, the result is agglutinated cells without germinative capacity. Teliospore agglutination without germination triggered by sugarcane arginase becomes the result of a false quorum signal that prevents teliospore infection.

5. Conclusions

Cytoskeleton reorganization is the trigger of displacement of *Nostoc* and *Sporisorium scitamineum* cells during exohabitant/endohabitant recognition. On one hand, movement of *S. scitamineum* teliospores occurs by means of continuous episodes of polymerization and depolymerization of the actin cytoskeleton, in collaboration with myosin. Fungal cells displace toward defensive sugarcane glycoproteins as part of a "suicidal behavior," since displacement finally results in cytoagglutination and cell death [15]. Chemotactic movement of teliospores was strongly inhibited by phalloidin and latrunculin A, which are involved in F-actin polymerization and depolymerization cycles, and by blebbistatin, which avoids the functionality of a contractile protein similar to a myosin II, responsible for the contraction-relaxation of the cytoskeleton. Migration of smut teliospores has been described as consistent with a jellyfish-like "swimming" mechanism.

On the other hand, interesting results presented by Díaz et al. [41] suggest a cytoskeletal-driven mode of cyanobacteria chemotaxis similar to those of eukaryotic cells responding to a chemoattractant gradient. It has been concluded that *Nostoc* chemotaxis toward arginase requires actin and myosin II-like proteins. Displacement implies a rearrangement of the cytoskeleton causing cell polarity, which is, in turn, inhibited by phalloidin and latrunculin A, as revealed by confocal microscopy.

F-actin reorganization in response to extracellular chemotactic signaling has been amply studied. Migration is typically linked to the formation of external structures that promote movement. However, similar results in such different systems (lichen and plant pathogen) indicate that this mechanism of cytoskeletal reorganization, which induces cell chemotaxis in absence of lamellipodia/filopodia formation, is conserved in different organisms for recognition between species.

Author details

Elena Sánchez-Elordi[1], Eva María Díaz[1], Carlos Vicente[1,2]* and María Estrella Legaz[1]

1 Intercellular Communication in Plant Symbiosis Team, Faculty of Biology, Madrid, Spain

2 Complutense University, Madrid, Spain

*Address all correspondence to: cvicente@bio.ucm.es

IntechOpen

© 2018 The Author(s). Licensee IntechOpen. This chapter is distributed under the terms of the Creative Commons Attribution License (http://creativecommons.org/licenses/by/3.0), which permits unrestricted use, distribution, and reproduction in any medium, provided the original work is properly cited. (cc) BY

References

[1] Leung TLF, Poulin R. Parasitism, commensalism, and mutualism: Exploring the many shades of symbioses. Life Environment. 2008;**58**: 107-115

[2] Martin CE, Schmitt AK. Unusual water relations in the CAM atmospheric epiphyte *Tillandsia usneoides* L. (Bromeliaceae). Botanical Gazette. 1989;**150**:1-8

[3] Montaña C, Dirzo R, Flore A. Structural parasitism of an epiphytic bromeliad upon *Cercidium praecox* in an intertropical semiarid ecosystem. Biotropica. 1997;**29**:517-521. DOI: 10.1111/j.1744-7429.1997.tb00046.x

[4] Bouaid K, Vicente C. Effects of lichen phenolics on defoliation of *Quercus rotundifolia*. Sauteria. 1998;**9**: 229-236

[5] Monso MA, Legaz ME, Vicente C. A biochemical approach to the hemiparasitic action of the epiphytic lichen *Evernia prunastri* on *Betula pendula*. Annales Botanica Fennici. 1993;**30**:299-303

[6] Legaz ME, Fontaniella B, Millanes AM, Vicente C. Secreted arginases from phylogenetically far-related lichen species act as cross-recognition factors for two different algal cells. European Journal of Cell Biology. 2004;**83**: 435-446. DOI: 0171-9335/04/83/0-1 $15.00/0

[7] Legaz ME, Díaz-Santos E, Vicente C. Lichen sustrates and urease production and secretion: A physiological approach using four Antarctic lichens. Biochemical Systematics and Ecology. 1986;**14**:375-379

[8] Rodríguez M, Vicente C. Water status and urease secretion from two ecotypes of *Xanthoria parietina*. Symbiosis. 1991;**11**:255-262

[9] Ahmadjian V. The Lichen Symbiosis. New York: Wiley; 1993. 250 p

[10] Joneson S, Armaleo D, Lutzoni F. Fungal and algal gene expression in early developmental stages of lichen-symbiosis. Mycologia. 2011;**103**: 291-306. DOI: 10.3852/10-064

[11] Athukorala SNP, Piercey-Normore MD. Recognition- and defense-related gene expression at 3 resynthesis stages in lichen symbionts. Canadian Journal of Microbiology. 2015;**61**:1-12. DOI: 10.1139/cjm-2014-0470

[12] Molina MC, Stocker-Wörgötter E, Turk R, Bajon C, Vicente C. Secreted, glycosylated arginase from *Xanthoria parietina* thallus induces loss of cytoplasmic material from *Xanthoria* photobionts. Cell Adhesion and Communication. 1998;**6**:481-490. DOI: 10.3109/15419069809010796

[13] Wang YY, Liu B, Zhang XY, Zhou QM, Zhang T, Li H, et al. Genome characteristics reveal the impact of lichenization on lichen-forming fungus *Endocarpon pusillum* Hedwig (Verrucariales, Ascomycota). Genomics. 2014;**15**:34 Available from: http://www.biomedcentral.com/1471-2164/15/34

[14] Sánchez-Elordi E, Contreras R, de Armas R, Benito MC, Alarcón B, de Oliveira E, et al. Differential expression of SofDIR16 and SofCAD genes in smut resistant and susceptible sugarcane cultivars in response to *Sporisorium scitamineum*. Journal of Plant Physiology. 2018;**226**:103-113. DOI: 10.1016/j.jplph.2018.04.016

[15] Sánchez-Elordi E, Morales de los Ríos L, Díaz EM, Ávila A, Legaz ME, Vicente C. Defensive glycoproteins from sugarcane plants induce chemotaxis, cytoagglutination and death of smut teliospores. Journal of Plant Pathology. 2016;**98**:493-501

[16] Sánchez-Elordi E, Morales de los Ríos L, Vicente C, Legaz ME. Sugar cane arginase competes with the same fungal enzyme as a false quorum signal against smut teliospores. Phytochemistry Letters. 2015;**14**:115-122. DOI: 10.1016/j.phytol.2015.09.013 1874-3900

[17] Galun M, Kardish N. Lectins as determinants of symbiotic specificity in lichens. Cryptogamic Botany. 1995;**5**: 144-148

[18] Molina MC, Muñiz E, Vicente C. Enzymatic activities of algal-binding protein and its algal cell wall receptor in the lichen *Xanthoria parietina*. An approach to the parasitic basis of mutualism. Plant Physiology and Biochemistry. 1993;**31**:131-142

[19] Vivas M, Sacristán M, Legaz ME, Vicente C. The cell recognition model in chlorolichens involving a fungal lectin binding to an algal ligand can be extended to cyanolichens. Plant Biology. 2010;**12**:615-621. DOI: 10.1111/j.1438-8677.2009.00250.x

[20] Díaz EM, Sacristán M, Legaz ME, Vicente C. Isolation and characterization of a cyanobacterium-binding protein and its cell wall receptor in the lichen *Peltigera canina*. Plant Signaling and Behaviour. 2009;**4**: 598-603

[21] Sacristán M, Millanes AM, Legaz ME, Vicente C. A lichen lectin specifically binds to the β-1,4-polygalactoside moiety of urease located in the cell wall of homologous algae. Plant Signaling & Behavior. 2006;**1**: 23-27

[22] Sacristán M, Millanes AM, Vicente C, Legaz ME. Synchronic production of fungal lectin, phycobiont lectin receptors and algal division in *Evernia prunastri*. Journal of the Hattori Botanical Laboratory. 2006;**100**:739-751

[23] Derewenda Z, Yariv J, Helliwell JR, Kaeb AJ, Dodson EJ, Papiz MZ, et al.

The structure of the saccharide binding site of Concanavalin a. The EMBO Journal. 1989;**8**:2189-2193

[24] Fontaniella B, Millanes AM, Vicente C, Legaz ME. Concanavalin A binds to a mannose-containing ligand in the cell wall of some lichen phycobionts. Plant Physiology and Biochemistry. 2004;**42**: 773-779. DOI: 10.1016/j.plaphy.2004.09.003

[25] Shoham M, Yonath A, Sussmann JL, Moult J, Traub W, Kalb J. Crystal structure of demetallized Concanavalin A: The metal binding region. Journal of Molecular Biology. 1979;**131**:137-155

[26] Geethanandan K, Abhilash J, Bharath SR, Sadasivan C, Haridas M. X-ray structure of a galactose-specific lectin from *Spatholobous parviflorous*. International Journal of Biological Macromolecules. 2011;**49**:992-998. DOI: 10.1016/j.ijbiomac.2011.08.021

[27] Marx M, Peveling E. Surface receptors in lichen symbionts visualized by fluorescence microscopy after use of lectins. Protoplasma. 1983;**114**:52-61

[28] Blanco Y, Arroyo M, Legaz ME, Vicente C. Isolation from *Gluconacetobacter diazotrophicus* cell walls of specific receptors for sugarcane glycoproteins, which act as recognition factors. Journal of Chromatography. A. 2005;**1093**:204-211. DOI: 10.1016/j.chroma.2005.07.019

[29] Blanco Y, Sacristán M, Legaz ME, Vicente C. Isolation of specific receptors from *Xanthomonas albilineans* cell walls for lectins-like glycoproteins of sugarcane. Journal of Plant Interactions. 2006;**1**:107-114. DOI: 10.1080/17429140600768759

[30] Legaz ME, Sánchez-Elordi E, Santiago R, de Armas R, Fontaniella B, Millanes AM, et al. Metabolic responses of sugar cane plants upon different plant–pathogen interactions. In: Ahmad P, Ahanger MA, Singh VP, Alam P,

editors. Plant Metabolites and Regulation under Environmental Stress. London: Academic Press; 2018. pp. 241-280. DOI: 10.1016/B978-0-12-812689-9.00013-3

[31] Zihni C, Mills C, Matter K, Balda MS. Tight junctions: From simple barriers to multifunctional molecular gates. Nature Reviews. Molecular Cell Biology. 2016;**17**:564-580. DOI: 10.1038/nrm.2016.80

[32] Su Y, Wang Z, Xu L, Peng Q, Liu F, Zhu Li Z, et al. Early selection for smut resistance in sugarcane using pathogen proliferation and changes in physiological and biochemical indices. Frontiers in Plant Science. 2016;**7**:art 1133. DOI: 10.3389/fpls.2016.01133

[33] Su Y, Xu L, Wang Z, Peng Q, Yang Y, Chen Y, et al. Comparative proteomics reveals that central metabolism changes are associated with resistance against *Sporisorium scitamineum* in sugarcane. BMC Genomics. 2016b;**17**:800-820. DOI: 10.1186/s12864-016-3146-8

[34] Kumar H, Kawai T, Akira S. Toll-like receptors and innate immunity. Biochemical and Biophysical Research Communications. 2009;**388**:621-625. DOI: 10.1016/j.bbrc.2009.08.062

[35] Millanes AM, Vicente C, Legaz ME. Sugarcane glycoproteins bind to surface, specific ligands and modify cytoskeleton arrangement of *Ustilago scitaminea* teliospores. Journal of Plant Interactions. 2008;**3**:95-110. DOI: 10.1080/17429140701861727

[36] Aguilar-Cuenca R, Llorente-Gonzalez C, Vicente C, Vicente-Manzanares M. Microfilament-coordinated adhesion dynamics drives single cell migration and shapes whole tissues. F1000Research. 2017;**6**(F1000 Faculty Rev):160. DOI: 10.12688/f1000research.10356.1

[37] King JS, Insall RH. Chemotaxis: Finding the way forward with *Dictyostelium*. Trends in Cell Biology. 2009;**19**:523-530. DOI: 10.1016/j.tcb.2009.07.004

[38] Vorotnikov AV. Chemotaxis: Movement, direction, control. Biochemistry. 2011;**76**:1528-1555. DOI: 10.1134/S0006297911130104

[39] Raftopoulou M, Hall A. Cell migration: Rho GTPases lead the way. Developmental Biology. 2004;**265**: 23-32. DOI: 10.1016/j.ydbio.2003.06.003

[40] Galun M. Lichenization. In: Galun M, editor. Handbook of Lichenology. Vol. II. Florida: CRC Press; 1988. pp. 153-169

[41] Insarova ID, Blagoveshchenskaya EY. Lichen symbiosis: Search and recognition of partners. Biology Bulletin. 2016;**43**:408-418. DOI: 10.1134/S1062359016040038

[42] Díaz EM, Vicente-Manzanares M, Sacristán M, Vicente C, Legaz ME. Fungal lectin of *Peltigera canina* induces chemotropism of compatible Nostoc cells by constriction-relaxation pulses of cyanobiont cytoskeleton. Plant Signaling & Behavior. 2011;**6**:1525-1536. DOI: 10.4161/psb.6.10.16687

[43] Hoiczyk E, Baumeister W. Envelope structure of four gliding filamentous cyanobacteria. Journal of Bacteriology. 1995;**177**:2387-2395. DOI: 10.1128/jb.177.9.2387-2395.1995

[44] Boissiere MC. Cytochemical ultrastructure of *Peltigera canina*: Some features related to its symbiosis. The Lichenologist. 1982;**14**:1-28. DOI: 10.1017/S0024282982000036

[45] Charras G, Paluch E. Blebs lead the way: How to migrate without lamellipodia. Nature Reviews. Molecular Cell Biology. 2008;**9**:730-736. DOI: 10.1038/nrm2453

[46] Usmanova A, Astier C, Méjean C, Hubert F, Feinberg J, Benyamin Y, et al.

Coevolution of actin and associated proteins: An alpha-actinin-like protein in a cyanobacterium (*Spirulina platensis*). Comparative Biochemistry and Physiology - Part B: Biochemistry & Molecular Biology. 1998;**120**:693-700. DOI: 10.1016/S0305-0491(98)10065-2

[47] Guerrero-Barrera AL, García-Cuéllar CM, Villalba JD, Segura-Nieto M, Gómez-Lojero C, Reyes ME, et al. Actin-related proteins in *Anabaena* spp. and *Escherichia coli*. Microbiology. 1996; **142**:1133-1140. DOI: 10.1099/13500872-142-5-1133

[48] Díaz EM, Vicente-Manzanares M, Legaz ME, Vicente C. A cyanobacterial β-actin-like protein, responsible for lichenized *Nostoc* sp. motility towards a fungal lectin. Acta Physiologiae Plantarum. 2015;**37**:249-260. DOI: 10.1007/s11738-015-2007-4

[49] Waller JM. Sugarcane smut (*Ustilago scitaminea*) in Kenya. II infection and resistance. Transactions of the British Mycological Society. 1970;**54**: 405-414. DOI: 10.1016/S0007-1536(70) 80155-3

[50] Alexander KC, Ramakrishnan K. Infection of the bud, establishment in the host and production of whips in sugarcane smut (*Ustilago scitaminea*) of sugarcane. Proceedings of the International Society of Sugarcane Technologist. 1980;**17**:1452-1455

[51] Santiago R, Alarcón B, de Armas R, Vicente C, Legaz ME. Changes in the cynnamyl alcohol dehydrogenases activities from sugarcane cultivars inoculated with *Sporisorium scitamineum* sporidia. Physiologia Plantarum. 2012; **145**:245-259. DOI: 10.1111/j.1399-3054.2012.01577.x

[52] Sánchez-Elordi E, Vicente-Manzanares M, Díaz E, Legaz ME, Vicente C. Plant–pathogen interactions: Sugar cane glycoproteins induce chemotaxis of smut teliospores by cyclic contraction and relaxation of the

cytoskeleton. South African Journal of Botany. 2016;**105**:66-78. DOI: 10.1016/j.sajb.2015.12.005

[53] Brand A, Gow NAR. Tropic orientation responses of pathogenic fungi. In: Pérez-Martin J, Di Pietro A, editors. Morphogenesis and Pathogenicity in Fungi. Berlin: Springer Verlag; 2012. pp. 21-41. DOI: 10.1007/978-3-642-22916-9

[54] McBride MJ. Bacterial gliding motility: Multiple mechanisms for cell movement over surfaces. Annual Review of Microbiology. 2001;**55**:49-75. DOI: 10.1146/annurev.micro.55.1.49

[55] Strange PG. Use of the GTPγS ([35S] GTPγS and Eu-GTPγS) binding assay for analysis of ligand potency and efficacy at G protein-coupled receptors. British Journal of Pharmacology. 2010; **161**:1238-1249. DOI: 10.1111/j.1476-5381.2010.00963.x

[56] Peterson DA, Peterson DC, Reeve HL, Archer SL, Wei EK. GTP (γS) and GDP(βS) as electron donors: New wine in old bottles. Life Sciences. 1999;**65**: 1135-1140. DOI: 10.1016/S0024-3205 (99)00347-1

[57] Rodriguez OC, Schaefer AW, Mandato CA, Forscher P, Bement WM, Waterman-Storer CM. Conserved microtubule–actin interactions in cell movement and morphogenesis. Nature Cell Biology. 2003;**5**:599-609. DOI: 10.1038/ncb0703-599

[58] Sánchez-Elordi E, Baluška F, Echevarría C, Vicente C, Legaz ME. Defence sugarcane glycoproteins disorganize microtubules and prevent nuclear polarization and germination of *Sporisorium scitamineum* teliospores. Journal of Plant Physiology. 2016;**200**: 111-123. DOI: 10.1016/j.jplph.2016.05.022

[59] Fischer R, Zekert N, Takeshita N. Polarized growth in fungi – Interplay between the cytoskeleton, positional

markers and membrane domains.
Molecular Microbiology. 2008;**68**:
813-826. DOI: 10.1111/
j.1365-2958.2008.06193.x

[60] Baumann S, Pohlmann T, Jungbluth
M, Brachmann A, Feldbrugge M.
Kinesin-3 and dynein mediate
microtubule-dependent co-transport of
mRNPs and endosomes. Journal of Cell
Science. 2012;**125**:2740-2752. DOI:
10.1242/jcs.101212

[61] Xiang X, Plamann M. Cytoskeleton
and motor proteins in filamentous
fungi. Current Opinion in Microbiology.
2003;**6**:628-633. DOI: 10.1016/j.
mib.2003.10.009

[62] Gupta K, Dey A, Gupta B. Plant
polyamines in abiotic stress responses.
Acta Physiologiae Plantarum. 2013;**35**:
2015-2036. DOI: 10.1007/s11738-013-
1.5239-4

Chapter 2

Hemorheological Evaluation and Cytokine Production in Dogs Naturally Infected with Anaplasmataceae

Saulo Pereira Cardoso, Giane Regina Paludo,
José Nivaldo da Silva, Adenilda Honório-França
and Eduardo Luzia França

Abstract

In this chapter, we describe that naturally infected dogs with Anaplasmataceae show altered rhreological parameters. Also, we have showed that lower viscosity correlated with the lower erythrocyte number and release of IFN-γ. The rheometry of the fresh blood samples was measured by using the Modular Compact Rheometer—MCR 102 (Anton Paar® GmbH, Ostfildern, Germany), and the graphs were obtained using Rheoplus software. Blood count data were obtained by analysis in a private laboratory. Diagnostic confirmation was obtained by molecular PCR technique that was used to determine the groups of not infected and infected by Anaplasmataceae. Serum cytokines were dosed by flow cytometry (FACScalibur BD®) using BD® Biosciences Cytometric Bead Array (CBA) Human Th1/Th2/Th17 Cytokine kits. The results showed a correlation between blood viscosity ($p < 0.05$, $r = 0.73$) and shear rate ($p < 0.05$; $r = -0.676$) with IFN-γ in the group of infected dogs that presented anemia, as well as correlations of shear rate with erythrocytes ($p < 0.05$; $r = -0.88$). Thus, IFN-γ appears to play an important role in the immunomodulation of the rheological behavior of naturally infected dogs to Anaplasmataceae. The alterations in cytokines profile and their relationship with blood viscosity and hematological parameters was related in this study the first time of dogs naturally infected with Anaplasmataceae.

Keywords: Anaplasmataceae, rheology, immunomodulation, cytokines, dogs

1. Introduction

In the environment, animals can naturally suffer from co-infections with more than one pathogen, primarily high-incidence diseases such as invertebrate vector-borne hemoparasites, which multiply in short cycles. The diseases caused by microorganisms of the Anaplasmataceae family, transmitted by the *Rhipicephalus sanguineus* ectoparasite vector, such as *Ehrlichia canis* and *Anaplasma platys* [1] are highly prevalent in Brazil and worldwide [2, 3].

E. canis is a causative bacterium of Canine Monocytic Ehrlichiosis (CME) that infects mononuclear cells, mainly found in monocytes, where they develop and replicate using the cellular apparatus, and subsequently spread and infect new cells [4]. The *A. platys* only infects platelets leading to transient thrombocytopenia [5] without developing severe dog disease, known as Canine Cyclic Thrombocytopenia [6].

Infectious diseases may alter the hematological parameters of the affected individuals and, consequently, there is alteration of hemorheological behavior [7–9]. In addition, immunological factors are also responsible for the change in blood viscosity. On the other hand, cytokines may play an important role in the immunomodulation of hemorheological behavior. Cytokine IL-17 has immunomodulatory effect on blood viscosity of human patients infected with *Plasmodium vivax*, such response may be important for maintaining erythrocyte integrity [7].

The therapeutic use of cytokines may help in the treatment of individuals with changes in blood viscosity [7]. In addition, it can modulate Th1 type responses [10, 11].

Studies on the hemorheological behavior of dogs with infectious diseases, as well as the immunomodulation of this process help to understand the immunophysiopathological mechanisms [7, 9].

This chapter deals with cytokines involved in the immunomodulation of hematological and rheological parameters of the blood of dogs naturally infected by bacteria from Anaplasmataceae family.

1.1 Etiology, occurrence, and distribution

The microorganisms of the Anaplasmataceae family belong to the order Alphaproteobacteria and to the class Rickettsiales. They are gram negative, intracellular-obligatory [12]. They have coccoid or rod shapes, varying in size from 0.2 to 0.5 micrometers (μm) in diameter and 0.8–2.0 μm in length. They are found forming colonies within intracytoplasmic vacuoles. These colonies are surrounded by a membrane that delimits them, being this colony-vacuole set called morula [13].

The Rickettsiales class microorganisms have an infective form, the dense nucleus cell. After infection, it develops the vegetative form, the reticulated cell, which multiplies by binary fission. In the process of infection, they are phagocytized by the host cell and remain inside vacuoles or phagosomes, where fusion with lysosomes does not occur, and develop there and form the morula. After vegetative forms mature, they can become infectious forms and be released from the cytoplasm by exocytosis or lysis of host cells, thereby infecting new cells [4].

The Anaplasmataceae family comprises the following species reported as infectious agents of dogs: *E. canis, E. ewingii, E. chaffeensis, A. phagocytophilum, A. platys,* and *Nanophyetus helminthoeca* [14, 15]. There are also reports of *E. risticii* infection [16]. However, to date in the Brazilian territory, the clinically important species for pets that cause hematological disorders in dogs are *E. canis and A. platys* [17, 18]. *E. canis* has mononuclear cell tropism, mainly monocytes, whereas *A. platys* infects platelets [19]. *E. ewingii* infections in dogs can also cause hematological changes and other signs of hemoparasitosis [2].

Prevalence studies of Anaplasmataceae show that these infectious agents are widely distributed in tropical and subtropical countries [20]. Dogs with suspected CME have high rates of positivity for Anaplasmataceae infections [1, 21], whereas in domestic cats, this rate is low [22].

Most studies involving the Anaplasmataceae family aim not only to identify the taxonomic family of agents, but also to try to identify genus and species. Thus, the epidemiology of *E. canis and A. platys*, which are the main species of this family that affect dogs in Brazil, will be presented below.

1.1.1 Ehrlichia canis

In the year 1935, researchers first detected a rickettsial microorganism parasitizing dog mononuclear cells [23]. Only in 1945 did Mashkovsky reclassify this agent as *E. canis* [24]. However, it has become known worldwide as a causative agent of CME in an outbreak of infection with a high mortality rate in German shepherd dogs used by the US military during the Vietnam War [25]. In Brazil, it had its first report in dogs in the 1970s [26].

Dogs infected with *E. canis* develop CME, a worldwide disease found in different continents: South America, Central America, Europe, Asia, Oceania [27], North America [28], and Africa [29]. They are in the tropical and subtropical regions of these continents where there is the ectoparasite vector *R. sanguineus* and the highest prevalence rates of CME [27, 30].

The genus *Ehrlichia* is widely distributed in Brazil [17], being positive for 20% of dogs seen in the country [31]. In 1996, in Venezuela, the first report of chronic *E. canis* infection in humans occurred [32]. There are also reports in humans in the United States causing a chronic disease that can be fatal [33, 34]. Clinical signs are variables such as fever, weakness, muscle and bone pain, headache, nausea, vomiting, abdominal pain, arthralgia, and rash. Hematological parameters present anemia, thrombocytopenia, and leukopenia [32]. Thus, *E. canis* infection can also be treated as a public health issue and not just veterinary [27, 35].

1.1.2 Anaplasma platys

A. platys is the causative agent of Canine Cyclic Thrombocytopenia (CRT), which colonizes and replicates in dog platelets. Its first description was in the 1970s, Florida-USA, as a *Rickettsia*-like organism capable of infecting dog platelets [6]. In addition to reporting the visualization of this agent in blood smears, Harvey et al. [6] reproduced the infection experimentally in other dogs. No animal showed macroscopic alteration, the only alteration being a transient thrombocytopenia, without causing evident hemorrhages in the infected ones [6].

In different countries in Europe, the prevalence of this agent can range from 0.4 to 70.5% according to molecular research using blood samples from dogs, age, animal breed or gender does not appear to influence the development of CRT [36, 37].

In Brazil, the prevalence of *A. platys* infection in dogs varies in different regions, being higher in the northeast [1, 2, 22, 38–40].

Molecular studies have also detected *A. platys* in humans in the United States and Venezuela, indicating potential risk of zoonosis [41, 42].

1.1.3 Coinfecção por E. canis e A. platys

E. canis and *A. platys* coinfection using molecular detection in dogs are reported in Brazil [43], with prevalence ranging from 5.5 to 53.3% [1, 44, 45].

In other countries, co-infections with these bacteria also occur in dogs. In the USA, they found a 5% prevalence in dogs with a history of tick exposure [46]. This same rate was found by Yabsley et al. [47, 48] in blood samples from dogs from Granada, Spain.

1.2 Transmission

The microorganisms of the Anaplasmataceae family are transmitted to their hosts mainly by vectors that inoculate them in susceptible animals. The increase in the number of cases of infections in dogs by these bacteria in a given region is linked to the presence of the transmitting vector in the environment and its behavior of feeding on mammalian blood, with a preference for canids. Infection occurs at the moment when the tick *R. sanguineus* performs hematophagy and ends up injecting saliva contaminated with Anaplasmataceae at the bite site [47, 48].

Both larvae and nymphs, as well as adult forms of the *R. sanguineus* tick infected by *E. canis*, are capable of transmitting it to the host [47, 48]. There is no transovarian transmission from adult ticks to their larval forms in the reproduction process of *R. sanguineus* [27]. Ticks only become infected when they feed on infected animals that are in the bacteremia phase of the disease [49]. Although vector transmission of *E. canis* is the main mode of infection, it can also occur in cases of blood transfusion from an infected to an uninfected host [50, 51].

Regarding *A. platys* transmission, it is not clear how it occurs. It is suspected to be similar to *E. canis* by ticks, but the process has not yet been confirmed experimentally [52, 53]. Some more recent studies point to possible vertical transmission from mother to pups, but the transmission process has not been confirmed [53, 54].

The *R. sanguineus* ectoparasite (Acari: Ixodida), known as the brown dog tick, is the main vector of *E. canis* [55]. It is also believed to serve as a vector for *A. platys*, although the infection has not been reproduced in the laboratory so far. One of the main evidence of this possibility is the discovery of *A. platys* DNA in female *R. sanguineus* using molecular technique [44, 56]. This tick has a cosmopolitan distribution in tropical regions and, taking advantage of global warming, proliferates in regions of temperate climate, but under conditions of shelter that provides its development [47, 48].

Once infected with *E. canis*, this vector becomes a source of lifelong infection. Thus, a larva may remain infected even after undergoing changes in its life cycle, maintaining trans-state transmission [57]. *E. canis* colonizes oral salivary gland cells and is also found in vector cells, called hemocytes, and tick intestinal cells [58].

Other ticks like Ixodes spp. and *Dermacentor* ssp. are also capable of transmitting the Anaplasmataceae family pathogens to susceptible hosts at the time of the bite [59, 60].

1.3 Immunological response and mechanisms of immune evasion of microorganisms from Anaplasmataceae family

Host resistance to the *Anaplasma* genus is linked to IFN-γ production [61]. This protective effect is potentiated by TNF-α [62]. On the other hand, there is a description that TNF-α may favor the aggravation of the clinical condition of dogs, as observed in cases of distemper [63].

The process of immune response to members of the Anaplasmataceae family can lead to tissue damage in the liver of the infected host regardless of the bacterial load in their body, due to a simple induction of proinflammatory mechanisms that induce a cellular response that develops such damage. These lesions are generally more severe than those directly induced by the infectious agent itself, as observed in a study with experimental *A. phagocytophilum* infection in mice [64].

Ehrlichia-infected monocytes have a slower response to LPS when compared to uninfected monocytes, as this pathogen inhibits activation of the nuclear factor kappa beta (NF-κβ) transcription factor. This infection also disrupts toll-like receptor expression (TLR 2 and 4) and inhibits other signaling pathways that rely on monocyte activation receptors [65]. In addition, infection induces inhibition of gene transcription for IL-12, IL-15, and IL-18 production [66].

In persistent *Ehrlichia* infections, it has been experimentally demonstrated in mice that the host maintains its survival when there is increased IFN-γ production by CD4 + and CD8 + T lymphocytes, low concentration of TNF-α and antibody production to *Ehrlichia*, mainly IgG2 [67].

The survival of the genus *Ehrlichia* in monocytes depends on the mechanisms that this bacterium uses to block the fusion of phagosomes with lysosomes, inhibiting cell apoptosis to utilize its nutrients and energy longer [68].

Susceptibility to the development of CME has immunomodulatory mechanisms involved in the process. Experimental infections in mice with *E. muris*, intracellular mononuclear leukocyte parasite demonstrated high concentration CD8 + T production of TNF-α as well as systemic inflammatory response mediated by this cytokine and inhibition of Th1 profile T CD4 proliferation [67].

Regarding *E. canis*, NK cells play their role in the immune response, but are not primordial in the host resistance process [69]. Although some animals with CME have bone marrow cell depletion in the chronic phase, subclinical neutropenia and transient lymphopenia in the acute phase, it was found in an experimental study that in the acute and subacute phases of the disease, *E. canis* was not able to induce immunosuppression in young dogs, up to 1 year old on average [69].

One study showed that dogs experimentally infected with *E. canis* had elevated TNF-α production by splenocytes and leukocytes during acute CME, followed by high levels of IL-10 for both cell lines and, finally, only the leukocytes showed IFN-γ production in small scale [70]. TNF-α production at high levels in the experimental infection with *E. canis* was also verified by Rikihisa and Tajima [5]. Since in naturally infected dogs, Lima et al. [71] found elevated levels of TNF-α and IL-10, but the analysis found no difference between the means of groups infected and uninfected for both cytokines.

Studies report that specific immune response to *A. platys* is innovative. Research involving *Anaplasma* genus and its immune response mostly describe the species *A. phagocytophilum*, which infects granulocytes of different animal species [72], or *A. marginale* which infect red blood cells and bovine monocytes [73].

The control of infection by *A. phagocytophilum* in humans and other animals, including the dog, is dependent on the IFN-γ production and macrophage activation, which leads to the control of a recent bacteremia [74]. This occurs in an initial immune response, with the role of NK cells to produce IFN-γ, but that is not important for eliminating the infectious agent.

Contrary to expectation, the immune response to *A. phagocytophilum* is not dependent Th1 cytokines such as IL-12 and IFN-γ, but CD4 + effector T cells are also strictly necessary for the eradication of the pathogen [75].

A. marginale infections induce CD4 T cell proliferation as well as a humoral response with high levels of IgG1 and IgG2. This bacterium has great ability to generate variant forms by converting gene segments, which allows an escape from the immune response [76].

Intracellular organisms have different mechanisms of escape from the immune response to maintain their survival and multiply. Some may induce non-fusion of phagosome with lysosome, while others escape from phagosome to cytosol. By using their structural apparatus to disrupt the phagosome environment and inhibit its fusion to lysosomes, these pathogens gain time to take on a more resistant form to the acid and proteolytic environment and perpetuate within the infected cell [77].

In many cases, these infectious agents may induce a Th2-type cellular response. IL-10 secretion by Th2 inhibits Th1 response and macrophage activation by the classical pathway [78]. Intracellular organisms may also inhibit IL-12 production by infected macrophages [79].

1.4 Pathophysiology of CME and CRT and clinical signs

E. canis uses different strategies from other traditional intracellular bacteria in the process of infection because is a bacterium with deficiency of structural membrane components such as peptidioglicanos and LPS. Its genome has genes that encode proteins responsible for evasion to the immune system and for playing an important role in parasite-host interaction. Surface proteins present in the genus *Ehrlichia* with repeats of serine and threonine components are responsible for membrane attack and host cell entry [80]. Twelve tandem repeating proteins, three specific for *E. canis*, were identified, demonstrating a variability of membrane protein repertoire, which facilitates escape to the immune system [81].

The manifestations and clinical signs in positive dogs can variable and are observed in the different phases of the CME. The acute phase occurs after an incubation period ranging from 8 to 20 days [82]. The subclinical course of infection, which occurs when no clinical signs of the disease are observed, may develop after an acute course of course in dogs that have not cleared the agent. And finally, there is the chronic course phase with signs of severe disease [83].

Significant low platelet count in CME is the main sign observed in the hematological parameters of dogs [84]. Such a fall is linked to different factors: excessive platelet consumption due to endothelial lesions, destruction by immunological action, and an increased splenic sequestration of these platelets [85]. It has been reported that there is a platelet migration inhibiting factor that favors splenic sequestration [86].

In CRT, the mechanism of platelet reduction occurs by phagocytosis of these blood components that have been damaged by the bacteria or destroyed in an immunomediated manner [6]. In addition, it has been shown that *A. platys* infection can occur in platelet-generating myeloid precursors, such as promegakaryocytes and megakaryocytes [87].

1.4.1 Fase aguda da CME

During the acute phase of CME, there is an elevation of inflammatory cytokines linked to the immune response, such as TNF-α, IL-10, and IFN-γ [70]. However, Lima et al. [71] reported in their work that TNF-α and IL-10 are not associated with early-stage clinical signs of CME. Some dogs may present in the acute phase thrombocytopenia and anemia; however, thrombocytopenia is also detected in dogs in the subclinical phase when the animal is not treated [84], and leukopenia may also occur [88]. In the acute phase, there are the appearances of several nonspecific clinical signs such as anorexia, fever, weight loss, lymphadenomegaly, splenomegaly, and apathy, also occurring vasculitis [83].

In the study by Sousa et al. [89], dogs with *E. canis* infection showed nonspecific clinical signs, such as apathy, anorexia, fever, and mucosal pallor. They also presented ophthalmic disorders, tendencies to hemorrhage and splenomegaly. Other studies reported diarrhea, emesis, hematemesis, abdominal pain, dilation of the abdomen, difficulty in walking [90].

Ophthalmologic lesions can occur at any stage of CME and include anterior uveitis, retinal or subretinal hemorrhage with detachment, chorioretinitis, and blindness [91].

Clinical and laboratory findings consist of an increase or decrease in the number of leukocytes (neutrophils and lymphocytes) and platelets and predominantly anemia [89]. It also presents anemia as the most frequent hematological disorder, followed by thrombocytopenia [90].

1.4.2 Subclinical phase of CME

The chronic course can last up to 5 years, in a subclinical state, until the serious disease develops. In the subclinical phase, there is thrombocytopenia [88], high antibody production, mainly due to hypergammaglobulinemia, but with hypoalbuminemia [88, 92].

1.4.3 Chronic phase of CME

In the severe phase, weight loss, wasting, lymphadenopathy, fevers, hemorrhages, non-regenerative anemia, thrombocytopenia, spinal cord pancytopenia, and death are observed [88, 93, 94]. Hyperglobulinemia is also observed and may favor the development of blood hyperviscosity [95]. Animals die due to bleeding or septicemia caused by *E. canis* [88].

1.4.4 Acute phase of TRC

TRC caused by *A. platys* has an acute and cyclic phase following an incubation period of 1–2 weeks, with a parasitemia occurring every 10 to 14 days causing a transient thrombocytopenia accompanied by fever [96]. One study has shown that experimental *A. platys* infection has developed lymph node enlargement in dogs [96]. However, many dogs present asymptomatic TRC [97].

In Europe and the Middle East, there are descriptions of *A. platys* strains that are more virulent and cause disease with clinical signs similar to dogs with CME [98, 99]. Thus, dogs with infection with virulent *A. platys* strains may show clinical signs of abdominal pain, splenomegaly, high fever, thrombocytopenia, hypoproteinemia, large platelets, monocytosis, and low hematocrit [88, 100]. Another study found dogs naturally infected with *A. platys* with acute clinical signs of anorexia, depression, weight loss, transient epistaxis, pale mucosae, severe thrombocytopenia, anemia, leukopenia, and hyperproteinemia [98].

1.4.5 Chronic phase of TRC

In Brazil, TRC does not develop severe clinical signs in dogs, only a decrease in platelet counts in general. Dogs that have *A. platys* infection have cyclic thrombocytopenia, but do not have bleeding episodes as in dogs with CME [101].

The chronic phase demonstrates an adaptation of the infected animal's organism to infection. At this stage, infected dogs have a cyclic period of low parasitemia accompanied by moderate thrombocytopenia [102].

2. Diagnostic methods

2.1 Parasitological diagnosis

Pathogen identification can be done using blood smears. In the acute phase of the disease, *E. canis* morulae can be observed inside mononuclear cells or, in the case of *A. platys*, on platelets. However, these agents may not be found in many of these cases, as they are more commonly found in dogs sick in the febrile phase [103].

Direct visualization of the agent in mononuclear cells, especially lymphocytes, seen in blood smears is known to be a definitive diagnosis of CME, as visualization of morulae with correct morphological characterization is considered a pathogno-monic sign of the disease [103]. However, there are other agents that infect mono-nuclear cells, and differential diagnosis should be made correctly in order to avoid false-negative diagnosis [104].

2.2 Serologic diagnosis

For the detection of CME, there are several diagnostic methods. At the veteri-nary clinic, a rapid test with only one drop of blood is routinely performed based on the serum evaluation of anti-*Ehrlichia* antibodies [88]. Similarly, there are kits for detection of *A. platys* and *A. phagocytophilum* [105].

Indirect immunofluorescence a serological test used more in research, marks the specific target with antibodies to be viewed and can be used as a definitive diagnosis [55, 106].

2.3 Culture and isolation

Members of the Rickettsialles family, such as *Ehrlichia*, can be cultured in cultured cells under controlled conditions, but proliferation time is prolonged. This, in addition to the fact that many techniques depend on purification of the agent relative to the host cell component of the culture, makes the process even more difficult and time consuming [107].

2.4 Molecular diagnosis

The definitive diagnosis can also be performed by molecular examinations by detecting genetic material from microorganisms in the samples [108, 109] and specificity [110]. Over the years, it has become an increasingly modern and improved technique for pathogen identification and safe against possible contami-nation, such as quantitative PCR (qPCR) [111].

2.5 Clinical and laboratory diagnosis

The presumptive clinical diagnosis of CME made by the professional in the vet-erinary office can be performed by observing clinical signs; however, there is a high chance of giving a different result than the real one, since CME has a multisystemic character and nonspecific clinical signs, thus requiring other tools [35].

In clinical and laboratory analyzes, thrombocytopenia presented by dogs with clinical signs suggestive of CME helps to rule out other diseases, being this param-eter used in routine veterinary clinics as a strong suspicion of being positive for *E. canis* [112]. Other signs such as anemia, leukocytosis, and leukopenia are observed in dogs with CME, which helps in the diagnosis [89]. Observation of isolated thrombocytopenia without other clinical signs are suggestive of CRT [6].

2.6 Differential diagnosis

The clinical and laboratory signs presented observed in CME and CRT can be observed in other diseases caused by other infectious agents, especially those transmitted by ticks. Infections such as hepatozonosis, babesiosis, and distemper may present similar clinical signs and should be considered in the differential diagnosis [113]. Another disease to be considered is canine visceral leishmaniasis (CVL) in cases of thrombocytopenia, anemia, medular aplasia, and hemorrhages [114], especially in regions endemic for CVL [113].

2.7 Hemorheological diagnosis

Animals infected with hematozoa, including Anaplasmataceae, may present changes in hematological parameters [89]. However, hematozoa can also lead to alteration of the rheological behavior of the blood, as a work that demonstrated alteration of blood viscosity of humans infected with *Plasmodium* ssp. [7], and another that demonstrated changes in blood viscosity of dogs infected with *Leishmania* ssp. [9].

Rheometry is an auxiliary tool that allows the measurement of the fluid viscosity curve, as well as the blood, and can be used to monitor these altered parameters in dogs with hematological and rheological disorders, thus serving as an ally in the therapeutic monitoring of sick dogs. Such a tool has been used experimentally to measure blood viscosity in both *Plasmodium* ssp. infected humans [7], as in dogs infected with *Leishmania* ssp. [9].

2.8 Rheology

Rheometric blood analysis or hemoremometry is a technique for measuring blood viscosity that helps in understanding the pathogenesis of diseases affecting the blood [9]. Blood functions as a viscous fluid, with different viscosities depending on the amount of cells, platelets, and other blood solutes [114, 115], so if a disease alters the amount of cells, the deformability erythrocyte or serum components, the viscosity also changes.

Rheometry allows the measurement of blood viscosity using the rheometer, a device that measures the ability of a liquid to flow based on its resistance to dissipation when pressure is applied to it [116]. To understand how immunomodulation of blood rheological behavior occurs in metabolic or infectious diseases, the change in blood viscosity can be compared between sick and healthy, and these data correlate with cytokine profile for investigation of the immunophysiopathological process, as demonstrated by França et al. [8] and Scherer et al. [7].

This branch of science allows an understanding of how hemorheological behavior is influenced by cellular components and blood plasma on blood viscosity, peripheral resistance, circulating volume, and blood pressure. The capacity of erythrocyte deformation is influenced by blood pressure, and this phenomenon is important for maintaining macro tantone blood flow as well as microcirculation [114]. Blood viscosity is also influenced by blood cell count. Patients with anemia demonstrate decreased blood viscosity [117].

The increased amount of leukocytes and platelets disturbs the normal flow of erythrocytes, especially in microcirculation. Another phenomenon that impairs this flow is when the erythrocytes lose their capacity for deformation, or when the pressure of the blood vessels is increased, making it difficult to pass, such as diabetes mellitus, changes in the physical characteristics of erythrocytes are observed [114].

Viscosity and blood flow become compromised to cellular and plasma changes that occur in various diseases. Metabolic diseases such as diabetes mellitus lead to erythrocyte changes [118], in addition to other factors such as increased serum osmolarity [119] and endothelial lesions lead to blood hyperviscosity syndrome [120]. In infectious diseases, such as those caused by obligate intracellular parasites, increased blood viscosity occurs, as observed in dogs with Canine Visceral Leishmaniasis [9] and in humans with malaria [7].

This technique has been used in research to help understand diseases by blood parasites such as *Plasmodium* spp., causative agent of malaria. Infected individuals showed elevated blood viscosity and high levels of IFN-γ and IL-17, as well as low TGF-β concentration compared to uninfected ones [7]. In addition to infectious diseases, metabolic diseases such as diabetes melittus lead to changes in blood viscosity [8]. Thus, blood viscosity may also be influenced by the action of substances present in serum such as cytokines.

Rheometry, considered as a low-cost auxiliary technique, can be used as a tool for monitoring the hematological condition and haemorrheological behavior of animals infected with infectious diseases, as shown in a study that evaluated dogs naturally infected with *Leishmania* sp. [9].

3. Metodology aspects, results, and discussion

The procedures were previously approved by the Animal Use Ethics Committee-CEUA/UFMT, Brazil, and collection of clinical samples was authorized by the dog owners by signing the informed consent form.

Blood samples were collected from 72 dogs, regardless of males and females, of different ages and breeds, during the 19 months in Barra do Garças—MT (52.2599 15° 53' 35 South, 52° 15' 36" Oeste), Midwest region of Brazil to analyze the rheometry parameters and cytokines concentrations. Diagnostic confirmation was obtained by molecular Polymerase Chain Reaction (PCR) technique that was used to determine the groups of not infected and infected by Anaplasmataceae. The rheometry of the fresh blood samples was measured by using the Modular Compact Rheometer—MCR 102 (Anton Paar® GmbH, Ostfildern, Germany), and the graphs were obtained using Rheoplus software. Blood count data were obtained by analysis in a private laboratory. Serum cytokines were dosed by flow cytometry (FACScalibur BD®) using BD® Biosciences Cytometric Bead Array (CBA) kits.

For the statistical analysis of the concentration of cytokines, rheological and hematological parameters used the Student t test. For the correlation analyses, the Pearson correlation test was used. Data were expressed as mean ± standard error. Values less than 0.05 ($p < 0.05$) were considered significant.

Thus, serological screening was initially performed to check for natural infection using the SNAP 4DX Plus of IDEXX ELISA test for detection of both *Ehrlichia* ssp. and *Anaplasma* spp. High rates of infection (75%) with Anaplasmataceae were observed (**Table 1**). Interestingly, studies on dogs with suspected infection also had high rates of infection with these bacteria [21].

Seroprevalence of 51% (29/57) for *Ehrlichia* spp. was higher in dogs evaluated when compared with other studies [1, 21, 55]. In the literature, there are data on seroprevalence of *A. platys* in Brazil and worldwide [2, 3]. In this work, the prevalence of *Anaplasma* spp. was 25%, whereas in other studies in Brazil and Asia were showed lower prevalence [2, 3].

Diagnostic confirmation was performed by PCR molecular examination using the primer oligonucleotides shown in **Table 2**. The results showed a prevalence of 52% of Anaplasmataceae infection, which is slightly lower compared to other similar work also developed in Mato Grosso [1]. Such high rates are also found in a

	Negative	**Anaplasmataceae**	**Ehrlichia spp.**	**Anaplasma spp.**	**Ehrlichia + Anaplasma**	**Total**
Number	14	43	29	14	12	57
Prevalence (%)	25	75	51	25	21	

Table 1.
*Detection of specific antibody for Anaplasmataceae family (*Ehrlichia *ssp. and* Anaplasma *spp.) using SNAP 4DX Plus of IDEXX ELISA test in dogs from the city of Barra do Garças—MT.*

Identification	Sequence 5'-3'	Author	Primer
Anaplasmataceae	GGTACCYACAGAAGAAGTCC	Inokuma et al. [121]	EHR16sd
	TAGCACTCATCGTTTACAGC	Inokuma et al. [121]	EHR16sr
E. canis	CAATTATTTATAGCCTCTGGCTATAGGA	Murphy et al. [122]	ECAN5
	TATAGGTACCGTCATTATCTTCCCTAT	Murphy et al. [122]	HE3
A. platys	GATTTTTGTCGTAGCTTGCTATG	Lima et al. [22]	PLATYS
	TAGCACTCATCGTTTACAGC	Lima et al. [22]	EHR16sr

Table 2.
Primers used in the PCR tests of the present study.

seroprevalence study in northeastern Brazil that shows to be greater than 50% in the Alagoas state [17].

In contrast, in the amplification of the *E. canis* and *A. platys* DNA gene16S, there were prevalences of 28 and 32%, respectively. Regarding *E. canis*, other authors found a prevalence of 38.4–59% [1, 21]. Studies with *A. platys* using molecular techniques in Mato Grosso revealed 26.2% [1]. However, higher prevalence of infection has been reported in other regions of Brazil [11, 123].

Coinfection by *A. platys* and *E. canis* are also commonly found in dogs in areas containing the *R. sanguineus* vector [34]. In the animals evaluated in this study, it was observed a prevalence of 20% of coinfection (**Table 3**).

Table 4 presents the results of the mean values of erythrogram, leukogram, platelet, and total protein parameters that were analyzed in the samples of negative dogs positive for Anaplasmataceae. Blood count showed a significant difference between mean erythrocyte values (p = 0.03) in the group of animals infected with Anaplasmataceae, suggesting a mild to severe anemia in these animals. Reduction in erythrocyte count showed a strong positive correlation (p = 0.013; r = 0.7) with blood viscosity, but was more evident in a negative erythrocyte correlation with shear rate in this same group (p = 0.0001; r = −0.88).

Dogs naturally infected by Anaplasmataceae showed changes in blood viscosity compared to uninfected dogs (**Table 5**). Viscosity values were inversely proportional to shear rate in both groups studied (**Figure 1**). Also, there were differences in shear rate (p = 0.008). Previous work on dogs infected with Leishmania also showed changes in blood viscosity [9]. Blood flow curves and their respective hysteresis areas in infected animals revealed lower shear rates compared to uninfected animals (**Figure 2**).

The mean viscosity and shear rate values in both groups revealed significant differences for both parameters (**Table 5**). There were differences in shear rate (p = 0.008) and also in viscosity (p < 0.0001). There was no difference in the averages analyzed between the groups regarding the leukocyte, platelet, and total protein concentrations.

The serum profile of inflammatory, anti-inflammatory, and regulatory cytokines, IL-2, IL-4, IL-6, IL-10, TNF-α, IFN-γ, IL-17A were evaluated according to Scherer et al. [7] and Silva et al. [9]. Among the cytokines, the only one that showed difference between the infected and uninfected groups was IL-10 (**Table 6**). The serum concentration of this interleukin was lower in the infected group when compared to dogs Anaplasmataceae negative.

The hemogram, rheometry, and serum cytokines parameters were correlated using Pearson's correlation test (**Figure 3**). There was an inversely proportional correlation between viscosity and shear rate, shear rate and erythrocytes, and shear

	Negative	Anaplasmataceae	*E. canis*	*A. platys*	*E. canis + A. platys*
Number	12	13	7	8	5
Prevalence (%)	48	52	28	32	20

Table 3.
Results of PCR tests for detection of Anaplasmataceae, E. canis *and* A. platys *bacteria.*

	Negative	Anaplasmataceae	Statistical
Erythrocytes (tera/L)	7.5 ± 1.09	5.76 ± 1.91	$p < 0.05$
Hemoglobin (g/dL)	17.18 ± 2.46	13.09 ± 4.19	$p < 0.05$
Hematocrit (%)	50.3 ± 6.77	38.4 ± 12.7	$p < 0.05$
Leukocytes(1/μL)	10.92 ± 2.40	11.81 ± 5.29	$p > 0.05$
Neutrophils (1/μL)	6.57 ± 1.87	8.02 ± 3.98	$p > 0.05$
lymphocytes (1/μL)	2.87 ± 0.98	2.5 ± 1.7	$p > 0.05$
Monocytes (1/μL)	0.42 ± 0.25	0.4 ± 0.24	$p > 0.05$
Platelets (1/μL)	177.16 ± 81.74	191.58 ± 103.56	$p > 0.05$
Total Protein (g/dL)	6.83 ± 0.86	6.15 ± 1.2	$p > 0.05$

Table 4.
Hemogram and total protein values of dogs negative and positive for Anaplasmataceae bacteria.

	Negative	Anaplasmataceae	Stastitical
Viscosity (Pa/s)	$7.44 \pm 5.8 \times 10^{-3}$	$5.5 \pm 5.67 \times 10^{-3}$	$p < 0.05$
Share rate (1/s)	405.68 ± 51.09	592.56 ± 223.24	$p < 0.05$

Table 5.
Mean and standard deviation of the rheology of healthy dogs and dogs naturally infected by bacteria of the Anaplasmataceae.

rate and IFN-γ. We also observed directly proportional correlations between erythrocytes and blood viscosity, IFN-γ and blood viscosity, and IFN-γ and erythrocytes.

Dogs naturally infected by Leishmania have altered blood viscosity related to decreased erythrocytes [9]. In this study, there was a negative correlation between shear rate and hematocrit ($p = 0.0004$; $r = -0.85$).

The explanation for the occurrence of hemorheological alterations observed in dogs infected by Anaplasmataceae in this study may be related to alteration of erythrocyte morphology which, in turn, leads to alteration of blood viscosity as a systemic disease. Diseases caused by infectious agents that parasitize erythrocytes or monocytes lead to changes in the rheological properties of blood [7, 9, 124].

Infectious agents of the Anaplasmataceae family cause diseases with systemic manifestations in dogs, with morphological changes in erythrocytes and anemia in dogs with CME are common [21].

Morphological changes in leukocytes, platelets, and erythrocytes have also been described in cattle infected with a variety of agents including Anaplasmataceae bacteria, protozoa, and filaroid parasites [125]. Dogs with different types of anemia also have morphological changes, including anemia secondary to systemic inflammatory disease [126].

Dogs infected with *Leishmania* showed no correlation between blood viscosity or shear rate and leukocyte, platelet, total protein and globulin parameters [9]. In this study, dogs naturally infected by bacteria of the Anaplasmataceae showed no

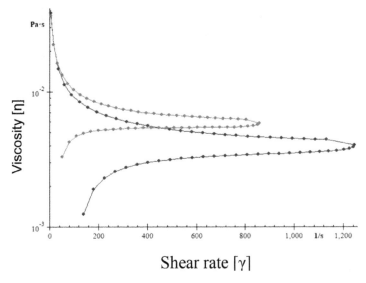

Figure 1.
Viscosity curves of dog whole blood infected or not by bacteria of Anaplasmataceae.

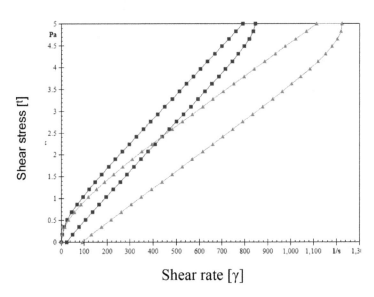

Figure 2.
Histerese area of flow curve of dog whole blood infected or not by bacteria of Anaplasmataceae.

correlation between viscosity and leukocytes, platelets and interleukins (IL-2, IL-4, IL-6, IL-10, TNF-α, and IL-17a).

The cytokine TNF-α may aggravate the clinical signs in animals infected by Anaplasmataceae [63], but in this study no correlations of this cytokine with altera-tion of viscosity, anemia or leukocytes were found. The data presented corroborate the one presented by Lima et al. [71] who found no correlation of anemia with TNF-α and IL-10 in dogs naturally infected with *E. canis*.

Total proteins were strongly correlated with blood viscosity in relation to the group of animals infected by Anaplasmataceae bacteria (p = 0.0007; r = 0.84). Studies by Silva et al. [9] found no correlation between these parameters in

Cytokines	Anaplasmataceae (−)	Anaplasmataceae (+)
IL-2	67.1 ± 10.6	73.0 ± 14.7
IL-4	31.2 ± 9.9	34.5 ± 4.9
IL-6	31.3 ± 11.6	32.0 ± 3.8
IL-10	32.7 ± 8.2	37.1 ± 3.7[*]
IL-17	371.7 ± 224.2	502.1 ± 379.1
TNF-α	533.8 ± 260.4	319.6 ± 245.4
IFN-γ	253.8 ± 172.5	256.2 ± 156.4

The results were expressed in mean and standard error.
[*]$P < 0.05.$

Table 6.
Cytokine concentrations in dogs non-infected and dogs with Anaplasmataceae.

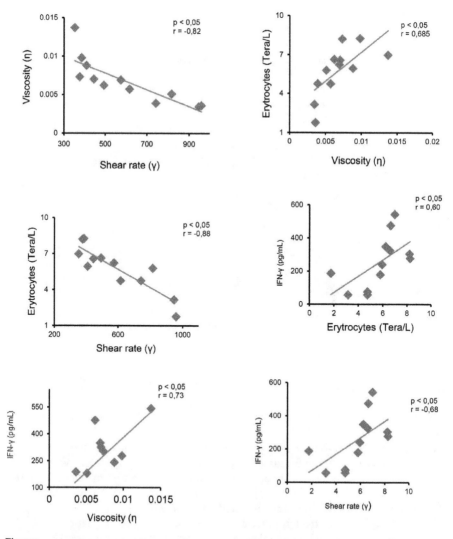

Figure 3.
Correlation between viscosity with erythrocytes, shear rates and IFN-γ; erythrocytes with shear rates and IFN-γ; and IFN-γ with shear rates of dogs infected with Anaplasmataceae.

Leishmania-positive dog samples, nor even a correlation between viscosity and immunoglobulins. However, it has been reported that fibrinogen binding may occur in erythrocytes due to increased serum fibrinogen concentration [127].

Interestingly, in this work, the serum IFN-γ concentration was promising. Regarding the group of animals infected by bacteria of the Anaplasmataceae family, this interleukin showed a strong positive correlation with blood viscosity (p = 0.007; r = 0.73), negative correlation with shear rate (p = 0.016; r = −0.68), which may indicate a modulation of hemorheological behavior, mainly a decrease in blood viscosity and, consequently, an increase in shear rate in animals infected by bacteria of the Anaplasmataceae family.

Cytokine immunomodulation is also reported in other mandatory intracellular parasite infections. Studies by Scherer et al. [7] demonstrated that in *P. vivax*-infected patients, IL-17a was the cytokine responsible for decreasing blood viscosity, which probably decreased erythrocyte rupture, as these cells demonstrated easy osmotic shock due to infection.

The possible correlation of IFN-γ with erythrocytes (p = 0.04; r = 0.6) in relation to the group of infected animals allows us to infer that IFN-γ was able to pathologically immunomodulate, aggravating the anemic condition in dogs. Martin et al. [61] described that IFN-γ is linked to the survival of the Anaplasmataceae infected patient, and this cytokine may have its effect increased in the presence of TNF-α [62]. No correlations were found between IFN-γ and TNF-α, even though there were serum concentrations of both cytokines in the blood of animals infected by bacteria from Anaplasmataceae family. Perhaps, TNF-α may influence the effect of IFN-γ on disease stage differences caused by Anaplasmataceae family bacteria in dogs.

Although IFN-γ is important in controlling infection with a Th1-type immune response [75], it can also be detrimental to erythrocytes in animals infected with Anaplasmataceae as it may lead to a severe decrease in cell count, if not immunoregulated by another cytokine.

Serum IL-10 levels showed a difference between the studied groups [**Table 6**], being relevant the increase of its concentration in dogs infected by Anaplasmataceae bacteria. Studies by Faria et al. [70] demonstrated that experimentally infected *E. canis* infected lymphocytes and splenocytes have high IL-10 and low IFN-γ production, indicating modulation to a Th2-like profile, as IL-10 negatively modulates IFN-γ production.

The use of IL-12 [11] and continuous use of IFN-γ [10] assist in the treatment of Leishmania infected animals, as the Th1 response profile is effective in eliminating the parasite. Experimental controlled use of anti-IL-10 antibodies also demonstrated improvement in Leishmania positive animals [128]. Thus, dogs undergoing treatment with Anaplasmataceae are likely to have a better chance of eliminating the agent using IFN-γ at controlled doses. In the case of dogs with anemia, perhaps the regulated use of IL-10 may immunomodulate the response and prevent the deleterious action of IFN-γ on erythrocytes.

4. Conclusion

Dogs naturally infected by Anaplasmataceae have serum concentration of different cytokines, but IFN-γ seems to be responsible for decreasing blood viscosity in these animals and causing disturbances in erythrocytes that are harmful. However, IFN-γ is also important in eliminating Anaplasmataceae by regulating the proliferation of these bacteria in infected dogs.

Alteration of blood rheology in dogs naturally infected with Anaplasmataceae probably occurs due to the systemic character of the infection that leads to erythrocyte alterations, which in turn disrupt the normal blood flow in these animals.

Thus, cytokine modulation reflects the hemorheological profile of infected animals and mainly the viscosity and shear rates.

It is not known which proteins could be involved in this process of viscosity alteration in dogs infected by bacteria of the Anaplasmataceae family. Thus, further studies are needed to understand which proteins are related to the decrease in viscosity in these animals.

It is proposed that the determination of blood rheological parameters as well as their therapeutic accompaniment may be important for dogs naturally infected with Anaplasmataceae. Controlled use of IFN-γ may be a tool to aid treatment, but anemia rates should be considered. In addition, infected dogs with moderate to severe anemia rates could benefit from IL-10 treatment.

Acknowledgement

This research received grants from the Mato Grosso Research Support Foundation (FAPEMAT No299032/ 2010), from the National Council for Scientific and Technological Development (CNPq No. 447218/ 2014-0 No. 308600/2015-0), in Brazil and Propes/IFMT (No. 36/2017).

Conflict of interests

The authors declare that there is no conflict of interest and non-financial competitors.

Author details

Saulo Pereira Cardoso[1,2], Giane Regina Paludo[3], José Nivaldo da Silva[1], Adenilda Honório-França[1*] and Eduardo Luzia França[1]

1 Institute of Biological and Health Sciences, Federal University of Mato Grosso, Barra do Garças, MT, Brazil

2 Federal Institute of Education, Science and Technology of Mato Grosso, Departament of Education, Barra do Garças, MT, Brazil

3 Faculty of Agronomy and Veterinary Medicine, Federal University of Brasilia, Brasilia, DF, Brazil

*Address all correspondence to: adenilda@ufmt.br

IntechOpen

© 2020 The Author(s). Licensee IntechOpen. This chapter is distributed under the terms of the Creative Commons Attribution License (http://creativecommons.org/licenses/by/3.0), which permits unrestricted use, distribution, and reproduction in any medium, provided the original work is properly cited. (cc) BY

References

[1] Almeida ABPF, Paula DAJ, Dutra V, Nakazato L, Mendonça AJ, Sousa VRF. Infecção por *Ehrlichia canis* e *Anaplasma platys* em cadelas e neonatos em Cuiabá, Mato Grosso. Archives of Veterinary Science. 2010;**15**:127-134

[2] Lasta CS, Santos AP, Messick JB, Oliveira ST, Biondo AW, Vieira RF, et al. Molecular detection of *Ehrlichia canis* and *Anaplasma platys* in dogs in southern Brazil. Revista Brasileira de Parasitologia Veterinária. 2013;**22**:360-366

[3] Yuasa Y, Tsai YL, Chang CC, Hsu TT, Chou CC. The prevalence of *Anaplasma platys* and a potential novel*Anaplasma* species exceed that of *Ehrlichia canis* in asymptomatic dogs and*Rhipicephalus sanguineus* in Taiwan. Journal of Veterinary Medical Science. 2017;**79**:1494-1502

[4] Pruneau L, Moumène A, Meyer DF, Marcelino I, Lefrançois T, Vachiéry N. Understanding Anaplasmataceae pathogenesis using "Omics" approaches. Frontiers in Cellular and Infection Microbiology. 2014;**4**:1-7

[5] Rikihisa Y. Diagnosis of emerging ehrlichial diseases of dogs, horses, and humans. Journal of Veterinary Internal Medicine. 2000;**14**:250-251

[6] Harvey JW, Simpson CF, Gaskin JM. Cyclic thrombocytopenia induced by rickettsi-like agent in dogs. The Journal of Infectious Diseases. 1978;**137**:182-188

[7] Scherer EF, Cantarini DG, Siqueira R, Ribeiro EB, Braga EM, Honório-França AC, et al. Cytokine modulation of human blood viscosity from vivax malaria patients. Acta Tropica. 2016;**158**:139-147

[8] França EL, Ribeiro EB, Scherer EF, Cantarini DG, Pessôa RS, França FL, et al. Effects of *Momordica charantia L.* on the blood rheological properties in diabetic patients. BioMed Research International. 2014;**2014**:1-8

[9] Silva JN, Cotrim AC, Conceição LAV, Marins CMF, Marchi PGF, Honório-França AC, et al. Immunohaematological and rheological parameters in canine visceral leishmaniasis. Revista Brasileira de Parasitologia Veterinária. 2018;**27**:211-217

[10] Murray HW. Effect of continuous administration of interferon-γ in experimental visceral leishmaniasis. The Journal of Infectious Diseases. 1990;**161**:992-994

[11] Murray HW, Montelibano C, Peterson R, Sypek JP. Interleukin 12 regulates the response to chemotherapy in experimental visceral leishmaniasis. The Journal of Infectious Diseases. 2000;**182**:1497-1502

[12] Correa ES, Paludo GR, Scalon MC, Machado JA, Lima ACQ, Pinto ATB, et al. Investigação molecular de *Ehrlichia* spp. e *Anaplasma platys* em felinos domésticos: alterações clínicas, hematológicas e bioquímicas. Pesquisa Veterinaria Brasileira. 2011;**31**:899-909

[13] Hackstadt T. The diverse habitats of obligate intracelular parasites. Current Opinion in Microbiology. 1998;**1**:82-87

[14] Ganta RR. Anaplasmataceae: *Anaplasma*. In: Mcvey DS, Melissa K, Chengappa MM, editors. Veterinary Microbiology. Chichester: John Wiley & Sons, Inc; 2013a. pp. 302-305

[15] Ganta RR. Anaplasmataceae: *Ehrlichia* and *Neorickettsia*. In: Mcvey DS, Melissa K, Chengappa MM, editors. Veterinary Microbiology. Chichester: John Wiley & Sons, Inc; 2013b. pp. 297-301

[16] Suksawat J, Hegarty BC, Breitschwerdt EB. Seroprevalence of *Ehrlichia canis*, *Ehrlichia equi*, and *Ehrlichia risticii* in sick dogs from North Carolina and Virginia. Journal of Veterinary Internal Medicine. 2000;**14**:50-55

[17] Vieira RFC, Biondo AW, Guimaraes MAS, Santos AP, Santos RP, Dutra LH, et al. Ehrlichiosis in Brazil. Revista Brasileira de Parasitologia Veterinária. 2011;**20**:1-12

[18] Ribeiro CM, Matos AC, Azzolini T, Bones ER, Wasnieski EA, Richini-Pereira VB, et al. Molecular epidemiology of *Anaplasma platys*, *Ehrlichia canis* and *Babesia vogeli* in stray dogs in Paraná, Brazil. Pesquisa Veterinária Brasileira. 2017;**37**:129-136

[19] Zobba R, Anfossia AG, Visco S, Sotgiu F, Dedola C, Pinna Parpaglia ML, et al. Cell tropism and molecular epidemiology of *Anaplasma platys*-like strains in cats. Ticks and Tick-borne Diseases. 2015;**6**:272-280

[20] Fontalvo MC, Braga IA, Aguiar DM, Horta MC. Serological evidence of exposure to *Ehrlichia canis* in cats. Ciência Animal Brasileira. 2016;**17**:418-424

[21] Dagnone AS, Souza AI, André MR, Machado RZ. Molecular diagnosis of Anaplasmataceae organisms in dogs with clinical and microscopical signs of ehrlichiosis. Revista Brasileira de Parasitologia Veterinária. 2009;**18**:20-25

[22] Lima MA, Aquino LC, Paludo GR. Evaluation of Anaplasmataceae family agents infection in domestic cats. Pakistan Veterinary Journal. 2017;**37**:201-204

[23] Donatien A, Lestoquard F. Existence en Algérie d'une *Rickettsia* du chien. Bulletin de la Société de Pathologie Exotique. 1935;**28**:418-419

[24] Machado RZ. Erliquiose canina. In: XIII Congresso Brasileiro de Parasitologia Veterinária & I Simpósio Latino-Americano de Rickettsioses. Revista Brasileira de Parasitologia Veterinária. 2004;**13**:53-57. Available from: https://docplayer.com. br/15106223-Xiii-congresso-brasileiro-de-parasitologia-veterinaria-i-simposio-latino-americano-de-ricketisioses-ouro-preto-mg-2004.html [Accessed on: 07 Feburary 2019]

[25] Huxsoll DL, Hildebrandt PK, Nims RM, Walker JS. Tropical canine pancytopenia. Journal of the American Veterinary Medical Association. 1970;**157**:1627-1632

[26] Costa JO, Silva M, Batista Júnior JA, Guimarães MP. *Ehrlichia canis* infection in dog in Belo Horizonte – Brazil. Arq Esc Vet Bela Horizonte. 1973;**25**:199-200

[27] Straube J. Canine Ehrlichiosis – From acute infection to chronic disease. CVBD: Digest. 2010;**7**:1-12

[28] Ojeda-Chi MM, Rodriguez-Vivas RI, Esteve-Gasent MD, Pérez de León AA, Modarelli JJ, Villegas-Perez SL. *Ehrlichia canis* in dogs of Mexico: Prevalence, incidence, co-infection and factors associated. Comparative Immunology, Microbiology and Infectious Diseases. 2019;**67**:101351

[29] Keefe TJ, Holland CJ, Salyer PE, Ristic M. Distribution of *Ehrlichia canis* among military working dogs in the world and selected civilian dogs in the United States. Journal of the American Veterinary Medical Association. 1982;**181**:236-238

[30] Hildebrandt PK, Conroy JD, Mckee AE, Nyindo MB, Huxsoll DL. Ultrastructure of *Ehrlichia canis*. Infection and Immunity. 1973;**7**:265-271

[31] Labarthe N, Pereira M, Barbarini O, Mckee W, Coimbra C, Hoskins J. Serologic prevalence of *Diroflaria immitis*,

Ehrlichia canis, and *Borrelia burgdorferi* infections in Brazil. Veterinary Therapeutics. 2003;**4**:67-75

[32] Perez M, Rikihisa Y, Wen B. *Ehrlichia canis*-like agent isolated from a man in Venezuela: antigenic and genetic characterization. Journal of Clinical Microbiology. 1996;**34**(9):2133-2139

[33] Dumler JS, Barbet AF, Bekker CP, Dasch GP, Palmer GH, Ray SC, et al. Reorganization of genera in the families Rickettsiaceae and Anaplasmataceae in the order Rickettsiales: Unification of some species of *Ehrlichia* with *Anaplasma*, *Cowdria* with *Ehrlichia* and *Ehrlichia* with *Neorickettsia*, descriptions of six new species combinations and designation of *Ehrlichia equi* and 'HGE agent' as subjective synonyms of *Ehrlichia phagocytophila*. International Journal of Systematic and Evolutionary Microbiology. 2001;**5**:2145-2165

[34] Mcquiston JH, Mccall CL, Nicholson WL. Ehrlichiosis and related infections. Journal of the American Veterinary Medical Association. 2003;**223**:1750-1756

[35] Neer TM, Harrus S. Ehrlichiosis, Neorickettsiosis, Anaplasmosis, and Wolbachia infection. In: Greene CE, editor. Infectious Diseases of the Dog and Cat. St Louis: Elsevier; 2006. pp. 203-232

[36] De La Fuente J, Torina A, Naranjo V, Nicosia S, Alongi A, Lamantia F, et al. Molecular characterization of *Anaplasma platys* strains from dogs in Sicily, Italy. BMC Veterinary Research. 2006;**2**:1-5

[37] De Caprariis D, Dantas-Torres F, Capelli G, Mencke N, Stanneck D, Breitschwerdt EB, et al. Evolution of clinical, haematological and biochemical findings in young dogs naturally infected by vector-borne pathogens. Veterinary Microbiology. 2011;**149**:206-212

[38] Rodrigues D, Daemon E, Rodirgues AFSF, Feliciano EA,

Soares AO, Souza AD. Levantamento de hemoparasitos em cães da área rural de Juiz de Fora, Minas Gerais, Brasil. Revista Brasileira de Parasitologia Veterinaria. 2004;**3**:371

[39] Ferreira RF, Cerqueira AMF, Pereira AM, Guimarães CM, Sá AG, Abreu FS, et al. *Anaplasma platys* diagnosis in dogs: Comparison between morphological and molecular tests. International Journal of Applied Research in Veterinary Medicine. 2007;**5**:113-119

[40] Ramos CAN, Ramos RAN, Araujo FR, Guedes DSJr., Souza IIF, Ono TM, Vieira AS, Pimentel DS, Rosas EO, Faustino MAG, Alves LC. Comparison of nested-PCR with blood smear examination indetection of *Ehrlichia canis* and *Anaplasma platys* in dogs. Revista Brasileira de Parasitologia Veterinária. 2009;**1**:58-62

[41] Maggi RG, Mascarelli PE, Havenga LN, Naidoo V, Breitschwerdt EB. Co-infection with *Anaplasma platys*, *Bartonella henselae* and *Candidatus Mycoplasma haematoparvum* in a veterinarian. Parasites & Vectors. 2013;**6**:103

[42] Arraga-Alvarado CM, Qurollo B, Parra OC, Berrueta MA, Hegarty BC, Breitschwerdt EB. Molecular evidence of *Anaplasma platys* infection in two women from Venezuela. The American Journal of Tropical Medicine and Hygiene. 2014;**91**:1161-1165

[43] Sousa VRF, Bomfim TCB, Almeida ABPF, Barros LA, Sales KG, Justino CHS, et al. Coinfecção por *Anaplasma platys* e *Ehrlichia canis* em cães diagnosticada pela PCR. Acta Scientiae Veterinariae. 2009;**37**:281-283

[44] Santos AS, Alexandre N, Sousa R, Nuncio MS, Bacellar F, Dumler JS. Serological and molecular survey of *Anaplasma* species infection in dogs with suspected tickborne disease

in Portugal. The Veterinary Record. 2009;**164**:168-171

[45] Silva GCF, Benitez NA, Girotto A, Taroda A, Vidotto MC, Garcia JL, et al. Occurrence of *Ehrlichia canis* and *Anaplasma platys* in household dogs from northern Parana. Revista Brasileira de Parasitologia Veterinaria. 2012;**21**:379-385

[46] Diniz PPVP, Beall MJ, Omark K, Chandrashekar R, Daniluk DA, Cyr KE, et al. High prevalence of tick-borne pathogens in dogs from an Indian reservation in northeastern Arizona. Vector Borne and Zoonotic Diseases. 2010;**10**:117-123

[47] Souza DMB, Coleto ZF, Souza AF, Silva SV, Andrade JK, Gimenez GC. Erliquiose transmitida aos cães pelo carrapato marrom (*Rhipicephalus sanguineus*). Ciência Veterinária nos Trópicos. 2012;**15**:21-31

[48] Yabsley MJ, Mckibben J, Macpherson CN, Cattan PF, Cherry NA, Hegarty BC, et al. Prevalence of *Ehrlichia canis*, *Anaplasma platys*, *Babesia canis vogeli*, *Hepatozoon canis*, *Bartonella vinsonii berkhoffii*, and *Rickettsia* spp. in dogs from Grenada. Veterinary Parasitology. 2008;**151**:279-285

[49] Piranda EM, Faccini JLH, Pinter A, Pacheco RC, Cançado PHD, LABRUNA MB. Experimental infection of *Rhipicephalus sanguineus* ticks with the bacterium *Rickettsia rickettsii*, using experimentally infected dogs. Vector-Borne and Zoonotic Diseases. 2011;**11**:29-36

[50] Sherding RG. Rickettsiosis, Ehrlichiosis, Anaplasmosis, and Neorickettsiosis. In: Birchard SJ, Sherding RG, editors. Manual Saunders of Small Animal Pratice. St Louis: Saunders Elsevier; 2006. pp. 178-185

[51] Borin S, Crivelenti LZ, Ferreira FA. Aspectos epidemiológicos, clínicos e

hematológicos de 251 cães portadores de mórula de *Ehrlichia* spp. naturalmente infectados. Arquivo Brasileiro de Medicina Veterinária e Zootecnia. 2009;**61**:566-571

[52] Harvey JW. Veterinary Hematology: A Diagnostic Guide and Color Atlas. Saunders: Elsevier; 2011. p. 368

[53] Matei IA, Stuen S, Modrý D, Degan A, D'amico G, Mihalca AD. Neonatal *Anaplasma platys* infection in puppies: Further evidence for possible vertical transmission. Veterinary Journal. 2017;**219**:40-41

[54] Latrofa MS, Dantas-Torres F, De Caprariis D, Cantacessi C, Capelli G, Lia RP, et al. Vertical transmission of *Anaplasma platys* and *Leishmania infantum* in dogs during the first half of gestation. Parasites & Vectors. 2016;**9**:149-269

[55] Silva JN, Almeida ABPF, Sorte ECB, Freitas AG, Santos LGF, Aguiar DM, et al. Soroprevalência de anticorpos anti-*Ehrlichia canis* em cães de Cuiabá, Mato Grosso. Revista Brasileira de Parasitologia Veterinaria. 2010;**19**:108-111

[56] Sanogo YO, Davoustb, Inokuma H, Camias JL, Parola P, Brouqui P. First evidence of *Anaplasma platys* in *Rhipicephalus sanguineus* (Acari: Ixodida) collected from dogs in Africa. The Onderstepoort Journal of Veterinary Research. 2003;**70**:205-212

[57] Bremer WG, Schaefer JJ, Wagner ER, Ewing SA, Rikihisa Y, Needham GR, et al. Transstadial and intrastadial experimental transmission of *Ehrlichia canis* by male *Rhipicephalus sanguineus*. Veterinary Parasitology. 2005;**131**:95-105

[58] Smith RD, Sells DM, Stephenson EH, Ristic MR, Huxsoll DL. Development of *Ehrlichia canis*, causative agent of canine Ehrlichiosis, in the tick

Rhipicephalus sanguineus and its differentiation from a symbiotic rickettsia. American Journal of Veterinary Research. 1976;**37**:119-126

[59] Breitschwerdt EB. Canine and feline anaplasmosis: Emerging infectious diseases. In: Breitschwerdt EB, editor. Proceedings of the 2nd Canine Vector-Borne Disease (CVBD) Symposium. Sícilia, Itália: CBVD World of Knowledge; 2007. pp. 6-14

[60] Welc-Faleciak R, Kowalec M, Karbowiak G, Bajer A, Behnke JM, Sinski E. Rickettsiaceae and Anaplasmataceae infections in Ixodes ricinus ticks from urban and natural forested areas of Poland. Parasites & Vectors. 2014;**7**:1-13

[61] Martin ME, Carspersen K, Dumler JS. Immunopathology and ehrlichial propagation are regulated by interferon-γ and interleukin-10 in a murine model of human granulocytic ehrlichiosis. The American Journal of Pathology. 2001;**158**:1881-1888

[62] Feng HM, Walker DH. Mechanisms of immunity to *Ehrlichia muris*: A model of monocytotropic ehrlichiosis. Infection and Immunity. 2004;**72**:966-971

[63] Beineke A, Markus S, Borlak J, Thum T, Baumgärtner W. Increase of pro-inflammatory cytokine expression in non-demyelinating early cerebral lesions in nervous canine distemper. Viral Immunology. 2008;**21**:401-410

[64] Scorpio DG, Von Loewenich FD, Göbel H, Bogdan C, Dumler JS. Innate immune response to *Anaplasma phagocytophilum* contributes to hepatic injury. Clinical and Vaccine Immunology. 2006;**13**:806-809

[65] Lin M, Rikihisa Y. *Ehrlichia chaffeensis* downregulates surface toll-like receptors 2/4, CD14 and transcription factors PU.1 and inhibits

lipopolysaccharide activation of NF-kB, ERK 1/2 and p38 MAPK in host monocytes. Cellular Microbiology. 2004;**6**:175-186

[66] Lee EH, Rikihisa Y. Protein kinase A-mediated inhibition of gamma interferon-induced tyrosine phosphorylation of Janus kinases and latent cytoplasmic transcription factors in human monocytes by *Ehrlichia chaffeensis*. Infection and Immunity. 1998;**66**:2514-2520

[67] Ismail N, Soong L, Mcbride JW, Valbuena G, Olano JP, Feng H-M, et al. Overproduction of TNF-a by CD8+ type 1 cells and down-regulation of IFN-g production by CD4+ Th1 cells contribute to toxic shock-like syndrome in an animal model of fatal monocytotropic ehrlichiosis. Journal of Immunology. 2004;**172**:1786-1800

[68] Zhang JZ, Sinha M, Luxon BA, Yu XJ. Survival strategy of obligately intracellular *Ehrlichia chaffeensis*: Novel modulation of immune response and host cell cycles. Infection and Immunity. 2004;**72**:498-507

[69] Hess PR, English RV, Hegarty BC, Brown GD. Breitschwerdt EB, Experimental *Ehrlichia canis* infection in the dog does not cause immunosuppression. Veterinary Immunology and Immunopathology. 2006;**109**:117-125

[70] Faria JLM, Munhoz TD, João CF, Vargas-Herández G, André MR, Pereira WAB, et al. *Ehrlichia canis* (Jaboticabal strain) induces the expression of TNF-α in leukocytes and splenocytes of experimentally infected dogs. Revista Brasileira de Parasitologia Veterinária. 2011;**20**:71-74

[71] Lima AL, Santos GJL, Roatt BM, Reis AB, Freitas JCC, Nunes-Pinheiro DCS. Serum TNF-α and IL-10 in *Ehrlichia* spp. naturally infected dogs. Acta Scientiae Veterinariae. 2015;**43**:1-7

[72] Dumler JS. The biological basis of severe outcomes in *Anaplasma phagocytophilum* infection. FEMS Immunology and Medical Microbiology. 2012;**64**:13-20

[73] Kocan KM, De La Fuente J, Blouin EF, Coetzee JF, Ewing SA. The natural history of *Anaplasma marginale*. Veterinary Parasitology. 2010;**167**:95-107

[74] Akkoyunlu M, Fikrig E. Gamma interferon dominates the murine cytokine response to the agent of human granulocytic ehrlichiosis and helps to control the degree of early rickettsemia. Infection and Immunity. 2000;**68**:1827-1833

[75] Birkner K, Steiner B, Rinkler C, Kern Y, Aichele P, Bogdan C, et al. The elimination of *Anaplasma phagocytophilum* requires CD4+ T cells, but is independent of Th1 cytokines and a wide spectrum of effector mechanisms. European Journal of Immunology. 2008;**38**:3395-3410

[76] Han S, Norimine J, Brayton KA, Palmer GH, Scoles GA, Brown WC. *Anaplasma marginale* infection with persistent high-load bacteremia induces a dysfunctional memory CD4+ T lymphocyte response but sustained high IgG titers. Clinical and Vaccine Immunology. 2010;**17**:1881-1890

[77] Desjardins M, Descoteaux A. Inhibition of phagolysosomal biogenesis by the *Leishmania* lipophosphoglycan. The Journal of Experimental Medicine. 1997;**185**:2061-2068

[78] Bogdan C, Rollinghoff M. The immune response to *Leishmania*: Mechanisms of parasite control and evasion. International Journal for Parasitology. 1998;**28**:121-134

[79] Sacks D, Sher A. Evasion of innate immunity by parasitic protozoa. Nature Immunology. 2002;**3**:1041-1047

[80] Popov VL, Yu X, Walker DH. The120 kDa outer membrane protein of *Ehrlichia chaffeensis*: Preferential expression on dense – Corecells and gene expression in *Escherichia coli* associated with attachment and entry. Microbial Pathogenesis. 2000;**28**:71-80

[81] Mavromatis K, Doyle CK, Lykidis A, Ivanova N, Francino MP, Chain P, et al. The genome of the Obligately intracellular bacterium *Ehrlichia canis* reveals themes of complex membrane structure and immune evasion strategies. Journal of Bacteriology. 2006;**188**:4015-4023

[82] Troy GC, Forrester SD. Canine ehrlichiosis. In: Greene CE, editor. Infectious Diseases of the Dog and Cat. Philadelphia: WB Saunders; 1990. pp. 404-418

[83] Harrus S, Waner T, Bark H. Canine monocytic ehrlichiosis – An update. Compendium on Continuing Education for the Practising Veterinarian. 1997b;**19**:431-444

[84] Waner T, Harrus S, Weiss DJ, Bar H, Keysary A. Demonstration of serum antiplatelet antibodies in experimental acute canine ehrlichiosis. Veterinary Immunology and Immunopathology. 1995;**48**:177-182

[85] Smith RD, Ristic M, Huxsoll DL, Baylor RA. Platelet kinetics in canine ehrlichiosis: Evidence for increased platelet destruction as the cause of thrombocytopenia. Infection and Immunity. 1975;**11**:1216-1221

[86] Abeygunawardena I, Kakoma, Smith RD. Pathophysiology of canine ehrlichiosis. In: Williams JC, Kakoma I, editors. Ehrlichiosis: A Vector-Borne Disease of Animals and Humans. Washington: Kluwer Academic Press; 1990. pp. 78-92

[87] De Tommasi AS, Baneth G, Breitschwerdt EB, Stanneck D,

Dantas-Torres F, Otranto D, et al. *Anaplasma platys* in bone marrow megakaryocytes of young dogs. Journal of Clinical Microbiology. 2014;**52**:2231-2234

[88] Nakaghi ACH, Machado RZ, Costa MT, André MR, Baldani CD. Canine Ehrlichiosis: Clinical, hematological, serological and molecular aspects. Ciência Rural. 2008;**38**:766-770

[89] Sousa VRF, Almeida ABPF, Barros LA, Sales KG, Justino CHS, Dalcin L, et al. Avaliação clínica e molecular de cães com erliquiose. Ciência Rural. 2010;**40**:1309-1313

[90] Bassi PB, Moreira TK, Silva CC, Bittar ER, Bittar JFF. Aspectos clínicos, epidemiológicos, hematológicos e sorológicos de animais diagnosticados com *Ehrlichia canis* no Hospital Veterinário de Uberaba-MG. Medvep - Revista Científica de Medicina Veterinária - Pequenos Animais e Animais de Estimação. 2011;**9**:678-680

[91] Harrus S, Waner T. Diagnosis of canine monocytotropic ehrlichiosis (*Ehrlichia canis*): An overview. Veterinary Journal. 2011;**187**:292-296

[92] Kataoka A, Santana AE, Seki MC. Alterações do proteinograma sérico de cães naturalmente infectados por *E. canis*. Ars Veterinaria. 2006;**22**:98-102

[93] Mcdade JE. Ehrlichiosis – A disease of animals and humans. The Journal of Infectious Diseases. 1990;**161**:609-617

[94] Kelly PJ. Canine ehrlichioses: An update. Journal of the South African Veterinary Association. 2000;**71**:77-86

[95] Shaw SE, Day MJ, Birtles RJ, Breitschwerdt EB. Tick-borne infectious diseases of dogs. Trends in Parasitology. 2001;**17**:74-80

[96] Gaunt SD, Baker DC, Babin SS. Platelet aggregation studies in dogs with acute *Ehrlichia platys* infection. American Journal of Veterinary Research. 1990;**51**:290-293

[97] Cardozo GP, Oliveira LP, Zissou VG, Donini IAN, Roberto PG, Marins M. Analysis of the 16S rRNA gene of *Anaplasma platys* detected in dogs from Brazil. Brazilian Journal of Microbiology. 2007;**38**:478-479

[98] Kontos VC, Papadopoulos O, French TW. Natural andexperimental canine infections with a Greek strain of *Ehrlichia platys*. Veterinary Clinical Pathology. 1991;**20**:101-105

[99] Harrus S, Aroch I, Lavy E, Bark H. Clinical manifestations of infectious canine cyclic thrombocytopenia. The Veterinary Record. 1997a;**141**:247-250

[100] Aguirre E, Tesouro MA, Ruiz L, Amusategui I, Sainz A. Genetic characterization of *Anaplasma* (*Ehrlichia*) *platys* in dogs in Spain. Journal of Veterinary Medicine. B, Infectious Diseases and Veterinary Public Health. 2006;**53**:197-200

[101] Dantas-Torres F. Canine vector-borne diseases in Brazi - review. Parasites & Vectors. 2008;**1**:1-17

[102] Harvey JW. Thrombocytotrophic anaplasmosis (*A. platys* [*E. platys*] infection). In: Greene CG, editor. Infectious Diseases of the Dog and Cat. St. Louis: Saunders Elsevier; 2006. pp. 229-231

[103] Elias E. Diagnosis of ehrlichiosis from the presence of inclusion bodies or morulae of *E. canis*. Journal of Small Animal Practice. 1991;**33**:540-543

[104] Mylonakis ME, Koutinas AF, Billinis C, Leontides LS, Kontos V, Papadopoulos O, et al. Evaluation of cytology in the diagnosis of acute canine

monocytic ehrlichiosis (*Ehrlichia canis*): A comparison between five methods. Veterinary Microbiology. 2003;**91**:97-204

[105] Bowman D, Little SE, Lorentzen L, Shields J, Sullivan MP, Carlin EP. Prevalence and geographic distribution of *Dirofilaria immitis*, *Borrelia burgdorferi*, *Ehrlichia canis*, and *Anaplasma phagocytophilum* in dogs in the United States: Results of a national clinic-based serologic survey. Veterinary Parasitology. 2009;**160**:138-148

[106] Davoust B, Parzy D, Vidor E, Hasselot N, Martet G. Ehrlichiose canine experimentale: étude clinique et terapeutique. Revue de Médecine Vétérinaire. 1991;**167**:33-40

[107] Mcclure EE, Chávez ASO, Shaw DK, Carlyon JA, Ganta RR, Noh SM, et al. Engineering of obligate intracellular bacteria: Progress, challenges and paradigms. Nature Reviews. Microbiology. 2017;**15**:544-558

[108] Martin AR, Brown GK, Dunstan RH, Roberts TK. *Anaplasma platys*: An improved PCR for its detection in dogs. Experimental Parasitology. 2005;**109**:176-180

[109] Aguiar DM, Saito TB, Hagiwara MK, Machado RZ, Labruma MB. Diagnóstico sorológico de erliquiose canina com antígeno brasileiro de *Ehrlichia canis*. Ciência Rural. 2007;**46**:796-802

[110] Nakaghi ACH, Machado RZ, Ferro JÁ, Labruna MB, Chryssafidis AL, André MR, et al. Sensitivity evaluation of a single-step PCR assay using *Ehrlichia canis* p28 gene as a target and its application in diagnosis of canine ehrlichiosis. Revista Brasileira de Parasitologia Veterinaria. 2010;**19**:75-79

[111] Doyle CK, Labruna MB, Breitschwerdt EB, Tang YW, Corstvet RE, Hegarty BC, et al. Detection of medically important *Ehrlichia* by quantitative

multicolor TaqMan real-time polymerase chain reaction of the dsb gene. The Journal of Molecular Diagnostics. 2005;**7**:504-510

[112] Mendonça CS, Mundim AV, Costa AS, Moro TV. Erliquiose Canina: Alterações hematológicas em cães domésticos naturalmente infectados. Bioscience Journal. 2005;**21**:167-174

[113] Birkenheuer AJ, Lvey MG, Breitschwerdt EB. Development andevaluation of a seminested PCR for detection and differentiationof *Babesia gibsoni* (Asian genotype) and *B. canis* DNA in canineblood samples. Journal of Clinical Microbiology. 2003;**41**:4172-4177

[114] Llera JL, López-García ML, Martín RE, De Vivar GR. Differential serological testing by simultaneous indirect immunofluorescent antibody test in canine leishmaniosis and ehrlichiosis. Veterinary Parasitology. 2002;**109**:185-190

[115] Baskurt OK, Meiselman HJ. Blood Reology and hemodynamics. Seminars in Thrombosis and Hemostasis. 2003;**29**:435-450

[116] Rosencraz R, Bogen SA. Clinical laboratory measurement of serum, plasma, and blood viscosity. American Journal of Clinical Pathology. 2006;**125**:78-86

[117] Mendlowitz M. The effect of anemia e polycythemia on digital intravascular blood viscosity. The Journal of Clinical Investigation. 1948;**27**:565-571

[118] Linderkamp O, Ruef P, Zilow EP, Hoffmann GF. Impaired deformability of erythrocytes and neutrophils in children with newly diagnosed insulin-dependent diabetes mellitus. Diabetologia. 1999;**42**:865-869

[119] Rizvi SI, Zaid MA. Intracellular reduced glutatione content in normal

and type 2 diabetic erythrocytes: Effect of insulin and (−) epicatechin. Journal of Physiology and Pharmacology. 2001;**52**:483-488

[120] Moutzouri AG, Athanassiou GA, Dimitropoulou D, Skoutelis AT, Gogos CA. Severe sepsis and diabetes mellitus have additive effects on red blood cell deformability. The Journal of Infection. 2008;**57**:147-151

[121] Inokuma H, Raoult D, Brouqui P. Detection of *Ehrlichia platys* DNA in Brown Dog Ticks (*Rhipicephalus sanquineus*) in Okinawa Island, Japan. The Journal of Clinical Microbiology. 2000;**38**:4219-4221

[122] Murphy GL, Ewing SA, Whitworth LC, Fox JC, Kocan AA. A molecular and serologic survey of *Ehrlichia canis*, *E. chaffeensis*, and *E. ewingii* in dogs andticks from Oklahoma. The Journal Veterinary Parasitology. 1998;**79**:325-339

[123] Ramos R, Ramos C, Araújo F, Oliveira R, Souza I, Pimentel D, et al. Molecular survey and geneticcharacterization of tick-borne pathogens in dogs in metropolitan Recife (North-Eastern Brazil). Parasitology Research. 2010;**107**:1115-1120

[124] Fedosov DA, Caswell B, Kamiadakis GE. Wall shear stress-based model for adhesive dynamics of red blood cells in malária. Biophysical Journal. 2011;**100**:2084-2093

[125] Al-Abadi BH, Al-Badrani BA. Cattle blood analyses for parasitic infestation in Mosul, Iraq. Research Opinions in Animal & Veterinary Sciences. 2012;**2**:535-542

[126] Schaefer DMW, Stokol T. The utility of reticulocyte indices indistinguishing iron deficiency anemia from anemia of inflammatory disease,portosystemic shunting, and breed-associated microcytosis in dogs. Veterinary Clinical Pathology. 2015;**44**:109-119

[127] Lominadze D, Dean WL. Involvement of fibrinogen specific binding in erythrocyte aggregation. FEBS Letters. 2002;**517**:41-44

[128] Murray HW, Lu CM, Mauze S, Freeman S, Moreira AL, Kaplan G, et al. Interleukin-10 (IL-10) in experimental visceral leishmaniasis and IL-10 receptor blockade as immunotherapy. Infection and Immunity. 2002;**70**:6284-6293

Chapter 3

Malarial Inflammation-Driven Pathophysiology and Its Attenuation by Triterpene Phytotherapeutics

Greanious Alfred Mavondo, Blessing Nkazimulo Mkhwanazi,
Mayibongwe Louis Mzingwane, Rachael Dangarembizi,
Blessing Zambuko, Obadiah Moyo, Patience Musiwaro,
Francis Farai Chikuse, Colline Rakabopa, Tariroyashe Mpofu
and Joy Mavondo

Abstract

Malaria driven pathophysiology inimically conjoined to systemic inflammation response cascade in a vicious feed-forward cycle destined to a terrible debilitation or demise of the host. The *Plasmodium* parasite initiates physiological changes when it is transmitted into the human host by intermediate host and vector. Sporozoites injection elicits immunological and inflammatory response suppression facilitating movement into the blood stream undetected, destined to hepatocyte. Subsequently, hepatocyte invasion culminates in intracellular growth and conversion of the parasites rapturing hepatocytes releasing merozoites into the extrahepatic circulation. Inflammatory and immunological response initiation results in overt malarial disease symptoms. Initially, inflammatory response alleviates and curtails infection. Activation of leukocytes, lymphocytes, monocytes, and phagocytes secretes inflammatory mediators, chemokines, cytokines cytoadhering molecules which accelerate infection patency. Hormonal processes influence disease tolerance without necessarily interfering with parasitemia. Current treatment is anti-parasitic. Phytotherapeutic intervention in malaria is anti-parasitic and anti-disease effects that terminate the vicious cycle and alleviating disease. The phytochemicals, in malarial experimental and clinical work, include asiatic acid, maslinic acid, oleanolic acid, and inflammatory and immunological aberrations evolving in malaria and the effects of phytochemical therapeutics in the alleviation of the disease to enable leverage of future treatment regimens through harnessing existing plants materials is explored.

Keywords: malaria inflammation, phytochemicals, Asiatic acid, Maslinic acid, Oleanolic acid, anti-parasitic, anti-disease, *Plasmodium falciparum*, *Plasmodium berghei*, pathophysiology

IntechOpen

1. Introduction

Malaria and inflammation seem to be intricately connected with the *Plasmodium* parasite having evolved mechanisms to evade its initiation before the parasite has set a strong and indelible foot print in either the intermediate (mosquito) or definitive (animal or human) hosts. Pathogen-driven tissue damage complements inflammatory response building a debilitating state against host fitness and survival [1, 2].

The disease is premised upon an immunological disease and a systematic inflammatory syndrome with a strong cachectic constituent driven by an endogenous cytokine milieu in the form of the pyrogens tumor necrosis factor alfa (TNF-α) and interleukin-1 (IL-1) [3, 4]. Eliciting and chaperoning this immunological-inflammatory response to malarial infection are the glycolipid glycosylphosphatidylinositol (GPI) moieties which are covalently connected to the antigens on the exterior topological aspect of malaria parasites or free in circulation. Whether linked to the parasite related proteins or free, GPI induce elevated levels of TNF-α and IL-1 from macrophages resulting in pyrexia, cachexia and, through their insulin memetic effect, regulate glucose homeostasis in adipocytes with profound hypoglycemia initiation [5]. In attends to these GPI-induced cytokine inflammatory effects and other malaria parasites by products like hemozoin, are the common malarial syndromes of severe malaria anemia (SMA), hypertriacylglycerolemia, hypotension, pulmonary vasculature hyperneutrophilia and acute respiratory distress syndrome (ARDS), diffuse intravascular coagulation, upregulated expression of endothelial cell and vascular cell intercell adhesion molecule 1 (ICAM1 and VCAM 1) [6, 7]. Mature parasites tend to recognize these molecules leading to their sequestration in cerebral malaria (CM) [8].

In a bid to neutralize the disease sequelae and induce disease tolerance (anti-disease effects), albeit without reduction in parasitemia (anti-infection effects) are the adrenal glands hormones which mediate immunological-inflammatory responses but do not affect the pathogen load [9]. Other hormones play a critical role in the amelioration of malarial inflammation.

Investigations and diagnosis of malarial-related inflammation and immunological aberrations have been vast owing to the importance of the tropical and subtropical disease. However, a lull in research has been experienced in the past making malaria one of the forgotten diseases. Interest has resurged in both disease investigations and management.

Malarial inflammatory response yields itself into the pathophysiology of malaria intimating that management needs to be directed at both the parasite and the disease, antiparasitic and anti-disease, respectively. The animal host develops disease tolerance through immunological and inflammatory response to a limited extent depending on the rate and duration of exposure to potent infection transmitting mosquito bites. Management of the disease with antiparasitic regimens alone or anti-disease management alone does not result in a radical cure but provides opportunity for future parasite recrudesces and drug resistance.

Phytotherapeutics and their derivatives have been administered in both experimental research and clinical practices with astonishing results. The drug artemisinin (extract from Chinese artemisinin *annua* herb) and its derivatives provide current mainstay of malaria treatment such that any meaningful parasite resistance to the drug will thrust the world into an era without effective malaria treatment. Anti-inflammatory activities have been reported for the drug. However, the proposed mode of action of the drug has been through a pro-oxidant capacity driven the endoperoxidase activity of the molecule which eventually is a compelling proinflammatory oriented outcome that rapidly kills the parasites. This process leaves behind an oxidative environment with possible fatal hemolytic episodes occurring days after successful treatment of the disease in what has been termed post artemisinin administration hemolytic diseases. Alternative and safer treatment regimens are urgently required.

Experimental phytotherapeutics administration in murine malaria, the likes of triterpenes Asiatic acid (AA), Maslinic acid (MA) [10] and Oleanolic acid (OA) have shown potential antiparasitic and anti-disease facultative propensities. Salvaging of inflammation-driven glucose homeostasis, acute renal injury (ARI), hyperlipidemias, hyperparasitemia, hyperinsulinemia, cerebral malaria, weight loss and reduced feeding disease patterns have been reported. Triterpenes have pleiotropic characteristics with both antioxidant and pro-oxidant properties dependent on the environmental homeostasis. A plethora of challenge bedevil malaria management. There is antimalaria multidrug resistance, high cost of antimalarials, poverty amongst those most affected by malaria, lack of 100% effectiveness of current antimalaria drugs, no efficacious vaccine against malaria in place yet and adverse drug related post treatment side effects are common constraints in malaria management. Therefore, it is imperative that alternative drugs, as suggested here, be explored or leads compounds with antimalarial disease alleviation properties be reported for either more work to be done or be implemented in human trials.

2. Malarial cycle and potential interventional areas

2.1 Parasitemia drives malarial inflammatory response

Malaria is a highly inflammatory condition characterized by acute periods of fever, headache and nausea which correspond to the release of merozoites into the blood stream as the erythrocytes rapture. Excessive erythrocyte rupture leads to anemia and high parasitemia. Molecules from the parasite and ruptured RBCs trigger host inflammatory responses [11]. The erythrocyte stage is characterized by up-regulation of inflammation-driving cytokines such as IL-1b, IL-6, IFN-g, TNF-a and IL-12 [12, 13], which may lead to excessive inflammation if not curtailed [14]. Some parasite molecules that have been associated with host inflammatory responses include glycosylphosphatidylinositol (GPI) anchors, hemozoin, uric acid and parasite DNA [5, 15–17].

In vitro studies showed induction of nitric oxide, TNF and IL-1β by parasite GPI-anchors while synthetic and purified [19] *Plasmodium* GPI had immunogenic properties in vivo. *Plasmodium* species produce hemozoin as they detoxify heme in pRBCs. The hemozoin induce IL-1β production by immune cells such as monocytes and macrophages once released into circulation during pRBCs lysis [20]. Hemozoin has been demonstrated to activate the inflammasome protein complex [21, 22] and injection of parasite-derived hemozoin in disease-free mice induce transcription of inflammatory genes [23]. Parasite DNA has also been shown to induce cytokine and chemokine responses by human plasmacytoid dendritic cells by the activating the TLR9-MyD88 signaling pathway [24].

Parasite DNA is also detected by several cytosolic DNA sensors in the cytoplasma upon release of phagolysosomal contents [25]. Uric acid derived from the parasite and from the rupture of infected pRBCs has also been reported to induce strong inflammatory responses in patients [11]. In vitro studies show that uric acid derived from the parasite promotes secretion of pro-inflammatory cytokines that include TNF, IL-1β and IL-6 by [26]. The uric acid levels are specifically elevated in periods correlating with parasitemia [27, 28]. Overall, the role of parasitemia and components of the parasite in pathological inflammation response is an on-going concern poised for novel target development for diagnosis and anti-inflammatory antimalarials.

2.2 Inflammatory cytokines in severe malaria

P. falciparum infection is associated with the release of proinflammatory cytokines which are crucial in mediating the control of parasite growth and sickness behaviors in the host e.g., lethargy, fever, anorexia, pain [7, 29, 30]. The excessive production of these mediators is implicated in host-harming effects associated with infection. However, the inflammatory response is a highly regulated response regulated, in part, by the production of cytokines. Apparently, malaria disease outcome depends on the delicate balance between proinflammatory and anti-inflammatory cytokines. Development of severe forms of the disease and death depends on the rapture of this balance [31–33].

During malarial infection, the recognition of different pathogen related molecules expressed by the parasite or released by the host stimulate the immune system and cytokine production. A glycolipid toxin of *P. falciparum*, glycosylphosphatidylinositol (GPI), is a potent pathogen associated molecular pattern (PAMP) expressed on the parasite whose interaction with the host immune system induces the expression of genes encoding pro- and anti-inflammatory cytokines including TNF-α, IL-1, IL-6, IL-12, IL4, IL10 and the enzyme inducible nitric oxide synthase (iNOS) [5, 34]. GPI interacts with toll like receptor (TLR)1/TLR2 and TLR2/TLR6 dimers, and possibly C-type lectins on dendritic cells and macrophages to produce proinflammatory cytokines. Hemozoin, a PAMP and detoxification crystal from hemoglobin binds to TLR9 and mediates the production of proinflammatory cytokines in dendritic cells and macrophages [35, 36].

Pure hemozoin is not a ligand for TLRs but acts a carrier molecule for malarial DNA which has the immunostimulatory effects [37–39]. The *P. falciparum* genome contains CpG motifs which act through the MYD-88-NFκβ to induce cytokine production. *P. falciparum* DNA also contains the highest AT content and the AT motifs induce the production of interferons [16]. Other proteins, sugars, RNA motifs and other phosphorylated non-peptidic antigens are known to be PAMPs with cytokine induction potential [7, 36, 40]. In addition to parasite expressed proinflammatory molecules, several host-derived molecules, commonly known as damage associated molecular patterns (DAMPs), are also involved in evoking the inflammatory response and cytokine release in severe malaria. These include nucleic acids and urate crystals, heme and microvesicles derived from platelets, endothelial cells and leukocytes [11, 41–43].

2.2.1 Tumor necrosis factor-α (TNF-α)

TNF-α is involved in the pathogenesis of malaria associated with disease severity and death. TNF-α is dramatically increased with up to two- and ten-fold concentrations in cerebral malaria (CM) and in fatal cases, respectively [44, 45]. TNF-α concentrations are associated with parasite clearance and blocking TNF-α function increases the risk of hyperparasitemia [46]. The administration of recombinant TNF also induce clinical manifestations characteristic of malarial pathology including fever, anemia and hypotension [47, 48].

The susceptibility of an individual to cerebral malaria is linked to the presence of a genetic variant of the gene that encodes the TNF promoter [49]. TNF-α exacerbates sequestration in cerebral blood vessels in the brain by increasing the expression adhesion molecules e.g., ICAM-1 in the endothelial cells [50]. However, there is contrary knowledge on the role of TNF-α in the pathogenesis of severe and cerebral malaria [51–53]. Blocking TNF-α using anti-TNF antibodies does not seem to reduce mortality in CM [54] although it successfully stops fever suggesting that the full biological effects of TNF may be a concerted effort with a complex network of other cytokines. TNF-α is produced quite early during infection and has a short half-life, hence the timing of TNF-α neutralization in inflammation has to be carefully considered. Blocking TNF-α when patients are already severely ill may be too late as an intervention to show anti-inflammatory efficacy of this process.

2.2.2 Lymphotoxin-α

Other cytokines demonstrate similar proinflammatory activity as TNF-α. Lymphotoxin-α (previously known as TNF-β) is a proinflammatory cytokine produced by lymphocytes which shares the same receptors with TNF and exhibits similar biological effects as TNF-α. Like TNF-α, lymphotoxin acts in synergy with IL-1 to increase the production of IL-6 and induce hypoglycemia; both are which are prominent clinical features in severe malaria [55]. Lymphotoxin also mediates the cell-mediated killing of *P. falciparum* parasites in infected erythrocytes [56].

2.2.3 Interferon γ

Another prominent proinflammatory cytokine in malarial pathology is IFNγ. IFNγ is produced by both CD4+ and CD8+ T lymphocytes during malarial infection. IFNγ activates macrophages and monocytes to produce other proinflammatory molecules including TNF, IL-1, IL-6, TGF-β and NO intermediates which help to kill the malarial parasite. As a result of its ability to induce TNF production, IFNγ has been implicated in the pathogenesis of cerebral malaria and blockage of IFNγ action was reported to prevent against cerebral malaria in murine models [57]. Additionally, IFNγ knockout mice showed resistance against cerebral malaria but were still susceptible to severe malaria and death. The release of IFNγ is controlled by IL-12 [58] and its relevance in severe disease may depend on the levels, timing and balance with other cytokines.

2.2.4 Interlukin-1

Interleukin-1 is a proinflammatory cytokine produced by macrophages, natural killer cells, B cells, dendritic cells and other immune cells. Serum concentrations of IL-1 correlate strongly with severity of disease with higher IL-1 levels observed in patients with CM and greater than in those in severe malarial anemia [59]. IL-1 has synergistic interactions with TNF-α and increases the expression of the adhesion molecule ICAM-1 in cerebral vasculature thus exacerbating sequestration.

2.2.5 Interleukin-6

IL-6 is proinflammatory cytokine released by monocytes/macrophages and Th2 cells. Serum concentrations of IL-6 vary with severity of disease with higher levels in CM than in severe and in uncomplicated cases [59]. IL-6 mediates TNF-α functions in severe malaria.

2.2.6 Interleukin-10

While proinflammatory cytokines play a critical role in the host immune defense against the malaria parasite, poorly regulated release of these chemical molecules results in the immunopathological response characteristic of severe malaria. Proinflammatory cytokines release is closely regulated by anti-inflammatory cytokines. IL-10 inhibits the release of Th1 type of cytokines but not Th2 showing its negative correlation with TNF-α, IL-1β and IL-8 [60].

Progression of malaria from uncomplicated to more severe forms is the functional balance of anti-inflammatory to proinflammatory cytokines than it is about individual cytokine levels. This explains why severe malaria does not occur in all cases where proinflammatory cytokine concentrations are very high. A downregulation of IL-10 coupled to the upregulation of TNF is usually associated with severe and CM. Thus, it is important to consider the ratio of IL-10 to TNF-α [61, 62].

2.2.7 Transforming growth factor-β (TGF-β)

TGF-β is an anti-inflammatory cytokine that immune-regulates malaria. A TGF-β neutralizing antibody in malaria infected mice is associated with dramatic increases in TNF-α and IFN-γ concentrations. TGF-β also upregulates IL-10 production while downregulating the expression of adhesion molecules, decreasing sequestration of pRBCs in severe malaria. Interestingly, at low concentrations TGF-β exhibits proinflammatory effects but has anti-inflammatory effects at high concentrations [63]. In malaria, the multifunctionality of TGF-β serves two important functions; (1) enhancing Th1 mediated parasite control during early infection, and (2) regulating the inflammatory response in later phases to prevent immunopathology [63].

3. Inflammation-induced mitochondrial dysfunction and cellular energy depletion in malaria

Parasitized red blood cells (pRBC's) agglutination to the endothelium causing blood vessels occlusion solely has been the ascribe process by which tissue hypoxia in malaria occurred. However, other mechanisms have since been elucidated as contributing to this phenomenon [64, 65]. Sepsis shares the same systemic pathology and disease presentation of tissue underlying tissue hypoxia with malaria but does not experience RBC's sequestration. Which may indicate other causes of the complication. In sepsis tissue oxygen tension is usually normal or elevated in the rat, patients or pigs [66]. This bring to the fore the aspect that poor oxygen utilization, compared to supply, as the major cause of malaria-related hypoxia.

Excessive reactive oxygen species (ROS), nitric oxide (NO) and peroxynitrite (ONOO$^-$), as seen in malaria, tend to cause mitochondria dysfunction. Proinflammatory cytokines induce excessive inducible nitric oxide synthase (iNOS) expression by monocytes and macrophages tend to increase NO and subsequently oxidative stress (OS). Increase OS reversibly inhibits cytochrome oxidase and aconitase [67, 68] with concomitant energy reduction with respiration fatigue and tissue hypoxia. Together or as separate phenomena, reduction in energy utilization potential and oxygen transportation, play a crucial role in the generation of hypoxic conditions of malaria in an escalating feed-forward mechanism.

Another mechanism for hypoxia in malaria involves the nuclear enzyme poly (ADP-ribose) polymerase (PARP). PARP catalyzes transfer of ADP-ribose units from β-nicotinamide adenine dinucleotide (NAD$^+$) to produce linear and branched polymers from a number of different proteins. The normal and malarial inflammation-driven DNA damages repair mechanism is the same mechanism that activates PARP. Activation of PARP invariably consumes NAD$^+$ and conversely leads to the depletion of ATP. Intriguingly, breaks of DNA strands may be initiated by oxygen free radicals or their NO reaction products ONOO$^-$ as OS. ROS and DNA strands breaks reigns supreme in malaria inflammation with consequential depletion of NAD$^+$ and decreased ATP generation without the critical NAD$^+$ [69]. Aerobic respiration is thus invariably compromised with the possibility of bioenergetics failure through increased glycolysis which generates insufficient energy and hyperlactemia. In malarial inflammation, there is increased generation of $ONOO^-$ through induction of iNOS and subsequently NO, which activates over expression of PARP through increased DNA damage. Concomitantly, a vicious cycle of mitochondrial dysfunction leading to ATP rundown predisposes to polymyopathy, hypoglycemia, hyperlactemia. The facets have been hitherto mostly attributed to poor oxygen delivery in malaria [70].

The solution to energy regeneration may be through prevention of PARP-induced energy rundown and may comprise of (i) increasing supply of NAD^+, (ii) PARP activation-inhibition, (iii) quenching the inflammatory drivers of PARP activation, i.e., NO and $ONOO^-$, or stopping DNA damages by other means [71]. However, supplementation with NAD^+ in sepsis or malaria is somewhat impractical; inhibition of PARP may have deadly effects if it was possible; elimination of DNA damage is impossible. Quenching the pro-oxidant drivers of activation of PARP through DNA damage seem the most plausible method to protect against both the inflammasome and energy rundown. Indeed, certain agents have been reported to protect against free radical oxidation inhibiting PARP activation salvaging brain ischemia, splanchnic ischemia and reperfusion [72–74], lipopolysaccharide-induced toxicity, local inflammation and brain pathology in mice, multi-organ failure in rats and sepsis of the pigs [75, 76].

The other fascinating feature in PARP is that transcription factor NF-kβ is intricately connected the activation of the nuclear enzyme. Also, NFkβ is involved in DNA repair, immunological response and apoptosis placing it pivotally in the expression of genes essential to systemic inflammatory disease mainly, TNF-α and interleukin-1 (IL-1), IL-1β, IL-6, IAM-1, E-selectin and iNOS [77–82].

Essentially, PARP activation through $ONOO^-$ as a result of inflammation, consumes NAD^+ causing poor energy utilization and energy depletion [69]. Subsequent to inflammation-driven PARP activation through $ONOO^-$, tissue hypoxia (from increased NAD^+ consumption) sets in causing more inflammation-induced tissue damage, increased inflammatory cytokines synthesis and more $ONOO^-$ production [69]. Coma and death are inevitable from the vicious cycle of severe inflammation breeding more of itself leading to multi-organ failure, ultimately [70]. As a result, anti-inflammatory agents like Asiatic acid may have indispensable roles, through inhibition of NF-kβ, in the assuagement of malarial disease which essentially is underscored by inflammatory processes.

4. Malarial oxidative stress-driven inflammatory response

Reactive oxygen species have destructive effects through their ability to increase oxidative stress. Malaria disease is able to orchestrate multi-organ injury and disintegration through the ROS's disparaging properties. Oxidative stress (OS) has a fundamental role in pRBC's influence to disease manifestation comprising of pRBC's vascular sequestration, AKI, CM, SMA and ARDS [83, 84]. The defense mechanism of ROS and reactive nitric oxide species (RNOS) against disease and their signal transduction capacities make them have a both beneficial and pathological role in malaria necessitating regulation.

Plasmodium parasites have contracted capacities to mobilize amino acids and depend on hemoglobin (Hb) breakdown, a process with a high potential to generate ROS. Hb breakdown yields heme and globin (protein), with the former being a highly toxic compound which generates high OS activity at very low concentrations. Hb-free heme contains ferri/ferroprotoporphyrin IX (FP-IX) a very reactive iron-containing compound which generates an OS environment. Detoxification of heme by the parasite to hemozoin (β-hematin) is necessary and critical [85, 86]. Failure to convert heme to its biocrystallization or biomineralization form will oxidize the parasite food vacuole membranes destroying it in the process. Chloroquine and other 4-aminoquinolines use this principle to dislocate parasite proliferation by inhibiting heme biocrystallization in pRBC's and increasing OS [85–89].

There is a high overall oxidative load that the host cell immune response to parasitemia likewise yields to the pRBC. Nevertheless, the parasite has developed mechanisms for amplified antioxidant capacity, which may only be overcome by an extremely oxidative agent [83, 90–93]. Agents that inhibit hemozoin creation from heme have since been rendered impotent through multidrug resistance (MDR) processes that extrude the drug from the food vacuole protecting the parasite from possible oxidative stress.

On the other hand, ROS may be deliberately generated and targeted at certain parasite enzymes and membranes, as what is witnessed in the use of endoperoxidase antimalarials, with higher chances of faster parasitemia clearance although with higher tissue inflammation induction as well [94].

Antioxidants may have an anti-inflammatory effect in malaria where inflammation is generated from OS. However, OS is beneficial in malarial parasite eradication. Pleiotropic characteristics of triterpenes, antioxidant and pro-oxidant, seem to be very ideal properties for combating malaria. Indeed, it has since emerged that certain phytotherapeutics do eradicate parasitemia while ameliorating the pathophysiology of malaria like inflammation [95] and severe malaria anemia [96]. Buttressing the antioxidant capacity of triterpene phytotherapeutics are findings that oral administration of Asiatic acid (20 mg/kg) in streptozotocin-induced diabetic rats up-regulated both enzymatic and non-enzymatic antioxidants with subsequent lipid peroxidation abating [97] and salvaged diabetic rats [98] where increased OS is common. Of note is that superoxide dismutase (SOD), catalase (CAT), glutathione peroxidase (GPx) and glutathione-S-transferase (GST), ascorbic acid and reduced glutathione (GSH) tend to be elevated in the phytochemical is administered animal experimental DM [97–99]. Moreover, severe malaria is accompanied by marked lipid peroxidation, prevention of which by triterpenes testifies their efficacy against OS driven inflammation in malaria and acute renal injury [100].

5. Hormonal anti-inflammatory processes in malaria mediate glucose homeostasis

Complications of malaria including CM, SMA, placental malaria, hypoglycemia, ARDS are not efficaciously resolved despite the effective parasitemia inhibition by current antimalarial agents [9]. Parasite infection and/or exaggerated immune reaction [101] contribute to malarial complications necessitating treatment emphasis on more than just pathogen clearance but extending it to host defense mechanism that do not interfere with parasitemia load. The malarial disease tolerance or anti-disease process has been linked to heme oxygenase [102] and to Fe^{3+} sequestration protein ferritin [103] and some novel phytotherapeutics [96]. Glucocorticoids (GC), cortisol in the human and corticosterone in rats and mineral corticoids (MC) are adrenal gland cortex products and the adrenaline-noradrenaline combination are from the adrenal medulla. Adrenal cortex responds to the circadian rhythm, when the hypothalamus-pituitary–adrenal axis is activated, in stress/trauma situations, infection or systemic inflammation [104] by producing hormones to influence metabolism, immunity, bone remodeling, cardiovascular function, reproduction and cognitive processes [105].

GC's have anti-inflammatory properties and differential effects on numerous leukocytes phenotypes [106, 107]. In response to GC's, liver, muscle, adipose tissue increase gluconeogenesis, protein catabolism and lipolysis, respectively, to increase glucose directly or indirectly [108]. Upon human malarial (*P. falciparum* or *P. vivax*) infection, GC's (cortisol) are the only hormones of the adrenal gland [109]. Malaria infection and pregnancy-associated corticosterone concentration increases cause the loss malarial immunity and recrudescence [110–112] with adrenalectomy reducing survival in mice infected with *P. berghei* K173 parasite [113]. Infection of adrenal-ectomized mice causes lethal hypoglycemia of insulin- and TNF-α-independent type with increased inflammation [9]. The phenotype is characterized by exhausted hepatic glycogen stores, no increase in glucogenesis and is rescued by dexametha-sone administration. This shows that GC's are essential for malarial disease tolerance through modulation of inflammatory mediators. Notably, raised cytokine concentra-tion tend to be observed in both the circulation and the brain; adrenal hormones differentially disturb inflammation in the brain and circulation compared to liver and lungs. Together with inflammation, marked hypoglycemia sufficient to cause functional brain failure and coma, has been observed with rapid brain death [114]. Hypoglycemia is a major life threat in malaria and glycemia correlates with clinical scores negatively regular consistence. Moreover, plasma glucose concentrations negatively correlate with brain concentrations of mRNA's encoding TNF-α, IL-1β, IL-6, CCL2 and iNOS, signifying the possible linkage between hypoglycemia and expression of these pro-inflammatory markers. Plasma concentrations of chemo-kines, cytokines and with the exception of IL-4, tend to be negatively interrelated to plasma glucose concentration.   Notwithstanding hypoglycemia, hyperlactemia in acidosis, resulting from increased glycolytic flux, may complicate malarial infection.

After malaria infection, hepatic gluconeogenic transcriptional response is dimin-ished regardless of increases in GC concentration showing the importance of adrenal glands in maintaining blood glucose concentration in malaria. The classical glycemia-regulating principles of adrenal corticosteroids includes transcriptional induction of gluconeogenic response in the liver and increase plasma free fat acids concentrations.

In the absence of adrenal hormones, like in adrenalectomy, malaria causes com-plete exhaustion of hepatic glycogen stores. This creates irreversible severe hypogly-cemia that may not be rescued by glucose supplementation by oral or intraperitoneal (i.p.) injection route in mice. Parasitemia remains unaffected by glucose supple-mentation in such situations. Amazingly, even the neutralization of the most potent pro-inflammatory cytokine, TNF-α, does not seem to salvage from lethal hypoglyce-mia in the absence of adrenal glands. Also, adrenal hormone absence in malaria affect glycemia independent of insulin secretion. Overall, malaria infection is moderated by adrenal hormones to alleviate hypoglycemia which cannot be reversed by glucose administration, insulin blocking with clonidine, neutralizing of TNF-α but is rescued by dexamethasone, a GC analog [9]. A similar effect has been shown when triterpene phytotherapeutics, potent anti-inflammatory capacity, are administered in murine malaria [115] also showing inflammation involvement in malarial lethality.

6. Inflammation and the pathogenesis of cerebral malaria

Cerebral malaria is the most severe neurological complication of malaria. It is a clinical syndrome characterized by coma and other acute and or chronic neurological disturbances. In children, coma may develop with seizures often following weakness and prostration. Other neurological symptoms include encephalitis, intracranial hypertension, retinal changes and brainstem signs (impaired pupillary reflexes, posture problems and abnormal eye movements) [116, 117]. In adults, patients develop fever and headaches and progressive delirium and coma but seizures and retinal abnormali-ties are less common [116, 117]. Several neurological sequelae have been associated with cerebral malaria and these include; spasticity (hemiplegia, quadriparesis or quadriplegia), hypotonia, cranial nerve palsies, ataxia, visual disturbances, aphasias, neurocognitive deficits, epilepsy and some behavioral and neuropsychiatric distur-bances. These sequelae may occur in the short-term and resolve, or may persist long term [117].

The pathogenesis of cerebral malaria has been be explained according to two theories: (1) the occlusion theory, or (2) the inflammation theory. The occlusion theory, supported by vast scientific evidence, suggests that brain injury and the resultant neurological disturbances are the result of increased sequestration of blood cells to the brain microvasculature which reduces perfusion and may cause ischemia and tissue injury. Increased sequestration of infected red blood cells, leukocytes and platelets is well known to occur in cerebral malaria [118–120] but the occlusion theory does not adequately explain how some fatal cases of cerebral malaria occur with little to no sequestration. Additionally, although *P. vivax* is not likely to seques-ter in brain vasculature, there have been isolated cases of *P. vivax* infection-related cerebral malaria cases [121]. These gaps in our knowledge of the pathogenesis of cerebral malaria have led to an increased interest in other possible pathologic mecha-nisms which may work independently or together with occlusion to cause cerebral malaria and related neurological disturbances. Stimulation of a local inflammatory response in the brain has been coined as an alternative or accompanying mechanism in the pathogenesis of cerebral malaria and is summarized in **Figure 1**.

The blood brain barrier (BBB) endothelium responds to PAMPs, DAMPs and peripheral cytokines and is now regarded as an integral part of the neurovascular unit. In response to these immunostimulatory molecules, endothelial cells produce proinflammatory cytokines and chemokines that mediate leukocyte recruit-ment and thus trigger local inflammation [122, 123]. Leukocytes further release proinflammatory cytokines and thus set up a vicious inflammatory cycle which exacerbates local inflammation with the brain. As part of the BBB, the integrity of the endothelium is central to BBB function and brain protection. Inflammatory activation of the endothelium has been associated with increased BBB permeability through the induction of regulatory miRNAs that reorganize endothelial tight junc-tions [124, 125]. This renders the BBB leaky and allows passage of substances into neural tissue, leading to neurotoxicity. Clinically the progression of cerebral malaria has been closely associated with changes in BBB function as evidenced by hemor-rhages in cerebral malaria and loss of endothelial intercellular junctions in pediatric fatal cerebral malaria (**Figure 2**) [132].

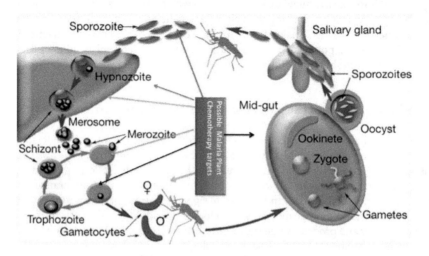

Figure 1.
Malaria Cycle and therapeutic possible cites [18].

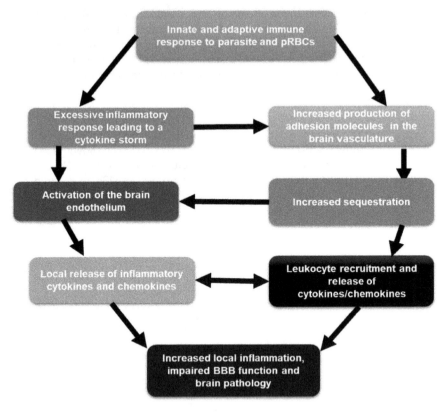

Figure 2.
Inflammatory events involved in the pathogenesis of cerebral malaria endothelial intercellular junctions in pediatric fatal cerebral malaria [126].

The production of proinflammatory cytokines in the brain could also be involved the development of encephalopathy. For example, TNF has been reported to regulate synaptic function and to cause glutamate neurotoxicity [127]; mechanisms which are closely linked to the development of seizures and neurocognitive deficits. IL-1 and TNF have also been shown to inhibit long term potentiation [128] and it is possible that high levels of these cytokines produced in severe malaria could be involved in the development of cognitive deficits associated with the disease.

7. Medicinal plants

Exposure to Plasmodium infection leads to elevation of pro-inflammatory markers such as TNF-α and interleukin-1 (IL-1) from macrophages and lymphocytes. Natural products have attracted interest due to their affordability to the general communities with low socio-economic status. Below is the description of the triterpenes that possess anti-inflammatory properties.

7.1 Synthetic oleanolic (SO) pentacyclic triterpenes derivatives

CDDO-EA (**Figure 3**) is a synthetic oleanolic derivative that has been shown to possess various biochemical activities which include efficacy against cerebral malaria (CM) [129]. The development of severe CM is associated with dysfunction of the immune system as shown by plasma levels of TNF-α and IFN-γ [59, 130]. A single injection dose of CCDO-EA (200 µmol/kg) lowered circulating levels of TNF-α and IFN-γ which improved mice survival and lowered inflammation [129]. Indeed, studies have indicated that the host's response to malaria is excess production of pro-inflammatory molecules which are thought to be central causes of inflammation in malaria.

7.2 Ursolic acid

Ursolic acid (3-hydroxy-urs-12-ene-28-oic acid, **Figure 4**) is triterpene which is widely distributed on different medicinal plants. UA has been shown to exhibit a number of pharmacological activities which include, anti-microbial [132], anti-malarial [133] and potent anti-inflammatory properties [134]. Although

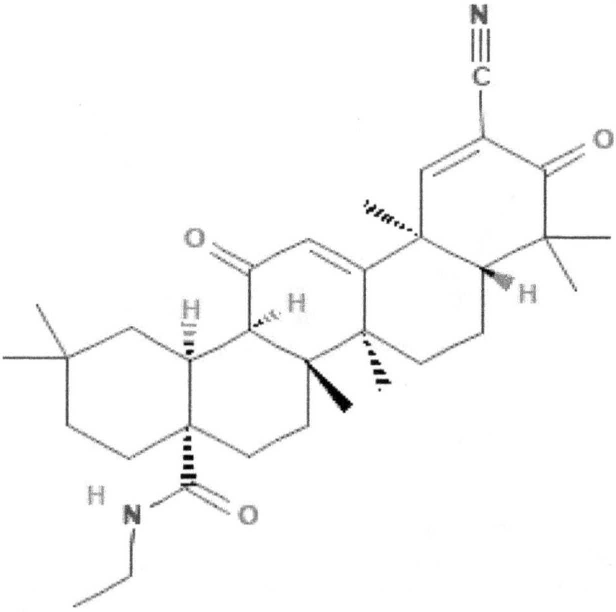

Figure 3.
Chemical structure of a synthetic oleanolae derivative [129].

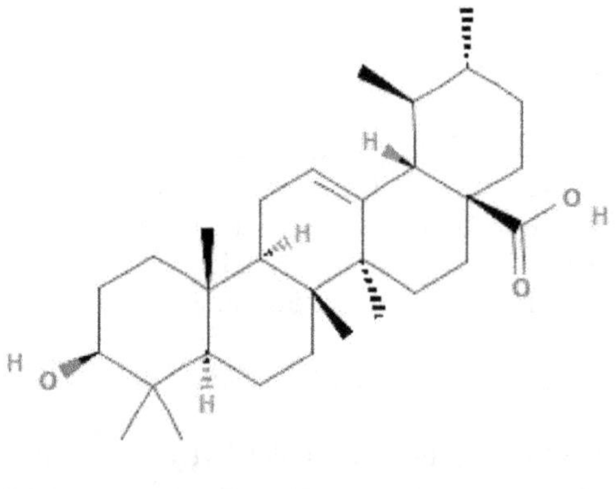

Figure 4.
2D chemical structure of ursolic acid [131].

no research has been done on anti-inflammatory properties of this triterpene in malaria rats, several studies have evaluated anti-inflammatory properties on other experimental models in vivo and in vitro [134]. However, several studies have evaluated the anti-inflammatory properties of the compounds in in-vitro and in vivo. Tsai and Yin's reports indicate that UA and oleanolic acid (OA) alleviate inflammation through reduction of IL-6 and TNF-α [135]. Additionally, studies also validate the anti-inflammatory potency of UA by reducing the production of IL-2 and through activation of T-helper cells [136]. Liu et al., have shown that UA suppressed T cell responses including NF-kB inhibition at 25 mM while Bharata et al. demonstrated the efficacy against a lowers dose of UA IS enough to lower immune cells such as T-cells, B-cell, and macrophage activation. Apart from this, Xu et al. have shown that anti-inflammatory effects of UA are mediated through.

7.3 Maslinic acid (MA) and oleanolic acid (OA)

Maslinic acid and oleanolic acid are two triterpenes widely abundant in olive trees and *Syzygium* spp. Among many pharmacological properties, these triterpenes have demonstrated efficacy against malaria [133]. The triterpenoids are generally highly hydrophobic, which reduces their bioavailability and efficacy. Sibiya et al. showed that once off application of an-OA patch reduces parasitemia and TNF-α plasma levels [137]. Exposure of the host to malaria activates macrophages which in turn induces production of TNF-α and then the release of other cytokines such as IL-6 which initiate inflammation. Reports also indicate the efficacy of another promising pentacyclic triterpene (maslinic acid) to alleviate malaria and inflammation in general. Extensive in vivo and in vitro studies indicate that MA reduces inflammation by reducing lipopolysaccharides (LPS)-induced production of nitric oxide (NO) and INOS gene expression [132] Márquez et al. also indicated that MA reduces the production of interleukin-6 (IL-6) on peritoneal macrophages [132] (**Figure 5**).

7.4 Anti-inflammatory effects of Asiatic acid (AA) in malaria

Many parasitic and metabolic diseases are built upon inflammatory processes. Ample indications exist that phytopharmaceuticals may moderate innumerable inflammatory mediators, govern the production and action of second messengers, direct the expression of transcription factors and key pro-inflammatory mechanisms [1, 2, 95, 115, 138–141]. The fundamental machinery of anti-inflammatory activity for AA in malarial may comprise: (i) anti-oxidative and radical scavenging;

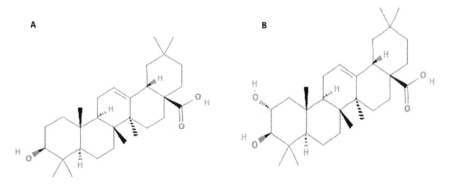

Figure 5.
2D chemical structure of oleanolic acid (A) and maslinic acid (B) adapted from the PubMed database [134].

(ii) inflammatory cellular components modulation (macrophages, lymphocytes neutrophils); (iii) modulation of expression and/or activity of pro-inflammatory enzymes such as phospholipase A2 (PLA2), cyclooxygenase (COX), lipooxygenase (LOX), iNOS and (iv) modulation of pro-inflammatory gene expression [138].

In malaria inflammation, the immune system-triggering-malaria-toxin is GPI which may be released pRBC rupture at erythrocytic schizogony [70]. GPI initiates TNF-α and lymphotoxin (formerly TNF-β) production [142], up-regulates ICAM-1 and IVCAM-1 [5, 143].

Hemopoietic mediators of inflammation comprise Th1/M1 cytokines largely TNF-α, IL-1, IL-6, IL-18 and Th2/M2 cytokines IL-4 and IL-10. When produced excessively as in severe malaria, Th1 cytokines may lead to the generation of fever, hypoglycemia, bone marrow suppression, coagulopathies, hypergammaglobulinemia, hypotension and elevated acute phase reactants [55, 144]. The works by Clark and Chaudhri [144], showing that TNF-α-induced dyserythropoiesis and erythrophagocytosis in malaria-infected animals, evidenced the association of SMA to inflammatory mediators and corroborated Peetre et al. who verified growth inhibition of culture hemopoietic cells [145].

Compounded, the anti-inflammatory outcome of AA may modify pro-inflammatory apparatuses in malaria in the same way it does in other inflammatory diseases. Indeed, AA displays a dose-dependent (10 and 20 μsg/kg AA) selective induction of selective mitochondria-dependent apoptosis in activated Th1 cells. This averted concanavalin (Con-A)-induced murine fulminant hepatitis in a fashion that disrupted mitochondrial transmembrane potential, released cytochrome c, activated caspases and cleaved poly(ADP-ribose) polymerase [PARP] [146].

In malaria, hematological differential counts display exaggerated leukocytosis. As inflammatory response is similar regardless of cause, AA may modify Th1 over expression in malaria by eradicating activated cells. Moreover, in a mouse model for pain and inflammation, AA blocked the activation of NF-kβ [147], a major transcription factor in the regulation of pro-inflammatory cells, cytokines and enzymes [148].

In unstimulated Th1 cells, NF-kβ subunit p65/p50, is sequestered in the cytoplasm bound to the inhibitory factor Ikβ-α. Proinflammatory signals in malaria comprising of GPI, cause the phosphorylation of Ikβ-α by Ikβ kinase (IKK) and its inactivation though the ubiquitin-mediated destruction. Liberated, NF-kβ translocate into the nucleus acting as pro-inflammatory mediator and transcription factor [70, 78, 148]. Eradication inflammatory responses is critical for overall health maintenance. AA may be able to inhibit GPI production or maintain inactivation of NF-kβ or both as this anti-inflammatory mechanism has been revealed in other diseases, and not malaria, when similar triterpenoid to AA, madecassoside (MA), was used [149–151].

By inhibiting activation of NF-kβ, AA may subsequently inhibit iNOS and COX-2 and reduce NO release. Moreover, AA (10 mg/kg) injected into Carrageenan-induced paw edema inhibited expression of iNOS, COX-2 and NF-kβ in mice [147]. This may mean, in malaria, reduction in unrestrained vasodilation related to vascular permeability, pulmonary edema or renal dysfunction. Toxic oxidative activities causing tissue injury may likewise be ablated by a NO reduction and possibly superoxide [$O_2^{\cdot-}$] [151]. Certainly, AA has been predicted by a computational model AutoDock v.3.05 to bind iNOS. This binding inhibits iNOS's strong affinity for arginine, exhibited as free energy binding (FEB) of -9.79 kcal.mol^{-1} [152–154].

Chemoattractant mediators hinging on NF-kβ activation may also be inhibited by AA resulting in abrogation of neutrophil-aggregation and inactivation of the linked oxidant and pro-inflammatory injury lytic enzymes [155]. Activation inhibition of peroxisome proliferator-activated gamma (PPAR-γ), which regulates inflammation through NF-kβ translocation, may be a route AA may confer anti-inflammatory activity. A similar process has been confirmed with curcumin, a multi-faceted phytopharmaceutical [156]. The consequent action of this activation will be up-regulation of CD36 in monocytes/macrophages for non-opsonic pRBC's phagocytosis with parasite extrusion or destruction [157].

Credence of AA anti-inflammatory capacity in malarial pathophysiology has been shown. Indeed, the anti-inflammatory effect of AA has been reported in a murine malaria model where C-reactive protein was shown to be significantly reduced in infected transdermal AA administered animals as compared to infected chloroquine-treated animals and non-treated controls [95].

8. Conclusion

The strong connection between malaria pathophysiology and systemic inflammation mobilizes various mediators, metabolic processes consummating in toxic cachexia, hypoglycemia, neuronal damage, coma and death. Numerous immunological and inflammatory response mediators drive the disease. Initial inflammatory response directed at alleviating and curtailing the infection through parasite killing turns around and aberrantly militates against the host. Hormonal involvement is crucial in maintain malaria tolerance by the host. The phytotherapeutics AA, Ma and OA intervention in malaria promises to engage the parasitic as well the inflammation salvaging glucose homeostasis, neuronal death and other disease effects in malaria terminating the vicious cycle and alleviating the disease. Potential alternative treatment regimens for malaria are thus in the offing.

Author details

Greanious Alfred Mavondo[1*], Blessing Nkazimulo Mkhwanazi[2],
Mayibongwe Louis Mzingwane[1], Rachael Dangarembizi[1], Blessing Zambuko[1],
Obadiah Moyo[3], Patience Musiwaro[1], Francis Farai Chikuse[4], Colline Rakabopa[5],
Tariroyashe Mpofu[1] and Joy Mavondo[6]

1 National University of Science and Technology (NUST), Bulawayo, Zimbabwe

2 University of KwaZulu Natal, Durban, South Africa

3 Chitungwiza General Hospital, Chitungwiza, Zimbabwe

4 Pathcare, Namibia

5 University of Zimbabwe, Harare, Zimbabwe

6 Imagegate Diagnostics (PL), Bulawayo, Zimbabwe

*Address all correspondence to: greanious.mavondo@nust.ac.zw

IntechOpen

© 2019 The Author(s). Licensee IntechOpen. This chapter is distributed under the terms of the Creative Commons Attribution License (http://creativecommons.org/licenses/by/3.0), which permits unrestricted use, distribution, and reproduction in any medium, provided the original work is properly cited. (cc) BY

References

[1] Mavondo GA, Kasvosve I. Antimalarial phytochemicals: Delineation of the triterpene asiatic acid malarial anti-disease and pathophysiological remedial activities—Part I. Journal of Infectious Disease and Pathology. 2017;**1**:104

[2] Mavondo GA, Kasvosve I. Antimalarial phytochemicals: Delineation of the triterpene asiatic acid malarial anti-disease and pathophysiological remedial activities—Part II. Journal of Infectious Disease and Pathology. 2017;**1**:103

[3] Dinarello CA. Interleukin-1 and the pathogenesis of the acute-phase response. The New England Journal of Medicine. 1984;**311**:1413

[4] Beutler B, Cerami A. Tumour necrosis factor, cachexia, shock, and inflammation: A common mediator. Annual Review of Biochemistry. 1988;**57**:505

[5] Schofield L, Hackett F. Signal transduction in host cells by a glycosylphosphatidylinositol toxin of malaria parasites. The Journal of Experimental Medicine. 1993;**177**:145-153

[6] Clark IA. Cell-mediated immunity in protection and pathology of malaria. Parasitology Today. 1987;**3**:300

[7] Schofield L, Grau GE. Immunological processes in malaria pathogenesis. Nature Reviews Immunology. 2005;**5**:722-735

[8] Hansen DS. Inflammatory responses associated with the induction of cerebral malaria: Lessons from experimental murine models. PLoS Pathogens. 2012;**8**(12):e1003045. DOI: 10.1371/journal.ppat.1003045

[9] Vandermosten L, Pham T-T, Knoops S, De Geest C, Lays N, Van der Molen K, et al. Adrenal hormones mediate disease tolerance in malaria. Nature Communications. 2018;**9**:4525. DOI: 10.1038/s41467-018-06986-5

[10] Moneriz C, Mestres J, Bautista JM, Diez A, Puye A. Multi-targeted activity of maslinic acid as an antimalarial natural compound. The FEBS Journal. 2011;**278**:2951-2961

[11] Gallego-Delgado J, Ty M, Orengo JM, van de Hoef D, Rodriguez A. A surprising role for uric acid: The inflammatory malaria response. Current Rheumatology Reports. 2014;**16**(2):401

[12] Dinko B, Pradel G. Immune evasion by *Plasmodium falciparum* parasites: Converting a host protection mechanism for the parasite's benefit. Advances in Infectious Disease. 2016;**6**(2):67759

[13] Artavanis-Tsakonas K, Tongren JE, Riley EM. The war between the malaria parasite and the immune system: Immunity, immunoregulation and immunopathology. Clinical and Experimental Immunology. 2003;**133**:145-152

[14] Dodoo D, Omer FM, Todd J, Akanmori BD, Koram K. Absolute levels and ratios of proinflammatory and anti-inflammatory cytokine production in vitro predict clinical immunity to *Plasmodium falciparum* malaria. The Journal of Infectious Diseases. 2002;**185**:971-979

[15] Griffith JW, Sun T, McIntosh MT, Bucala R. Pure hemozoin is inflammatory in vivo and activates the NALP3 inflammasome via release of uric acid. Journal of Immunology. 2009;**183**:5208-5220

[16] Sharma S, DeOliveira RB, Kalantari P. Innate immune recognition of an AT-rich stem-loop DNA motif in

the *Plasmodium falciparum* genome. Immunity. 2011;**35**:194-207

[17] Gowda NM, Wu X, Gowda DC. The nucleosome (histone-DNA complex) is the TLR9-specific immunostimulatory component of *Plasmodium falciparum* that activates DCs. PLoS One. 2011;**6**:e20398

[18] Winzeler EA. Malaria research in the post-genomic era. Nature. 2008;**455**:751-756. DOI: 10.1038/nature07361

[19] Naik RS, Branch OH, Woods AS. Glycosylphosphatidylinositol anchors of Plasmodium falciparum: Molecular characterization and naturally elicited antibody response that may provide immunity to malaria pathogenesis. The Journal of Experimental Medicine. 2000;**192**(11):1563-1576. DOI: 10.1084/jem.192.11.1563

[20] Olivier M, Van Den Ham K, Shio MT, Kassa FA, Fougeray S. Malarial pigment hemozoin and the innate inflammatory response. Frontiers in Immunology. 2014;**5**:25. DOI: 10.3389/fimmu.2014.00025

[21] Dostert C, Guarda G, Romero JF, Menu P, Gross O, Tardivel A. Malarial hemozoin is a Nalp3 inflammasome activating danger signal. PLoS One. 2009;**4**:e6510. DOI: 10.1371/journal.pone.0006510

[22] Shio MT, Eisenbarth SC, Savaria M, Vinet AF, Bellemare MJ, Harder KW. Malarial hemozoin activates the NLRP3 inflammasome through Lyn and Syk kinases. PLoS Pathogens. 2009;**5**:e1000559. DOI: 10.1371/journal.ppat.1000559

[23] Deroost K, Lays N, Pham T-T, Baci D, Van den Eynde K, Komuta M. Hemozoin induces hepatic inflammation in mice and is differentially associated with liver pathology depending on the *Plasmodium*

strain. PLoS One. 2014;**9**(11):e113519. DOI: 10.1371/journal.pone.0113519

[24] Pichyangkul S, Yongvanitchit K, Kum-arb U, Hemmi H, Akira S, Krieg AM. Malaria blood stage parasites activate human plasmacytoid dendritic cells and murine dendritic cells through a toll-like receptor 9-dependent pathway. Journal of Immunology. 2004;**172**:4926-4933. DOI: 10.4049/jimmunol.172.8.4926

[25] Gowda DC, Wu X. Parasite recognition and signaling mechanisms in innate immune responses to malaria. Frontiers in Immunology. 2018;**9**:3006. DOI: 10.3389/fimmu.2018.03006

[26] Orengo JM, Leliwa-Sytek A, Evans JE. Uric acid is a mediator of the *Plasmodium falciparum*-induced inflammatory response. PLoS One. 2009;**4**:e5194

[27] Lopera-Mesa TM, Mita-Mendoza NK, van de Hoef DL. Plasma uric acid levels correlate with inflammation and disease severity in Malian children with *Plasmodium falciparum* malaria. PLoS One. 2012;**7**:e46424

[28] Mita-Mendoza NK, van de Hoef DL, Lopera-Mesa TM. A potential role for plasma uric acid in the endothelial pathology of *Plasmodium falciparum* malaria. PLoS One. 2013;**8**:e54481

[29] Mackintosh CL, Beeson JG, Marsh K. Clinical features and pathogenesis of severe malaria. Trends in Parasitology. 2004;**20**(12):597-603

[30] Lyke K, Burges R, Cissoko Y, Sangare L, Dao M, Diarra I, et al. Serum levels of the proinflammatory cytokines interleukin-1 beta (IL-1β), IL-6, IL-8, IL-10, tumor necrosis factor alpha, and IL-12 (p70) in Malian children with severe *Plasmodium falciparum* malaria and matched uncomplicated malaria

or healthy controls. Infection and Immunity. 2004;**72**(10):5630-5637

[31] Crompton PD, Moebius J, Portugal S, Waisberg M, Hart G, Garver LS, et al. Malaria immunity in man and mosquito: Insights into unsolved mysteries of a deadly infectious disease. Annual Review of Immunology. 2014;**32**:157-187

[32] Dieye Y, Mbengue B, Dagamajalu S, Fall MM, Loke MF, Nguer CM, et al. Cytokine response during non-cerebral and cerebral malaria: Evidence of a failure to control inflammation as a cause of death in African adults. PeerJ. 2016;**4**:e1965

[33] Clark IA, Budd AC, Alleva LM, Cowden WB. Human malarial disease: A consequence of inflammatory cytokine release. Malaria Journal. 2006;**5**(1):85

[34] Tachado SD, Gerold P, McConville MJ, Baldwin T, Quilici D, Schwarz RT, et al. Glycosylphosphatidylinositol toxin of *Plasmodium* induces nitric oxide synthase expression in macrophages and vascular endothelial cells by a protein tyrosine kinase-dependent and protein kinase C-dependent signaling pathway. The Journal of Immunology. 1996;**156**(5):1897-1907

[35] Sherry BA, Alava G, Tracey KJ, Martiney J, Cerami A, Slater A. Malaria-specific metabolite hemozoin mediates the release of several potent endogenous pyrogens (TNF, MIP-1 alpha, and MIP-1 beta) in vitro, and altered thermoregulation in vivo. Journal of Inflammation. 1995;**45**(2):85-96

[36] Gazzinelli RT, Kalantari P, Fitzgerald KA, Golenbock DT. Innate sensing of malaria parasites. Nature Reviews Immunology. 2014;**14**(11):744

[37] Parroche P, Lauw FN, Goutagny N, Latz E, Monks BG, Visintin A, et al. Malaria hemozoin is immunologically inert but radically enhances innate responses by presenting malaria DNA

to toll-like receptor 9. Proceedings of the National Academy of Sciences. 2007;**104**(6):1919-1924

[38] Schwarzer E, Turrini F, Ulliers D, Giribaldi G, Ginsburg H, Arese P. Impairment of macrophage functions after ingestion of *Plasmodium falciparum*-infected erythrocytes or isolated malarial pigment. The Journal of Experimental Medicine. 1992;**176**(4):1033-1041

[39] Scorza T, Magez S, Brys L, De Baetselier P. Hemozoin is a key factor in the induction of malaria-associated immunosuppression. Parasite Immunology. 1999;**21**(11):545-554

[40] Liehl P, Zuzarte-Luís V, Chan J, Zillinger T, Baptista F, Carapau D, et al. Host-cell sensors for *Plasmodium* activate innate immunity against liver-stage infection. Nature Medicine. 2014;**20**(1):47

[41] Butt AN, Swaminathan R. Overview of circulating nucleic acids in plasma/serum: Update on potential prognostic and diagnostic value in diseases excluding fetal medicine and oncology. The Annals of the New York Academy of Sciences. 2008;**1137**(1):236-242

[42] Figueiredo RT, Fernandez PL, Mourao-Sa DS, Porto BN, Dutra FF, Alves LS, et al. Characterization of heme as activator of Toll-like receptor 4. The Journal of Biological Chemistry. 2007;**282**(28):20221-20229

[43] Mantel PY, Marti M. The role of extracellular vesicles in *Plasmodium* and other protozoan parasites. Cellular Microbiology. 2014;**16**(3):344-354

[44] Kern P, Hemmer CJ, Gallati H, Neifer S, Kremsner P, Dietrich M, et al. Soluble tumor necrosis factor receptors correlate with parasitemia and disease severity in human malaria. The Journal of Infectious Diseases. 1992;**166**(4):930-934

[45] Molyneux M, Engelmann H, Taylor TE, Wirima JJ, Aderka D, Wallach D, et al. Circulating plasma receptors for tumour necrosis factor in Malawian children with severe falciparum malaria. Cytokine. 1993;**5**(6):604-609

[46] Geraghty EM, Ristow B, Gordon SM, Aronowitz P. Overwhelming parasitemia with *Plasmodium falciparum* infection in a patient receiving infliximab therapy for rheumatoid arthritis. Clinical Infectious Diseases. 2007;**44**(10):e82-e84

[47] Spriggs D, Imamura K, Rodriguez C, Horiguchi J, Kufe D. Induction of tumor necrosis factor expression and resistance in a human breast tumor cell line. Proceedings of the National Academy of Sciences. 1987;**84**(18):6563-6566

[48] Creagan ET, Kovach JS, Moertel CG, Frytak S, Kvols LK. A phase I clinical trial of recombinant human tumor necrosis factor. Cancer. 1988;**62**(12):2467-2471

[49] McGuire W, Hill AV, Allsopp CE, Greenwood BM, Kwiatkowski D. Variation in the TNF-α and interleukin-1 (IL-1) promoter region associated with susceptibility to cerebral malaria. Nature. 1994;**371**(6497):508

[50] Berendt A, Simmons D, Tansey J, Newbold CI, Marsh K. Intercellular adhesion molecule-1 is an endothelial cell adhesion receptor for *Plasmodium falciparum*. Nature. 1989;**341**(6237):57

[51] Esamai F, Ernerudh J, Janols H, Welin S, Ekerfelt C, Mining S, et al. Cerebral malaria in children: Serum and cerebrospinal fluid TNF-α and TGF-β levels and their relationship to clinical outcome. Journal of Tropical Pediatrics. 2003;**49**(4):216-223

[52] Armah HB, Wilson NO, Sarfo BY, Powell MD, Bond VC, Anderson W, et al. Cerebrospinal fluid and serum biomarkers of cerebral malaria mortality in Ghanaian children. Malaria Journal. 2007;**6**(1):147

[53] Thuma PE, Van Dijk J, Bucala R, Debebe Z, Nekhai S, Kuddo T, et al. Distinct clinical and immunologic profiles in severe malarial anemia and cerebral malaria in Zambia. The Journal of Infectious Diseases. 2011;**203**(2):211-219

[54] van Hensbroek MB, Palmer A, Onyiorah E, Schneider G, Jaffar S, Dolan G, et al. The effect of a monoclonal antibody to tumor necrosis factor on survival from childhood cerebral malaria. The Journal of Infectious Diseases. 1996;**174**(5):1091-1097

[55] Clark I, Gray K, Rockett E, Cowden W, Rockett K, Ferrante A, et al. Increased lymphotoxin in human malarial serum, and the ability of this cytokine to increase plasma interleukin-6 and cause hypoglycaemia in mice: Implications for malarial pathology. Transactions of the Royal Society of Tropical Medicine and Hygiene. 1992;**86**(6):602-607

[56] Kumaratilake L, Ferrante A, Rzepczyk C. The role of T lymphocytes in immunity to *Plasmodium falciparum*. Enhancement of neutrophil-mediated parasite killing by lymphotoxin and IFN-gamma: Comparisons with tumor necrosis factor effects. The Journal of Immunology. 1991;**146**(2):762-767

[57] Grau GE, Heremans H, Piguet P-F, Pointaire P, Lambert P-H, Billiau A, et al. Monoclonal antibody against interferon gamma can prevent experimental cerebral malaria and its associated overproduction of tumor necrosis factor. Proceedings of the National Academy of Sciences. 1989;**86**(14):5572-5574

[58] Sedegah M, Finkelman F, Hoffman SL. Interleukin 12 induction of interferon gamma-dependent

protection against malaria. Proceedings of the National Academy of Sciences. 1994;**91**(22):10700-10702

[59] Mandala WL, Msefula CL, Gondwe EN, Drayson MT, Molyneux ME, MacLennan CA. Cytokine profiles in Malawian children presenting with uncomplicated malaria, severe malarial anemia, and cerebral malaria. Clinical and Vaccine Immunology. 2017;**24**(4):e00533-e00516

[60] Mahanta A, Kar SK, Kakati S, Baruah S. Heightened inflammation in severe malaria is associated with decreased IL-10 expression levels and neutrophils. Innate Immunity. 2015;**21**(5):546-552

[61] Othoro C, Lal AA, Nahlen B, Koech D, Orago AS, Udhayakumar V. A low interleukin-10 tumor necrosis factor-α ratio is associated with malaria anemia in children residing in a holoendemic malaria region in western Kenya. The Journal of Infectious Diseases. 1999;**179**(1):279-282

[62] Kurtzhals JA, Adabayeri V, Goka BQ, Akanmori BD, Oliver-Commey JO, Nkrumah FK, et al. Low plasma concentrations of interleukin 10 in severe malarial anaemia compared with cerebral and uncomplicated malaria. The Lancet. 1998;**351**(9118):1768-1772

[63] Omer F, Kurtzhals J, Riley E. Maintaining the immunological balance in parasitic infections: A role for TGF-β? Parasitology Today. 2000;**16**(1):18-23

[64] Bihari D, Smithies M, Gimson A, Tinker J. The effects of vasodilation with prostacyclin on oxygen delivery and uptake in critically ill patients. The New England Journal of Medicine. 1987;**317**:397-403

[65] Bersten A, Sibbald WJ. Circulatory disturbances in multiple systems organ failure. Critical Care Clinics. 1989;**5**:233-254

[66] Boekstegers P, Weidenhofer S, Kapsner T, Werdan K. Skeletal muscle partial pressure of oxygen in patients with sepsis. Critical Care Medicine. 1994;**22**:640-650

[67] Cleeter MW, Cooper JM, Darley-Usmar VM, Moncada S, Schapira AH. Reversible inhibition of cytochrome c oxidase, the terminal enzyme of the mitochondrial respiratory chain, by nitric oxide. Implications for neurodegenerative diseases. FEBS Letters. 1994;**345**:50-54

[68] Castro L, Rodriguez M, Radi R. Aconitase is readily inactivated by peroxynitrite, but not by its precursor, nitric oxide. The Journal of Biological Chemistry. 1994;**269**:29409-29415

[69] Szabo C. The pathophysiological role of peroxynitrite in shock, inflammation, and ischemia-reperfusion injury. Shock. 1996;**6**:79-88

[70] Clark IA, Cowden WB. The pathophysiology of *falciparum* malaria. Pharmacology and Therapeutics. 2003;**99**:221-260

[71] Khan AU, Delude RL, Han YY, Sappington PL, Han X, Carcillo JA, et al. Liposomal NAD(+) prevents diminished O_2 consumption by immunostimulated Caco-2 cells. The American Journal of Physiology. 2002;**282**:L1082-L1091

[72] Takahashi K, Pieper AA, Croul SE, Zhang J, Snyder SH, Greenberg JH. Post-treatment with an inhibitor of poly(ADP-ribose) polymerase attenuates cerebral damage in focal ischemia. Brain Research. 1999;**829**:46-54

[73] Jagtap P, Soriano FG, Virag L, Liaudet L, Mabley J, Szabo E, et al. Novel phenanthridinone inhibitors of poly(adenosine 5'-diphosphateribose) synthetase: Potent cytoprotective and antishock agents. Critical Care Medicine. 2002;**30**:1071-1082

[74] Mazzon E, Dugo L, De SA, Li JH, Caputi AP, Zhang J, et al. Beneficial effects of GPI 6150, an inhibitor of poly(ADP-ribose) polymerase in a rat model of splanchnic artery occlusion and reperfusion. Shock. 2002;**17**:222-227

[75] Koedel U, Winkler F, Angele B, Fontana T, Pfister HW. Meningitis-associated central nervous system complications are mediated by the activation of poly(ADP-ribose) polymerase. Journal of Cerebral Blood Flow and Metabolism. 2002;**22**:39-49

[76] Cuzzocrea S, Zingarelli B, Costantino G, Sottile A, Teti D, Caputi AP. Protective effect of poly(ADP-ribose) synthetase inhibition on multiple organ failure after zymosan-induced peritonitis in the rat. Critical Care Medicine. 1999;**27**:1517-1523

[77] Jimi E, Ghosh S. Role of nuclear factor-kappaB in the immune system and bone. Immunological Reviews. 2005;**208**:80-87

[78] Ogawa Y, Yoneda M, Tomeno W, Imajo K, Shinohara Y, Fujita K, et al. Peroxisome proliferator-activated receptor gamma exacerbates concanavalin A-induced liver injury via suppressing the translocation of NF-κB into the nucleus. 2012;**2012**:940384. DOI: 10.1155/2012/940384

[79] Janssens S, Tschopp J. Signals from within: The DNA-damage-induced NF-kappaB response. Cell Death and Differentiation. 2006;**13**(5):773-784

[80] Niu J, Shi Y, Tan T, Yang CH, Fan M, Pfeffer LM, et al. DNA damage induces NF-kB-dependent micro RNA-21 up-regulation and promotes breast cancer cell invasion. The Journal of Biological Chemistry. 2012;**287**:21783-21795

[81] Lawrence T. The nuclear factor NF-κB pathway in inflammation. Cold Spring Harbor Perspectives in Biology. 2009;**1**(6):a001651. DOI: 10.1101/cshperspect.a001651

[82] Hayden MS, West AP, Ghosh S. NF-kappaB and the immune response. Oncogene. 2006;**25**(51):6758-6780

[83] Becker K, Tilley L, Vennerstrom JL, Roberts D, Rogersone S, Ginsburg H. Oxidative stress in malaria parasite-infected erythrocytes: Host-parasite interactions. International Journal for Parasitology. 2004;**34**:163-189

[84] Descamps-Latscha B, Lunel-Fabiani F, Kara-Binis A, Druilhe P. Generation of ROS in whole blood from patients with acute *falciparum* malaria. Parasite Immunology. 1987;**9**:275-279

[85] Hempelmann E. Hemozoin biocrystallization in *Plasmodium falciparum* and the antimalarial activity of crystallization inhibitors. Parasitology Research. 2007;**100**:671-676

[86] Egan TJ. Haemozoin formation. Molecular and Biochemical Parasitology. 2008;**157**:127-136

[87] Goldberg DE. Haemoglobin degradation. Current Topics in Microbiology and Immunology. 2005;**295**:275-291

[88] Foley M, Tilley L. Quinoline antimalarials: Mechanisms of action and resistance and prospects for new agents. Pharmacology & Therapeutics. 1998;**79**:55-87

[89] Bonilla-Ramírez L, Galiano S, Quiliano M, Aldana I, Pabón A. Primaquine-quinoxaline 1,4-di-N-oxide hybrids with action on the exo-erythrocytic forms of *Plasmodium* induce their effect by the production of reactive oxygen species. Malaria Journal. 2019;**18**:201

[90] Hiller NL, Bhattacharjee S, van Ooij C, Liolios K, e a HT. A

host-targeting signal in virulence proteins reveals a secretome in malarial infection. Science. 2004;**306**:1934-1937

[91] Etkin NL, Ross PJ. Malaria, medicine and meals: A biobehavioral perspective. In: Romanucci-Ross L, Moerman DE, Tancredi LR, editors. The Anthropology of Medicine. New York: Praeger Publishers; 1997. pp. 169-209

[92] Etkin NL. Co-evolution of people, plants, and parasited: Biological and cultural adaptations to malaria. Proceedings of the Nutrition Society. 2003;**62**:311-317. DOI: 10.1079/PN2003244

[93] Etkin NL. Plants as antimalarial drugs: Relation to G-6-PD deficiency and evolutionary implications. In: MED LSG, editor. Adaptation to Malaria: The Interaction of Biology and Culture. New York: Gordon and Breach Publishers; 1997. pp. 139-176

[94] Olliaro PL, Haynes RK, Meunier B, Yuthavong Y. Possible modes of action of the artemisinin-type compounds. Trends in Parasitology. 2001;**17**:122-126

[95] Mavondo GA, Musabauane CT. Asiatic acid-pectin hydrogel matrix patch transdermal delivery system influences parasitaemia suppression and inflammation reduction in *P. berghei* murine malaria infected Sprague-Dawley rats. APJTM. 2016;**9**:1172-1180

[96] Mavondo GA, Mkhwananzi BN, Mabadla MV, Musabayane CT. Asiatic acid influences parasitaemia reduction and ameliorates malaria anaemia in *P. berghei* infected Sprague-Dawley male rats. BMC Complementary and Alternative Medicine. 2016;**16**:357. DOI: 10.1186/s12906-016-1338-z

[97] Ramachandran V, Saravanan R. Asiatic acid prevents lipid peroxidation and improves antioxidant status in rats with streptozotocin-induced diabetes. Journal of Functional Foods. 2013;**5**:1077-1087

[98] Ramachandran V, Saravanan R. Efficacy of asiatic acid, a pentacyclic triterpene on attenuating the key enzymes activities of carbohydrate metabolism in streptozotocin-induced diabetic rats. Phytomedicine. 2013;**20**:230-236

[99] Ramachandran V, Saravanan R. Antidiabetic and antihyperlipidemic activity of asiatic acid in diabetic rats, role of HMG CoA: *In vivo* and *in silico* approaches. Phytomedicine. 2014;**21**:225-232

[100] Mavondo GA, Musabayane CT. Transdermal drug delivery of asiatic acid influences renal function and electrolyte handling in *Plasmodium berghei*-infected Sprague-Dawley male rats. Journal Diseases and Medicinal Plants. 2017;**4**(1):18-29. DOI: 10.11648/j.jdmp.20180401.13

[101] Deroost K, Pham T-T, Opdenakker G, Van den Steen PE. The immunological balance between host and parasite in malaria. FEMS Microbiology Reviews. 2016;**40**:208-257

[102] Ferreira A, Marguti I, Bechmann I, Jeney V, Chora A, Palha NR, et al. Sickle hemoglobin confers tolerance to *Plasmodium* infection. Cell. 2011;**145**(3):398-409. DOI: 10.1016/j.cell.2011.03.049

[103] Gozzelino R, Andrade BB, Larsen R, Luz NF, Vanoaica L, Seixas E, et al. Metabolic adaptation to tissue iron overload confers tolerance to malaria. Cell Host & Microbe. 2012;**15**(5): 693-704. DOI: 10.1016/j.chom.2012.10.011

[104] Silverman MN, Sternberg EM. Glucocorticoid regulation of inflammation and its functional correlates: From HPA axis to glucocorticoid receptor dysfunction. Annals of the New York Academy of Sciences. 2012;**1261**:55-63

[105] Oakley RH, Cidlowski JA. The biology of the glucocorticoid receptor: New signaling mechanisms in health and disease. The Journal of Allergy and Clinical Immunology. 2013;**132**:1033-1044

[106] Cain DW, Cidlowski JA. Immune regulation by glucocorticoids. Nature Reviews. Immunology. 2017;**17**:233-247

[107] Coutinho AE, Chapman KE. The anti-inflammatory and immunosuppressive effects of glucocorticoids, recent developments and mechanistic insights. Molecular and Cellular Endocrinology. 2011;**335**:2-13

[108] Patel R, Williams-Dautovich J, Cummins CL. Minireview: New molecular mediators of glucocorticoid receptor activity in metabolic tissues. Molecular Endocrinology. 2014;**28**:999-1011

[109] Muehlenbein MP, Alger J, Cogswell F, James M, Krogstad D. The reproductive endocrine response to *Plasmodium vivax* infection in Hondurans. The American Journal of Tropical Medicine and Hygiene. 2005;**73**:178-187

[110] van Zon AA, Eling WM, Hermsen CC, Koekkoek AA. Corticosterone regulation of the effecto function of malarial immunity during pregnancy. Infection and Immunity. 1982;**36**:484-491

[111] van Zon A A, Eling W M, Hermsen C C, Van de Wiel T J, and Duives M E. (1983) Malarial immunity in pregnant mice, in relation to total and unbound plasma corticosterone. Bulletin de la Société de pathologie exotique et de ses filiales 76:493-502

[112] van Zon AA, Eling WM, Schetters TP, Hermsen CC. ACTH-dependent modulation of malaria immunity in mice. Parasite Immunology. 1985;7:107-117

[113] Herms V, Baumgart E, Kretschmar W. Effects of adrenalectomy and cortisone treatment on the course of malaria (*Plasmodium berghei*) in NMRI mice. Zeitschrift für Tropenmedizin und Parasitologie. 1968;**19**:389-400

[114] Cryer PE. Hypoglycemia, functional brain failure, and brain death. The Journal of Clinical Investigation;**117**:868-870

[115] Mavondo GA, Mkhwananzi BN, Mabandla MV, Musabayane CT. Asiatic acid influences glucose homeostasis in *P. berghei* murine malaria infected Sprague-Dawley rats. African Journal of Traditional, Complementary, and Alternative Medicines. 2016;**13**(5):91-101

[116] Idro R, Jenkins NE, Newton CR. Pathogenesis, clinical features, and neurological outcome of cerebral malaria. The Lancet Neurology. 2005;**4**(12):827-840

[117] Idro R, Marsh K, John CC, Newton CR. Cerebral malaria: Mechanisms of brain injury and strategies for improved neurocognitive outcome. Pediatric Research. 2010;**68**(4):267

[118] Berendt A, Tumer G, Newbold C. Cerebral malaria: The sequestration hypothesis. Parasitology Today. 1994;**10**(10):412-414

[119] Patnaik JK, Das BS, Mishra SK, Mohanty S, Satpathy SK, Mohanty D. Vascular clogging, mononuclear cell margination, and enhanced vascular permeability in the pathogenesis of human cerebral malaria. The American Journal of Tropical Medicine and Hygiene. 1994;**51**(5):642-647

[120] Grau GE, Mackenzie CD, Carr RA, Redard M, Pizzolato G, Allasia C, et al. Platelet accumulation in brain microvessels in fatal pediatric cerebral malaria. The Journal of Infectious Diseases. 2003;**187**(3):461-466

[121] Anstey NM, Russell B, Yeo TW, Price RN. The pathophysiology of vivax malaria. Trends in Parasitology. 2009;**25**(5):220-227

[122] Dunst J, Kamena F, Matuschewski K. Cytokines and chemokines in cerebral malaria pathogenesis. Frontiers in Cellular and Infection Microbiology. 2017;7:324

[123] Medana IM, Turner GD. Human cerebral malaria and the blood–brain barrier. International Journal for Parasitology. 2006;**36**(5):555-568

[124] Barker KR, Lu Z, Kim H, Zheng Y, Chen J, Conroy AL, et al. miR-155 modifies inflammation, endothelial activation and blood-brain barrier dysfunction in cerebral malaria. Molecular Medicine. 2017;**23**(1):24-33

[125] Lopez-Ramirez MA, Wu D, Pryce G, Simpson JE, Reijerkerk A, King-Robson J, et al. Micro RNA-155 negatively affects blood–brain barrier function during neuroinflammation. The FASEB Journal. 2014;**28**(6):2551-2565

[126] Brown H, Rogerson S, Taylor T, Tembo M, Mwenechanya J, Molyneux M, et al. Blood-brain barrier function in cerebral malaria in Malawian children. The American Journal of Tropical Medicine and Hygiene. 2001;**64**(3):207-213

[127] Pickering M, Cumiskey D, O'connor JJ. Actions of TNF-α on glutamatergic synaptic transmission in the central nervous system. Experimental Physiology. 2005;**90**(5):663-670

[128] Cunningham A, Murray C, O'neill L, Lynch M, O'connor J. Interleukin-1β (IL-1β) and tumour necrosis factor (TNF) inhibit long-term potentiation in the rat dentate gyrus in vitro. Neuroscience Letters. 1996;**203**(1):17-20

[129] Crowley VM, Ayi K, Lu Z, Liby KT, Sporn M, Kain KC. Synthetic oleanane triterpenoids enhance blood brain barrier integrity and improve survival in experimental cerebral malaria. Malaria Journal. 2017;**16**(1):463. DOI: 10.1186/s12936-017-2109-0

[130] Ho M, Sexton MM, Tongtawe P, Looareesuwan S, Suntharasamai P, Webster HK. Interleukin-10 inhibits tumor necrosis factor production but not antigen-specific lymphoproliferation in acute *Plasmodium falciparum* malaria. The Journal of Infectious Diseases. 1995;**172**(3):838-844. DOI: 10.1093/infdis/172.3.838

[131] National Center for Biotechnology Information. Ursolic acid, CID=64945, PubChem Database. Available from: https://pubchem.ncbi.nlm.nih.gov/compound/Ursolic-acid

[132] Marquez Martin A, de la Puerta Vazquez R, Fernandez-Arche A, Ruiz-Gutierrez V. Supressive effect of maslinic acid from pomace olive oil on oxidative stress and cytokine production in stimulated murine macrophages. Free Radical Research. 2006;**40**(3):295-302. DOI: 10.1080/10715760500467935

[133] Moneriz C, Marin-Garcia P, Garcia-Granados A, Bautista JM, Diez A, Puyet A. Parasitostatic effect of maslinic acid. I. Growth arrest of *Plasmodium falciparum* intraerythrocytic stages. Malaria Journal. 2011;**10**:82. DOI: 10.1186/1475-2875-10-82

[134] National Center for Biotechnology Information. Maslinic acid, CID=73659, PubChem Database. Available from: https://pubchem.ncbi.nlm.nih.gov/compound/Maslinic-acid

[135] Tsai SJ, Yin MC. Antioxidative and anti-inflammatory protection of oleanolic acid and ursolic acid in PC12 cells. Journal of Food Science. 2008;**73**(7):H174-H178. DOI: 10.1111/j.1750-3841.2008.00864.x

[136] Zeng G, Chen J, Liang QH, You WH, Wu HJ, Xiong XG. Ursolic acid inhibits T-cell activation through modulating nuclear factor-kappa B signaling. Chinese Journal of Integrative Medicine. 2012;**18**(1):34-39. DOI: 10.1007/s11655-011-0858-0

[137] Sibiya H, Musabayane CT, Mabandla MV. Transdermal delivery of oleanolic acid attenuates pro-inflammatory cytokine release and ameliorates anaemia in *P. berghei* malaria. Acta Tropica. 2017;**171**:24-29. DOI: 10.1016/j.actatropica.2017.03.005

[138] Bellik Y, Boukraâ L, Alzahrani HA, Bakhotmah BA, Abdellah F, Hammoudi SM, et al. Molecular mechanism underlying anti-inflammatory and anti-allergic activities of phytochemicals: An update. Molecules. 2013;**18**:322-353. DOI: 10.3390/molecules18010322

[139] Evans AG, Wellems T. Coevolutionary genetics of *Plasmodium* malaria parasites and their human hosts. Integrative and Comparative Biology. 2002;**42**:401-407

[140] Calixto JB, Otuki MF, Santos Adair RS. Anti-inflammatory compounds of plant origin. Part I. Action on arachidonic acid pathway, nitric oxide and nuclear factor κB (NF-κB). Planta Medica. 2003;**69**:973-983

[141] Gautam R, Jachak SM. Recent developments in anti-infammatory natural products. Medicinal Research Reviews. 2009;**29**:767-820

[142] Rockett KA, Awburn MM, Aggarwal BB, Cowden WB, Clark IA. In vivo induction of nitrite and nitrate by tumor necrosis factor, lymphotoxin, and interleukin-1-possible roles in malaria. Infection and Immunity. 1992;**60**:3725-3730

[143] Schofield L, Novakovic S, Gerold P, Schwarz RT, Mcconville MJ, Tachado SD. Glycosylphosphatidylinositol toxin of *Plasmodium* up-regulates intercellular adhesion molecule-1, vascular cell adhesion molecule-1, e-selectin expression in vascular endothelial cells, increases leukocyte and parasite cytoadherence via tyrosine kinase-dependent signal transduction. Journal of Immunology. 1996;**156**:1886-1896

[144] Clark IA, Chaudhri G. Tumour necrosis factor may contribute to the anaemia of malaria by causing dyserythropoiesis and erythrophagocytosis. British Journal of Haematology. 1988;**70**:99-103

[145] Peetre C, Gullberg U, Nilsson E, Olsson I. Effects of recombinant tumor necrosis factor on proliferation and differentiation of leukemic and normal hemopoietic cells in vitro. The Journal of Clinical Investigation. 1986;**78**:1694-1700

[146] Guo W, Liu W, Hong S, Liu H, Qian C, Shen Y, et al. Mitochondria-dependent apoptosis of Con A-activated T lymphocytes induced by asiatic acid for preventing murine fulminant hepatitis. PLoS One. 2012;7(9):e46018. DOI: 10.1371/journal.pone.0046018

[147] Huang SS, Chiu CS, Chen HJ, Hou WC, Sheu MJ, Lin YC, et al. Antinociceptive activities and the mechanisms of anti-inflammation of asiatic acid in mice. Evidence-based Complementary and Alternative Medicine. 2011;**2011**:895857

[148] Karin M, Ben-Neriah Y. Phosphorylation meets ubiquitination: The control of NF-κB activity. Annual Review of Immunology. 2000;**18**:621-663

[149] Baker RG, Hayden MS, Ghosh S. NF-kB, inflammation, and metabolic disease. Cell Metabolism. 2011;**15**:11-22

[150] Cao W, Li X-Q, Zhang X-N, Hou Y, Zeng A-G, Xie Y-h, et al. Madecassoside suppresses LPS-induced TNF-α production in cardiomyocytes through inhibition of ERK, p38, and NF-κB activity. International Immunopharmacology. 2010;**10**:723-729

[151] Hogg N. Free radicals in disease. Seminars in Reproductive Endocrinology. 1998;**16**(4):241-248

[152] Musfiroh I, Muhtadi NA, KartasasmitaRE,DaryonoHT,IbrahimS.In silico study of asiatic acid interaction with inducible nitric oxide synthase (iNOS) and cyclooxygenase (COX-2). International Journal of Pharmacy and Pharmaceutical Sciences. 2013;**5**(1):204-207

[153] Kartasasmitaa RE, Musfiroha I, Muhtadib A, Ibrahima S. Binding affinity of asiatic acid derivatives design against inducible nitric oxide synthase and ADMET prediction. Journal Applied Pharmaceutical Science. 2014;**4**(02):075-080. DOI: 10.7324/JAPS.2014.40213

[154] Lee SK, Lee IH, Kim HJ, Chang GS, Chung JE. The PreADME Approach: Web-based Program for Rapid Prediction of Physico-Chemical, Drug Absorption and Drug-Like Properties. Massachusetts: Blackwell Publishing; 2003. pp. 418-420

[155] Yoshikawa T, Naito Y. The role of neutrophils and inflammation in gastric mucosal injury. Free Radical Research. 2000;**33**(6):785-794

[156] Jain K, Sood S, Gowthamarajan K. Modulation of cerebral malaria by curcumin as an adjunctive therapy. The Brazilian Journal of Infectious Diseases. 2013;**17**(5):579-591. DOI: 10.1016/j.bjid.2013.03.004

[157] Serghides L, Kain KC. Peroxisome proliferator-activated receptor gamma-retinoid X receptor agonists increase CD36-dependent phagocytosis of *Plasmodium falciparum*-parasitized erythrocytes and decrease malaria induced TNF-alpha secretion by monocytes/macrophages. Journal of Immunology. 2001;**166**:6742-6748

Chapter 4

Clinical and Immuno-Pathology Aspects of Canine Demodicosis

Valéria Régia F. Sousa, Naiani D. Gasparetto
and Arleana B.P.F. Almeida

Abstract

Canine demodicosis is a common and often severe dermatopathy of dogs. It is caused mainly by *Demodex canis*, a parasitic mite of the skin of dogs of the genus *Demodex*, of the order *Acarina* and family *Demodecidae*. This study is aimed to review the clinical-pathological presentation of canine demodicosis and the cytokine-mediated immune response to the cutaneous density of the mite. Only dogs with a defective immune response will present the disease, whether localised or generalised. Microscopically, the dermal inflammatory response is similar among dogs. Localised and generalised demodicosis and pyoderma associated with a high cutaneous density of mites are factors associated with aggravation of lesions in both forms of disease presentation. In addition, the participation of cytokines has been investigated in the induction of the immune response in the different forms of the disease. Although different research groups have invested in studies aimed at elucidating the canine demodicosis pathogenesis, there is still insufficient data to understand the important role of the host immune system in triggering clinical signs and the reproductive management is still an effective preventive method for disease perpetuation.

Keywords: *Demodex canis*, parasite-host interaction, generalised demodicosis, localised demodicosis, dog

1. Introduction

Canine demodicosis is an inflammatory disease caused by a species of the genus *Demodex* frequently diagnosed in veterinary clinical routine [1–3] and is considered the most prevalent parasitic dermatopathy [4]. The genus *Demodex* belongs to the order *Acarina*, family Demodecidae, and *Demodex canis* is the species of greatest occurrence in dogs [5]. This relationship is considered commensal. The mites embed themselves in hair follicles, sebaceous ducts, and sebaceous glands, where they feed on cells, sebaceous material and epidermal debris [4, 6].

The clinical presentation of demodicosis occurs according to the extent of the affected area and may manifest in localised or generalised forms. These forms also differ among themselves in terms of disease progression, prognosis and therapeutic measures adopted [7].

IntechOpen

Peri-folliculitis, mural folliculitis and furunculosis are histopathological findings observed, with demodicosis in both clinical forms of the disease due to the action of the mite inside the hair follicles [8]. However, the severity of the lesions may vary depending on the presence and extent of secondary bacterial infection, characterised by pyoderma [9, 10].

Until now, it has not been fully understood why *D. canis*, a mite that is proven to be present in the canine skin [6], triggers demodicosis. In addition, the fact that some dogs develop the most severe form of the disease while others limit themselves to localised lesions only is still being elucidated.

Several factors such as genetic, structural and biochemical alterations of the skin, immunological disorders, hormonal status, race, age, fur length, endoparasitism, and debilitating disease have been considered as predisposing to the disease [11]. In addition, it is possible for mites to induce local immunosuppression, stimulating the onset of their proliferation [12]. Despite the multifactorial nature, studies suggest the dysfunctions of patients with clinical disease may be directly associated with the pathogenesis of demodicosis [7, 13–15].

The number of parasites in dogs seems to be lower in relation to humans [16]. This is likely because they are distributed throughout the fur and not concentrated in certain areas, as in the human face [6, 17]. Regarding the clinical manifestations of canine demodicosis, the number of mites on the skin of dogs determines the occurrence of clinical signs, but does not define the severity of the lesions [16].

A number of studies involving the immunopathogenic mechanisms of demodicosis have been performed and although there is no evidence of any abnormalities related to nonspecific or humoral immunity, functional immunodeficiency was observed in T lymphocytes [7, 18]. Furthermore, the role of proinflammatory and immunosuppressive cytokines in modulating the immune response of demodicosis has been investigated and the results demonstrate the active participation of these proteins in recruitment and activation, as well as the suppression, of host immune system cells [11, 19–26].

This study reviews the morphophylogenetic characterisation of the *Demodex canis* mite, discusses the clinical and pathological features that appear in dogs with demodicosis in order to understand the effects of the action of *D. canis* on the skin of dogs with localised and generalised demodicosis, as well as discusses the participation of the immune system, especially cytokine activity, in the development of clinical disease.

2. Methodological procedure

For understanding the main hypotheses related to the development of canine demodicosis, classical and modern data on the pathogenesis of the disease were gathered through systematic review. The articles were obtained from bibliographic databases. We were preferred to search for free terms, without the use of controlled vocabulary, to guarantee the recovery of most published works within the area of interest. Original articles related to mite Epidemiology, Morphology, Physiology and Pathogenesis; and Immunology, Clinical, Pathology and Genetics of sick dog were used to support this approach. Separate terms have been disregarded because they are not the purpose of the review. In addition, book chapters related to parasitological dermatopathies were used.

3. Morphophylogenetic characterisation of *Demodex canis*

Demodex canis [27], genus *Demodex*, order *Acarina*, family *Demodecidae*, is a mite described as inhabiting commensal in hair follicles, sebaceous ducts and sebaceous glands of dogs, found in small amounts in healthy animals [28, 29]. According to Scott et al. [7], the transmission of this mite occurs by direct contact of the mother with the neonates during the first 3 days of breast-feeding.

In its life cycle, the mite *D. canis* presents as an egg, larvae, protonymph, nymph, and adult (male and female), where all stages of the life cycle can be found in microscopic analysis of skin scalings [7, 28, 30]. The eggs in fusiform (length 81.5 ± 3.5 µm) hatch into small larvae (length 91 ± 5.9 µm) with three pairs of paws, next protonymphs (length of 130.7 ± 10.7 µm), then nymphs (length of 201.2 ± 21.9 µm) [30] and finally evolve into adult mites with four pairs of legs, which commonly measure from 40 to 300 µm [7].

In general, *Demodex* mites are described as small, with elongated bodies, having four pairs of legs. The body is separated into three distinct tagma: the gnathosoma, the small anterior segment with a trapezoidal or rectangular shape, containing mouth parts; the podosoma, which contains reduced and slightly projected legs beyond the podosoma line; and the opisthosoma, the posterior segment, elongated and formed by cuticular striae [31] (**Figure 1**). The morpho-biological characteristics of the adult mite *D. canis* are similar in several studies.

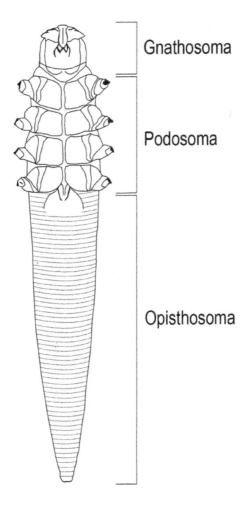

Figure 1.
Morphology of Demodex canis.

Tagmas	Nutting e Desch [30]	Tamuri et al. [32]	Izdebska e Fryderyk [31]	Rojas et al. [33]	Sivajothi et al. [34]
Gnathosoma (µm)	24	18.9	26.9	26.27	18.89
Podosoma (µm)	63.9	94.11	63.8	64.69	60.98
Opisthosoma (µm)	135.9	136.6	116.5	134.31	129.68
Total body lenght (µm)	224.3	229.7	195.2	224.80	214.32

Table 1.
Biometric means Demodex canis found in the literature.

Table 1 describes the biometric measurements of *D. canis* mite segments as described in the literature [30–34].

Although the *D. canis* mite is the most common species [7, 31, 35], two new species, *D. injai* [36] and *D.* sp. *cornei* [37–40], have also been documented causing dermatological alterations in dogs.

Rojas et al. [33], comparing the three species described in dogs, revealed inter-related but distinct populations in which *D. canis* presented with elongated opist-hosoma (ratio opisthosoma length/total length 0.59), and an absence of a band-like segmental plate between the fourth coxisternal plate and opisthosoma. *D. injai* presented opisthosoma comprising 70% of the total length (ratio 0.70) and *D.* sp. *cornei* presented with a segmental plate, nearly rectangular (ratio 0.47), between the fourth coxisternal plate and opisthosoma.

In addition to the morphobiometric characteristics, Rojas et al. [33], using molecular markers of mitochondrial DNA, 16S rDNA, and cytochrome oxidase I genes, suggested that these three species could be polymorphisms of the same species. However, Sastre et al. [41] in the sequencing analysis of 16S rDNA demonstrated that *D. canis* and *D. injai* present a genetic distance of 23.3%, therefore are different species, while *D.* sp. *cornei* is likely a variant of *D. canis*.

Although *D. canis* is a common commensal mite, Fondati et al. [29] in a microscopic analysis of the presence of *D. canis* in healthy dogs, emphasised that the presence of *D. canis* in the skin should not be considered as normal. However, Ravera et al. [6] using real time PCR demonstrated that mite DNA was present in all examined dogs, regardless of age, sex, breed, coat or clinical status, albeit in smaller numbers in healthy dogs. Regardless, the positivity increased when a greater number of areas were analysed. A similar result was observed by Gasparetto et al. [16], detecting a higher number of mites in dogs with clinical demodicosis (6.2 × 10^4 copies/µl of the parasite in the generalised form and 1.2 × 10^4 copies/µl in the localised form) compared to healthy dogs, (8.7 × 10^2 copies/µl of the parasite) using the same technique.

4. Pathological clinical aspects of canine demodicosis

Clinical changes in demodicosis may be induced by the excessive proliferation of mites associated with weakness in the immune system, or induced by the mites themselves [14, 17, 42]. Variables such as breed, age, nutrition, oestrus, pregnancy, stress, endoparasitism and debilitating diseases are predisposing factors for the disease. Purebred dogs appear to be more predisposed. Based on the autosomal recessive inheritance hypothesis, this would lead to immune dysfunction [15, 43].

Bowden et al. [44] found that dogs of the American pit bull and West Highland White Terrier breeds and those with allergic diseases were more predisposed to demodicosis. Likewise, Gasparetto et al. [8] verified that dogs with a defined breed were the most affected.

Regarding classification, demodicosis can be divided according to age of onset of clinical signs (juvenile or adult), or the extent of lesions (localised or generalised), though there is no consensus on the criteria [15]. Kumari et al. [26] suggest classifying as generalised demodicosis when there are lesions on more than 50% of the body surface with the involvement of two or more limbs, and classifying as localised demodicosis when there are alopecia, erythematous and desquamative lesions with hyperpigmentation on the face and one thoracic limb. Other authors have suggested that cases in which there are four or fewer lesions (with a diameter less than 2.5 cm), including a maximum of one focal lesion on any limb, be classified as localised demodicosis and cases with extensive multiple limb lesions, be classified as generalised demodicosis [44–46].

In a retrospective study investigating demodicosis in an US region, dogs with juvenile onset of lesions had a mean age of 7.6 months, having a predominance of the generalised form (74.2%). Dogs with adult onset (over 48 months) of demodicosis were also more likely classified as generalised, with 87.1% of the cases [44]. In Brazil, a study involving 46 dogs, 24 males and 22 females showed generalised demodicosis (60.9%) was more common than localised (39.1%) with a mean age of onset of 23 months [8].

Dogs that develop lesions such as alopecia or erythema as juveniles, are not usually pruritic, have spontaneous remission of clinical signs, and progression to the generalised form is rare. Only in cases of external earwax associated with localised demodicosis, a rare form of the disease, will dogs require therapy [15].

Unlike the localised disease, the generalised form of demodicosis can reach serious proportions and clinical signs such as alopecia, desquamation and erythema (**Figure 2**) are particularly intense [8]. Secondary bacterial infection is often due to the proliferation of opportunistic microorganisms, mainly *Staphylococcus pseudintermedius* and *Pseudomonas* [47, 48], which progress from superficial folliculitis to severe cases of furunculosis and cellulitis [7, 10, 49]. Gasparetto et al. [8] observed pyoderma in 95.5% of dogs with generalised demodicosis and half presented with pruritus, indicating bacterial pyoderma and an immunological reaction against *Demodex* [9, 50]. In more severe cases, lymphadenopathy, fever, anorexia and lethargy associated with secondary bacterial infection may occur [51, 52]. Pododemodicosis, which affects the interdigital, palmar and/or plantar regions, has a poor prognosis. It manifests with severe erythema, oedema and fistulous tracts that cause intense localised pain, requiring prolonged periods of treatment [10, 15, 49].

In histopathological examination, mites are frequently observed in hair follicles that induce folliculitis, peri-folliculitis and furunculosis, as well as sebaceous gland hyperplasia [53]. According to Gasparetto et al. [8], hyperkeratosis was the most frequent epidermal alteration with either form of demodicosis. Mild to moderate interstitial and perivascular exudate containing lymphocytes, plasma cells and macrophages. Dogs with generalised demodicosis and pyoderma had lymphocytes, macrophages and plasma cells associated with the neutrophilic exudate. In chronic cases of generalised demodicosis, follicular hyperkeratosis predominates, and mononuclear inflammation of sudoriferous glands and sebaceous glands is present [9, 10].

Peri-folliculitis occurs in the early stage of the inflammatory process evidenced by the presence of macrophages and lymphocytes around the hair [7]. This finding is apparent both in dogs with the localised disease and in those with more severe

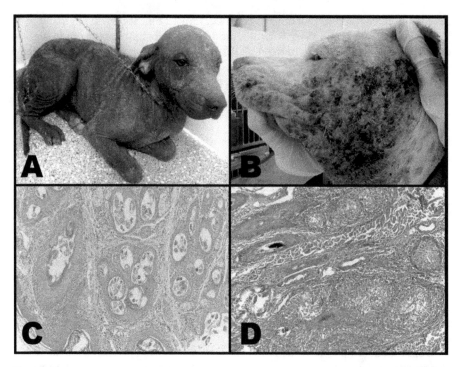

Figure 2.
(A) Generalised demodicosis in dog with cutaneous hyperpigmentation, alopecia and desquamation.
(B) Pyoderma and generalised demodicosis in facial region of dog. (C) Demodex in the interior of the hair
follicles and folliculitis. H&E, 10×. (D) Furunculosis. H&E, 10×.

clinical lesions [8]. As the disease progresses, mural folliculitis occurs due to the infiltration of lymphocytes and histiocytes into the follicular wall, causing injury to follicular keratinocytes. Hydropic degeneration, follicular keratinocyte apoptosis and follicular exocytosis occurs [9, 50]. Mural folliculitis, which has been reported most frequently in dogs with the localised disease [8], is observed to be a consistent and an important lesion pattern of active demodicosis. The histological lesion generated is often associated with diseases in which immune response is recognised as important in its pathogenesis [10, 50, 54, 55].

Finally, multiplication of *Demodex* in the interior of the hair follicles induces follicle dilation causing rupture and releasing mites into the dermal interstitium [10]. The observation of mural folliculitis and multifocal pyogranulomatous furunculosis more frequently in dogs with localised demodicosis indicates that the histological stages of follicular inflammation may have similar severity in the different clinical forms of the disease [8].

5. Host-Parasite Interaction, *Demodex canis versus* dog

Because they are natural inhabitants of the skin of mammals, mites of the genus *Demodex* usually do not generate adverse reactions to the host due to the capacity of the animal's immune system [6, 11, 17, 26, 56]. This is due to the recognition of mite chitin by host keratinocytes through their toll-like receptors (TLR), specifically TLR2, triggering an innate immune response. In addition, studies report that the immune systems of healthy dogs are especially effective at detecting the lipases and proteases secreted by *Demodex* mite, possibly stimulating the adaptive immune response, which is more specific and effective for the control of the *Demodex* mite [17, 57].

The reason for the progressive evolution of the disease in some dogs has not been completely elucidated. The most accepted hypothesis is that immune system dysfunctions play an important role in the manifestation of clinical signs of the disease in its different forms [7, 11, 13–15]. The proposition that the host immune system is the main mediator in the overpopulation of *Demodex* is sustained by the occurrence of the disease in patients who have undergone prolonged treatments with immunosuppressive drugs, in addition to clinical signs in immunodeficient mice, as well as in people and animals with chronic degenerative diseases [17, 56, 57]. However, studies in dogs indicate that immunosuppression occurs at various times in the course of the disease and may be induced by the action of the mite itself on the hair follicles and/ or sebaceous glands and not as a primary trigger for parasitic proliferation [14, 17, 32, 42, 57]. This explains why not all immunosuppressed dogs develop clinical demodicosis and indicates that the manifestation of the disease may involve more than one factor.

Unlike humans, there is little evidence of humoral immune response being involved in canine demodicosis and although Ravera et al. [58] have shown the existence of immunoglobulin (Ig) G against *D. canis* with generalised juvenile demodicosis, the real meaning of this response remains unclear. On the other hand, dogs with generalised demodicosis tend to present functional immunodeficiency in T lymphocytes [7, 18]. Many of the studies indicate that the main mechanism of *Demodex* population control is cell mediated. When mite proliferation occurs, it is probable that there is impaired cellular immunity [7, 57].

This immune dysfunction is defined by the exhaustion of T cells. This type of depletion is not uniform and is generally characterised by high levels of suppressor cytokines such as interleukin (IL)-10 and transforming growth factor (TGF)-β, low production of stimulatory interleukins, such as IL-2 and IL-21 and a reduction in circulating CD4+ [17].

Higher serum levels of IL-10 were observed in dogs with relapsing demodicosis, compared to healthy dogs and those with first manifestation. This change culminates in T cell suppression and antigen presentation ability by inhibiting the synthesis of cytokines and helper 1 T cells (Th1) [22].

Lemarié et al. [59] observed a reduction in the expression and in vitro production of IL-2 resulting from a decrease in Th1 cell response and pointed to a functional irregularity of this class of lymphocytes, directly affecting the balance between Th1 and Th2 responses during the course of the disease. The establishment and perpetuation of demodicosis was attributed to suppression of the Th1 response to Th2, resulting in an inflammatory process capable of inducing tissue damage but not eliminating or containing the proliferation of the mite.

The decrease in transcription of cytokines TNF-α and IFN-γ, and the unprecedented increase in IL-5, as evidenced by Tani et al. [20], appears to be due to Th2 lymphocyte overexpression in the presence of *Demodex* [59]. In addition, Yarim et al. [23] and Tani et al. [20] demonstrated an increase in circulating TGF-β concentrations in dogs with generalised disease compared to healthy animals. Elevated TGF-β levels may compromise the regulation of various biological processes, such as tissue homeostasis, angiogenesis, and cell differentiation, especially in cases of chronic disease, allowing the evolution of localised to generalised demodicosis [56].

Considering that most of these previously described changes were observed in dogs with generalised demodicosis, a recent study investigated the serum levels of a selection of proinflammatory cytokines in dogs with localised and generalised demodicosis in order to observe the levels of certain proteins. There was no difference in serum cytokine levels between groups of diseased animals, but IL-6 was significantly higher in dogs with localised disease than in healthy animals. Thus, characterising the nonspecific inflammatory reaction that occurs shortly after tissue injury precedes the acquired immune response in the acute phase of the disease [16].

Moreover, a modern approach supports the involvement of the cholinergic pathway in the immunopathogenesis of canine demodicosis. In addition to acting as a neurotransmitter, acetylcholine (Ach) plays an important role as a mediator in the inflammatory process by inhibiting the release of certain proinflammatory cytokines, without affecting the production of inhibitory cytokines such as IL-10. The increased activity of its indirect biomarker, acetylcholinesterase, in the serum of dogs with demodicosis, has established the overproduction of Ach in diseased dogs, resulting in immunosuppression [26, 56].

Finally, it is known that TLR receptors play an important role in the identification and control of *Demodex* proliferation in the skin of healthy dogs [17]. However, in a recent study involving animals with demodicosis, important changes in the function of these receptors were detected. Kumari et al. [60] showed elevated expression of mononuclear type 2 TLRs (lymphocytes and monocytes), as well as a decrease in the expression of TLR types 4 and 6. These effects were directly attributed to the action of the mites, but it is not yet known how the mite stimulates or decreases the production of TLR receptors in the disease process [12, 60].

6. Conclusion

Although the *D. canis* mite is considered a commensal inhabitant of dog's skin, demodicosis is one of the most frequent parasitic diseases in this species. Clinical signs such as alopecia, desquamation, erythema and crusting are common in dogs with localised and generalised demodicosis and may be aggravated by secondary bacterial infection. Pyoderma produces severe dermal microscopic inflammation; however, the histopathological findings of dogs with localised and generalised disease tend to be similar. In addition, the increase in the parasitic load of mites in the canine tegument induces the clinical disease, but does not define the severity of the lesions, indicating that the predisposing factor for the mite proliferation likely relates to the immunocompetence of the host.

Low production of stimulating cytokines and high levels of suppressor cytokines coupled with reduced numbers of CD4+ lymphocytes are invariably observed in dogs that develop clinical signs of demodicosis, indicating T-cell depletion. However, due to the multifactorial nature of the disease, immunological mechanisms that allow the excessive growth of the parasites in the dog skin is still misunderstood and this limitation in the understanding of the host-mite interaction makes that the impediment of diseased animals reproduction prevail as the main strategy of control until now.

Currently, research groups from different countries have suggested several mechanisms to understand the immunopathogenesis of demodicosis and although the various hypotheses raised are not yet enough to establish the determining cause of clinical disease development, observed together they allow for new hypotheses that may serve as starting points for subsequent studies in the area.

Author details

Valéria Régia F. Sousa*, Naiani D. Gasparetto and Arleana B.P.F. Almeida
Universidade Federal de Mato Grosso, UFMT, Mato Grosso, Brazil

*Address all correspondence to: regia@ufmt.br

IntechOpen

© 2019 The Author(s). Licensee IntechOpen. This chapter is distributed under the terms of the Creative Commons Attribution License (http://creativecommons.org/licenses/by/3.0), which permits unrestricted use, distribution, and reproduction in any medium, provided the original work is properly cited. (cc) BY

References

[1] Sischo WM, Ihrke PJ, Franti CE. Regional distribution of ten common skin diseases in dogs. Journal of the American Veterinary Medical Association. 1989;**195**:752-756

[2] Larsson CE. Dermatoparasitoses de cães e gatos: Patogenia, diagnóstico diferencial e saúde pública. Revista Brasileira de Parasitologia Veterinária. 1995;**4**(2):216-270

[3] Gasparetto ND, Trevisan YPA, Almeida NB, Neves RCSM, Almeida ABPF, Dutra V, et al. Prevalência das doenças de pele não neoplásicas em cães no município de Cuiabá, Mato Grosso. Pesquisa Veterinaria Brasileira. 2013;**33**:359-362

[4] Larsson CE, Lucas R. Tratado de Medicina Externa: Dermatologia Veterinária. 1a. edição ed. São Paulo: Editora Interbook; 2016. p. 888

[5] Foreyt WJ. Veterinary Parasitology Reference Manual. 5a ed. Iowa: Blackwell Publishing; 2001. p. 248

[6] Ravera I, Altet L, Francino O, Sánchez A, Roldán W, Villanueva S, et al. Small *Demodex* populations colonize most parts of the skin of healthy dogs. Veterinary Dermatology. 2013;**24**:168-172

[7] Scott D, Miller W, Griffin C. Parasitic skin diseases. In: Muller & Kirk's: Small Animal Dermatology. 6th ed. Philadelphia: W.B. Saunders; 2001. pp. 423-516

[8] Gasparetto ND, Bezerra KS, Soares LMC, Makino H, Oliveira ACS, Colodel EM, et al. Aspectos clínicos e histológicos da demodicose canina localizada e generalizada. Pesquisa Veterinaria Brasileira. 2018a;**38**(3):496-501

[9] Hargis AM, Ginn PE. The integument. In: McGavin MD, Zacchary JF, editors. Pathologic Basis of Veterinary Disease. 4th ed. Saint Louis: Mosby; 2007. pp. 1107-1261

[10] Gross TL, Ihrke PJ, Walder EJ, Affolter VK. Doenças de pele do cão e do gato: Diagnóstico clínico e histopatológico. 2a. edição ed. São Paulo: Editora Roca; 2009. p. 904

[11] Singh SK, Dimri U. The immuno-pathological conversions of canine demodicosis. Veterinary Parasitology. 2014;**203**:1-5

[12] Akilov O, Mumcuoglu K. Immune response in demodicosis. Journal of the European Academy of Dermatology and Venereology. 2004;**18**:440-444

[13] Healey MC, Gaafar SM. Immunodeficiency in canine demodectic mange I. Experimental production of lesions using antilymphocyte serum. Veterinary Dermatology. 1977;**3**:121-131

[14] Barriga OO, Al-Khalidi NW, Martin S, Wyman M. Evidence of immunosupression by *Demodex canis*. Veterinary Immunology and Immunopathology. 1992;**32**:37-46

[15] Gortel DVM. Updates in canine demodicosis. The Veterinary Clinics of North America. Small Animal Practice. 2006;**36**:229-241

[16] Gasparetto ND, Almeida ABPF, Nakazato L, França EL, França ACH, Fagundes DLG, et al. Density measure-ment of *Demodex canis* by qPCR and analysis of sérum cytokine levels in dogs with different clinical forms of demodicosis. Veterinary Parasitology. 2018b;**257**:1-4

[17] Ferrer L, Ravera I, Silbermayr K. Immunology and pathogenesis of canine demodicosis. Veterinary Dermatology. 2014;**25**:427-e65

[18] Tizard IR. Imunologia Veterinária. 9a. edição ed. São Paulo: Editora Elsevier; 2014. p. 1217

[19] Lemarié SL, Horohov DW. Evaluations of interleukin-2 production and interleukin2 expression in dogs with generalized demodicosis. Veterinary Dermatology. 1996;7:213-129

[20] Tani K, Morimoto M, Hayashi T, Inokuma H, Ohnishi T, Hayashiya S, et al. Evaluation of cytokine messenger RNA expression in peripheral blood mononuclear cells from dogs with canine demodicosis. The Journal of Veterinary Medical Science. 2002;64:513-518

[21] Singh SK, Dimri U, Sharma MC, Sharma B, Saxena M. Determination of CD4+ and CD8+ T cells in the peripheral blood of dogs with demodicosis. Parasitology. 2010;13:1921-1924

[22] Félix AOC, Guiot EG, Stein M, Felix SR, Silva EF, Nobre MO. Comparison of systemic interleukin 10 concentrations in healthy dogs and those suffering from recurring and first time *Demodex canis* infestations. Veterinary Parasitology. 2013;193:312-315

[23] Yarim GF, Yagci BB, Ciftci G. Increased circulating concentrations of PDGF-BB and TGF-β1 in canine generalized demodicosis. Revista de Medicina Veterinaria. 2013;164:13-17

[24] Oliveira CD, Larsson CE, Camargo MM. Longitudinal assessment of T lymphocyte subpopulations during generalized demodicosis in dogs and their relationship with remission. Veterinary Dermatology. 2015;26:18-22

[25] Yarim GF, Yagci BB, Yarim M, Sozmen M, Pekmezci D, Cenesiz S, et al. Serum concentration and skin tissue expression of insulin-like growth factor 2 in canine generalized demodicosis. Veterinary Dermatology. 2015;26(6):421-5, e99

[26] Kumari P, Nigam R, Singh A, Nakade UP, Sharma A, Garg SK, et al. *Demodex canis* regulates cholinergic system mediated immunosuppressive pathways in canine demodicosis. Parasitology. 2017;144(10):1412-1416

[27] Leydig F. About hair follicle mites and itch mite. Arch Nature. 1859;1:338-354

[28] Nutting WB. Hair follicle mites (*Demodex* spp) of medical and veterinary concern. The Cornell Veterinarian. 1976;66:214-231

[29] Fondati A, De Lucia M, Furiani N, Monaco M, Ordeix L, Scarampella F. Prevalence of *Demodex canis*-positive healthy dogs at trichoscopic examination. Veterinary Dermatology. 2010;21:146-151

[30] Nutting WB, Desch CE. *Demodex canis* redescription and reevaluation. The Cornell Veterinarian. 1978;68:139-149

[31] Izdebska JN, Fryderyk S. Diversity of three species of the genus *Demodex* (Acari, Demodecidae) parasiting dogs in Poland. Polish Journal of Environmental Studies. 2011;20(3):565-569

[32] Tamura Y, Kawamura Y, Inoue I, Ishino S. Scanning eléctron microscopy description of a new species of *Demodex canis* spp. Veterinary Dermatology. 2001;12:275-278

[33] Rojas M, Riazzo C, Callejón R, Guevara D, Cutillas C. Molecular study on three morphotypes of *Demodex* mites (Acarina: Demodicidae) from dogs. Parasitology Research. 2012;111:2165-2172

[34] Sivajothi S, Sudhakara Reddy B, Rayulu VC. Demodicosis caused by *Demodex canis* and *Demodex cornei*

in dogs. Journal of Parasitic Diseases. 2015;**39**(4):673-676

[35] Pekmezci GZ, Pekmezci D, Bolukbas CS. Molecular characterization of *Demodex canis* (Acarina: Demodicidae) in domestic dogs (*Canis familiaris*). Kocatepe Veterinary Journal. 2018;**11**(4):430-433

[36] Desch CE, Hillier A. *Demodex injai*: A new species of hair follicle mite (Acari: Demodecidae) from the domestic dog (Canidae). Journal of Medical Entomology. 2003;**40**(2):146-149

[37] Scarff D. Morphological differences in *Demodex* spp. In: Proceedings of the Fifth Annual Congress of the European Society of Veterinary Dermatology. London: ECVD–ESVD; 1988. p. 23

[38] Mason KV. A New Species of Demodex Mite with *D. canis* Causing Canine Demodecosis: A Case Report. San Diego: Annual Member's Meeting of the American Academy of Veterinary Dermatology and the American College of Veterinary Dermatology; 1993. p. 92

[39] Chesney CJ. Short form of *Demodex* species mite in the dog: Occurrence and measurements. The Journal of Small Animal Practice. 1999;**40**:58-61

[40] Saridomichelakis MA, Koutinas E, Papadogiannakis M, Papazachariadou M, Llapitrakas D. Adult-onset demodicosis in two dogs due to *Demodex canis* and a short-tailed demodectic mite. The Journal of Small Animal Practice. 1999;**40**:529-532

[41] Sastre N, Ravera I, Villanueva S, Altet L, Bardagí M, Sánchez A, et al. Phylogenetic relationships in three species of canine *Demodex* mite based on partial sequences of mitochondrial 16S rDNA. Veterinary Dermatology. 2012;**23**:509-e101

[42] Delayte EH, Otsuka M, Larsson CE, Castro RCC. Eficácia das lactonas macrocíclicas sistêmicas (ivermectina e moxidectina) na terapia da demodicidose canina generalizada. Arquivo Brasileiro de Medicina Veterinária e Zootecnia. 2006;**58**:31-38

[43] Muller GH, Kirk RW, Scott DW. Parasitic skin diseases. In: Ibid, editor. Muller & Kirk's Small Animal Dermatology. 6th ed. Philadelphia: W.B. Saunders, PA; 2001. pp. 457-474

[44] Bowden DG, Outerbridge CA, Kissel MB, Baron JN, White SD. Canine demodicosis: A retrospective study of a veterinary hospital population in California, USA (2000-2016). Veterinary Dermatology. 2018;**29**(1):19-e10

[45] Muller WH, Griffi CE, Campbell KL. Small Animal Dermatology. Muller and Kirk's. St. Louis: Elsevier; 2013. pp. 304-313

[46] Mueller RS, Bensignor E, Ferrer L, Holm B, Lemarie S, Paradis M, et al. Treatment of demodicosis in dogs: 2011 clinical practice guidelines. Veterinary Dermatology. 2012;**23**(2):86-96

[47] Wilkinson GT, Harvey RG. Doença parasitária: Demodicose. In: Ibid, editor. Atlas Colorido de Dermatologia dos Pequenos Animais: Guia para o diagnóstico. 2a edição ed. Editora Manole: São Paulo; 1998. pp. 73-79

[48] Herni JA, Boucher JF, Skogerboe TL, Tarnacki S, Gajewski KD, Lindeman CJ. Comparison of efficacy of cefpodoxime proxetil and cephalexin in treating bacterial pyoderma in dogs. International Journal of Applied Research in Veterinary Medicine. 2006;**4**:85-93

[49] Santarém V. Demodicose canina: Revisão. Clínica Veterinária. 2007;**69**:86-96

[50] Caswell JL, Yager JA, Parker WM, Moore PF. A prospective study of the immunophenotype and temporal changes in the histologic lesions of canine demodicosis. Veterinary Pathology. 1997;**34**(4):279-287

[51] Quinn PJ, Donnely WJC, Carter ME, Markey BKJ, Torgenson PR, Breathnach RMS. Microbial and Parasitc Diseases of the Dog and Cat. London: W.B. Saunders; 1997. p. 362p

[52] Medleau L, Hnilica KA. Dermatites parasitárias. In: Medleau L, Hnilica KA, editors. Dermatologia de Pequenos Animais. São Paulo: Editora Roca; 2003. pp. 59-88

[53] Sood NK, Mekkib B, Singla LD, Gupta K. Cytopathology of parasitic dermatitis in dogs. Journal of Parasitic Diseases. 2012;**36**(1):73-77

[54] Caswell JL, Yager JA, Ferrer L, Weir MAM. Canine Demodicosis: A reexamination of the histopathologic lesions and description of the immunophenotype of infiltrating cells. Veterinary Dermatology. 1995;**6**(1):9-19

[55] Day M. An Immunohistochemical study of the lesions of demodicosis in the dog. Journal of Comparative Pathology. 1997;**116**(2):203-216

[56] Cen-Cen CJ, Bolio-González ME, Rodríguez-Vivas R. Principales hipótesis inmunológicas de la demodicosis canina. Revista Ciencia y Agricultura. 2018;**15**(2):61-69

[57] Ravera I. Deconstructing canine demodicosis. Tese de Doutorado. Facultade de Medicina Veterinária, Departamento de Medicina e Cirurgia Animal, Universidade Autônoma de Barcelona. 2015

[58] Ravera I, Ferreira D, Gallego LS, Bardagí M, Ferrer L. Serum detection of IgG antibodies against *Demodex canis* by western blot in healthy dogs and dogs with juvenile generalized demodicosis. Research in Veterinary Science. 2015;**101**:161-164

[59] Lemarié SR, Foil CS, Horohov DW. Evaluation of interleukin-2 production and interleukin-2 receptor expression in dogs with generalized demodicosis. Veterinary Dermatology. 1996;7:213-219

[60] Kumari P, Nigam R, Choudhury S, Singh SK, Yadav B, Kumar D, et al. *Demodex canis* targets TLRs to evade host immunity and induce canine demodicosis. Parasite Immunology. 2018;**40**(3):1-5

Protein-Protein Interactions in Malaria: Emerging Arena for Future Chemotherapeutics

Rahul Pasupureddy, Sriram Seshadri, Rajnikant Dixit and Kailash C. Pandey

Abstract

Malaria is one of the most deadly diseases infecting humans. Advances in elimination and vector control have reduced the global malaria burden in the past decade; however, the emerging threat of drug resistance and suboptimal vaccine efficacies threaten global eradication efforts. Unlocking novel drug and vaccine targets while simultaneously mitigating spread of resistant strains seems to be the need of the hour. Protein-protein interactions (PPIs), an integral part of host-pathogen cross-talk and parasite survival, have only recently emerged as promising drug targets. Large PPI networks (interactome) are being developed to better our understanding of various parasite biochemical pathways. In this chapter, we throw light on several newly characterized protein-protein interactions between the host (humans) and parasite (plasmodium) in key processes such as hemoglobin degradation, enzyme regulation, protein export, egress, invasion, and drug resistance and further discuss their viability for development as novel chemotherapeutic targets.

Keywords: malaria, proteases, drug resistance, protein-protein interactions, host-parasite interactions, interactome

1. Introduction

Malaria is one of the deadliest diseases to affect humans, with the latest WHO reports indicating ~445,000 deaths in 2017 alone [1]. More alarmingly, despite decades of advances in controlling the malaria epidemic, death rates caused by malaria seem to have plateaued in the past 3 years, indicating drug resistance and re-emergence. Drug resistance to the current frontline antimalarials have been confirmed by many recent studies and steadily observed over increasing geographic coverage [2]. Thus, it is of utmost importance to develop novel antimalarials, with different modes of action and distinct targets, if possible in conjunction, to check the onslaught of malaria. This chapter looks at such potential scope for antimalarial drug development: disruption of protein-protein interactions in the malaria parasite *Plasmodium*, crucial for survival and proliferation.

2. PPIs: the basics

Protein-protein interactions (PPIs) constitute the fundamental backbone required for occurrence of any biological event. They are defined as the residue level interactions between either the same protein (dimers, trimers, or other multimers) or diverse proteins (protein complexes). These basic interactions are necessary for a myriad of functions such as kinase signaling, receptor binding, proteolytic digestion, apoptosis regulation, and antigen-antibody interactions [3, 4]. Disruptions in the protein interaction networks (PINs) as a result of PPI inhibition have been shown to cause several diseases where either single or multiple biochemical pathways are affected [5]. Owing to their fundamental roles in almost every process imaginable, PPIs have emerged as attractive therapeutic targets in several diseases. Several forms of cancer were also shown to have dysregulated protein interaction networks (PINs) [6]. Similarly, PPI disruptions have been observed in several autoimmune as well as parasitic diseases. Small peptides that infiltrate cellular defenses and specifically bind to target structures are already in development. Taken together, targeting PPIs though challenging can provide a novel understanding of biochemical processes as well as uncover new ways to combat diseases like malaria.

PPIs can be generally categorized into several groups depending on their function or the type of interactions. They include internal (hot-spots) or external (surface), obligate (permanent) or non-obligate (transient), stabilizing or destabilizing, ability to induce conformational changes in either of the partner molecules, peptide-protein or peptide-peptide interactions, and contiguous or discontiguous epitope binding [7] (**Figure 1**).

Some types of PPIs such as membrane PPIs can be difficult to characterize. While dedicated techniques like the split-ubiquitin membrane yeast two-hybrid (MYTH) system were developed to specifically detect membrane protein interactions [8], these techniques are still considered time-consuming and labor-intensive. Such bottlenecks make it hard to generate a complete picture of the membrane interactome. Even for reliable bioinformatic models for detection of membrane

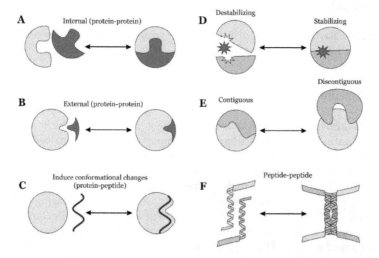

Figure 1.
Categorization of PPIs based on types of interactions. (A) Internal, where the site of interaction lies buried inside such as "hot-spots", (B) external, where proteins interact at the surface, (C) where a peptide could induce conformational changes upon binding, (D) interactions can be stabilized or dissociated based on the type of cofactor/compound binding, (E) whether the epitope binding is contiguous or not, and (F) if both interacting partners are peptides/small molecules.

PPIs to be developed, there need to be large sets of positive, false-positive, as well as negative data to accurately train such models, which are currently unavailable for membrane PPIs [9]. Thus, decoding membrane PPIs even through bioinformatic approaches remains challenging.

3. PPIs in malaria

Malaria traditionally has been treated using inhibitors which target the broad spectrum proteasome offering several advantages as compared to specific protein inhibitors. Specific inhibitors had comparatively low efficacy in vivo. Also, inhibitors targeting a specific protein/ligand could potentially inhibit parasite growth only in stages when the target proteins are expressed. Broad spectrum antimalarials, such as the current frontline drugs artemisinins (ARTs) and their combination therapies (ACTs), target and break down various cellular pathways including but not limited to hemozoin formation, DNA repair, and mitochondria machinery, which make them highly potent within short exposure times [10, 11]. However, exposure to various cellular targets leads to the rapid development of drug resistance. While resistance to chloroquine worldwide was observed after ~40 years of continued use, resistance to ARTs was achieved in a relatively short span of a decade, from its inception in late 1990s to the first reported resistance in 2008 [12]. While this rapid emergence resistance was partially attributed to suboptimal drug regimens and poor administrative practices, the same could be attributed to earlier drugs as well. Thus, compounds that are specific/flexible to the target protein are the need of the hour. This section deals with and summarizes current knowledge about crucial PPIs in various biochemical pathways of the malaria parasite *Plasmodium falciparum*.

3.1 Hemoglobin hydrolysis

Hemoglobin hydrolysis is one of the most targeted pathways for treatment as it is fundamental for parasite survival and involves numerous proteins [13]. Majority of earlier and currently used drugs disrupt multiple protein interactions. Several studies have been conducted recently that target individual PPIs and design inhibitors based on those interactions. Our lab has previously identified a "hot-spot" region in falcipains, the principal hemoglobinases of *P. falciparum* [14]. Falcipains contain a pro and a mature domain, with the pro domain bound to and blocking access to the active site in the mature domain. The interactions between these two domains, termed "hot-spot" interactions, dissociate under acidic conditions and are essential for hemoglobinase activity. This specific hot-spot was identified at the interface of pro and mature domains in falcipain-2 (FP2) and falcipain-3 (FP3). The study further demonstrated that synthetic compounds, NA01 and NA03, specifically bound to this hot-spot region and stabilized these interactions. Thus, even in the presence of an acidic environment (pH - 5.5), pro-mature domains remained intact, rendering them inactive [15].

Falcipains, owing to their crucial role in Hb degradation, are considered as attractive chemotherapeutic targets. Several inhibitors were designed based on the interactions of the FP2 and the active site inhibitor E64. Molecular dynamics (MD) simulations indicated that two sets of residues, namely, recruiter groups A (rgA) and B (rgB) (rgA (D170, Q171, C168, G169, A151, and G230); rgB (K76, N77, and N81)) of FP2 are primarily involved in the initial binding with E64 about 80% and 14% of the time, respectively, before finally proceeding to bind with the active site residues [16]. Efforts elsewhere have focused on selective inhibition of falcipains rather than indiscriminate inhibition including its human host cathepsin isoforms.

While the S1 and S3 subsite residues have been conserved across *Plasmodium* and human cysteine proteases, the P2 residue in the S2 pocket in falcipains contained an acidic amino acid (Asp234 in FP2 and Glu243 in FP3) as compared to neutral residues in cathepsins (Leu209 in Cat-K, Ala215 in Cat-L, and Phe211 in Cat-S). A class of peptidomimetic amino-nitrile compounds known to inhibit cysteine proteases was further engineered to exploit the P2-region charge differences and inhibit falcipains specifically [17, 18].

Falcipains also contain a domain at their C-terminal called the hemoglobin binding domain (Hb domain), a β-hairpin loop which protrudes away from the active site. Deletion of this 14 amino acid domain ablated the ability of falcipains to degrade Hb, thus indicating a necessary role of this domain in Hb capture prior to degradation at the active site [19]. Our lab recently published another study that identified crucial protease-substrate PPIs within this domain. A functionally conserved single amino acid position in both falcipains (Glu185 in FP2 and Asp194 in FP3) was found to be essential for Hb interactions, with activated falcipain mutants unable to degrade Hb even with accessibility to the active site. Molecular docking results indicated both the residues interacted with Hb-α as well as Hb-β subunits with interactions mediated primarily through this position (**Figure 2**). A specific inhibitor which could target this position could have potential applications in arresting the parasite hemoglobin degradome [20].

Hemoglobin degradation as a source for parasite growth was also shown to be dependent on the hemoglobin tetramer composition. Children (<5 years) have different Hb subunits (HbF, $\alpha_2\gamma_2$) as compared to adults (HbA, $\alpha_2\beta_2$), and malaria mortality rates have consistently indicated child mortality to be higher (61% of

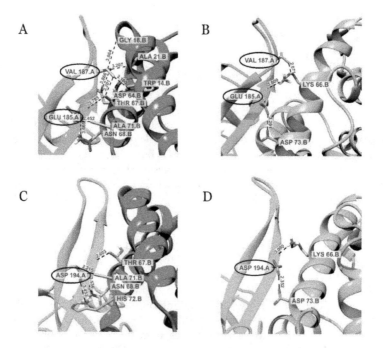

Figure 2.
Interactions of falcipains (FP2, FP3) with Hb (α, β) chains. A residue level interaction map of the interactions between Hb-binding motif of FP2 (green) with Hb α chain (a; red) and Hb β chain (B; orange) of hemoglobin. Similarly, a view of interactions between C-terminus Hb-binding motif of FP3 (blue) with Hb α chain (C; red) and Hb β chain (D; orange). Bond lengths of interactions have been indicated in angstrom units (Å). Adapted and modified from [20].

deaths in 2017) [20]. The essential amino acid isoleucine (I) was found to be a main differentiating factor as it is absent in both α and β chains but present in γ subunit and makes up to 99% of encoded proteins in *P. falciparum* proteome [21]. Thus, compounds that interfered with the isoleucine acquiring pathways, such as targeting the two *P. falciparum* isoleucyl tRNA synthetases (IRSs), have been described. The compound thiaisoleucine, where γ-methylene of isoleucine was substituted by a sulfur atom, was found to potently inhibit cytosolic IRS, while another compound, mupirocin, a known inhibitor of methicillin-resistant *S. aureus* (MRSA) IRS, inhibited the apicoplast-localized IRS [22]. Of the 36 putative aminoacyl tRNA synthetases present in *P. falciparum*, nearly 5 have been targeted with potent inhibitors, and more are being tested [23, 24].

3.2 Invasion/egress

Both invasion and egress are important events in the erythrocytic stage and are responsible for the malaria symptoms including chills and fever. The process of invasion requires a host of proteins to be secreted from its apical organelles including rhoptry bodies and micronemes, among others, and is precisely coordinated. The parasite initially aligns the merozoite apical region toward the host erythrocyte and forms a tight junction at the apex, progressing as the moving junction (MJ) pushes the parasite into the erythrocyte, with the erythrocyte surface forming a ring around the engorged parasite, which would later become the parasitophorous vacuolar membrane (PVM) [25].

While the process of moving junction (MJ) formation and important players involved in the process were well elucidated in *P. falciparum*, the other major causative agent of malaria, *P. vivax*, remains poorly understood, partially owing to difficulties in culturing *P. vivax* in vitro. Recombinant *P. vivax* rhoptry neck protein 2 (PvRON2), based on literature evidence of involvement of PfRON2 in MJ formation and invasion, showed that both rhoptry proteins PvRON2 and PvRON4 bound preferentially to CD71-labeled human reticulocytes rather than normocytes [26]. More importantly, the cysteine-rich C-terminal PvRON2 region strongly interacts with PvAMA1 domains II and III, similar to earlier reports of PfRON2-PfAMA1 interactions [27].

The *P. falciparum* genome encodes 10 aspartic proteases termed plasmepsins, a few of which including PMIX and PMX have remained functionally uncharacterized until recently. Conditional knockdown (KD) using TetR-aptamer regulators inserted at PMIX and PMX loci using CRISPR-Cas9 gene editing tools indicated a drastic decrease in parasite that could egress in PMIX-KD and role of PMX-KD in both invasion and egress. Further, PMX was found to be involved in the processing of a semi-proenzyme PfSUB1 to mature protein, a step crucial in both egress and invasion and also in the final processing step of a known egress protein, SERA5 [28]. Another study was simultaneously published that attempted to inhibit the activity of both PfPMIX and PfPMX. A hydroxyl-ethyl-amine (HEA) scaffold-based compound, 49c, was shown to potently inhibit both the proteases in vitro and in vivo at nanomolar concentrations and reiterated the role of these two proteases in egress and invasion [29]. MD simulations indicated that the flap tip and hinge regions present in both the plasmepsins were very well stabilized by the rigid structure of compound 49c, leading to higher-binding free energy as compared to control plasmepsin inhibitor pepstatin [30].

For a *Plasmodium* parasite to successfully invade different types of cells at different life stages, it must display multiple families of receptor molecules on its surface to perform various functions such as gliding and traversal between hepatocyte cells or other motile functions. To successfully egress from erythrocytes, the parasite expresses a merozoite-thrombospondin-related anonymous protein (MTRAP) which interacts with the tetrameric glycolytic enzyme, fructose-1,6-bisphosphate aldolase, for powering the actomyosin motors required for movement [31]. However, continuous detachment and reattachment of these two enzymes are required for proper gliding motility. Therefore, compounds have been described that specifically stabilize MTRAP-aldolase interactions thereby rendering the parasite immotile. Of the 400 Medicines for Malaria Venture's (MMV) Malaria Box inhibitor library, a single compound (C4) was found to significantly inhibit hepatocyte invasion and led to abnormal gliding movements in a dose-dependent manner. A structure of C4 bound to the TRAP-aldolase complex could provide better insight into the key interactions of the inhibitor and help design more potent compounds [31].

3.3 Protein export

The protein export element (PEXEL) comprising of the conserved sequence RxLxE/Q/D is found in the N-terminus of ~300 proteins bound for export in the *Plasmodium* proteome. The aspartic protease plasmepsin V (PMV) was shown to be the sole protease involved in the cleavage of the PEXEL domain at the ER, specifically cleaving after the leucine residue (RxL$^{\downarrow}$xE/D/Q). The first, third, and fifth conserved positions were thoroughly probed for role in protease activity and showed that the first Arg and third Leu are essential for PMV recognition and cleavage, while the fifth E/Q/D position was shown not to be essential for cleavage but for trafficking out of PVM [32]. Owing to the importance of PMV, peptidomimetic compounds that resembled PEXEL were developed. While statin-based compounds were the traditional inhibitors of aspartic proteases, inhibitors based on HEA moiety were also shown to be strong inhibitors of aspartic proteases. A compound named LG20 consisted of PEXEL-like motif R-L-[L-HEA-A]-E-A, where the L-HEA-A mimics the aspartic protease transition state, while HEA motif is proteolytically uncleavable by PMV. Overall, the compound successfully inhibited PMV activity with concentrations in the picomolar range [33].

PfEMP1 is one the most studied exported protein as it is one of the exported in abundant quantities to the outer surface and thus is an attractive target along with others such as circumsporozoite protein (CSP). Immunoprecipitation (IP) and mass spectrometry studies of a GFP-tagged minimal section of PfEMP1 (PfEMP1B) identified novel targets in different cellular components including parasitophorous vacuole (PV), Maurer's clefts, the plasmodium translocon of exported proteins (PTEX) translocon, and a novel exported protein-interacting complex (EPIC). Several new interacting partners including parasitophorous vacuole protein-1 (PV1), PV2, and exported protein-3 (EXP3) have been identified, all of whom localized to the newly described EPIC [34]. Finally, a comprehensive pathway of PfEMP1 export has been suggested, where PfEMP1 is initially translocated to the ER and then trafficked to PTEX machinery and out of PVM with the aid of EPIC, where finally it is received by host erythrocytic chaperonin complex, the TCP-1 ring complex (TRiC), and transported to erythrocyte surface [34].

IP assays coupled with truncated-construct interaction assays have helped identify few prominent PMV-partner PPIs. The *P. falciparum* ortholog of signal peptidase complex 25 (PfSPC25) was found to interact with PMV as well as PfSec61 and PfSec62 translocon. Together, the PfSPC25-PfSec61-PfSec62 interactome along with PMV was found to regulate the entry of the effector cargo into the ER [35]. Apart from export, protein-protein interactions during autophagy, where different cellular components are engulfed and fused with vacuoles or lysozymes, can be considered as important PPI targets. The *P. falciparum* autophagy-related protein 8 (PfAtg8) upon activation binds to PfAtg3 through a thioester bond, and this complex promotes the membrane assembly for the formation of autophagosomes. Solved crystal structure of the PfAtg3-PfAtg8 complex identified an additional region, called the A-loop, having very low sequence similarity to that of humans, thus providing a new avenue for drug development [36]. MD simulations revealed several crucial PPIs including H-bonds, van der Walls contacts, and other electrostatic interactions that are crucial for their interactions. Crucially, a peptidomimetic compound mimicking the PfAtg3 segment WLLP that interacts with PfAtg8 was identified to achieve maximum potency [37].

3.4 PPIs mediating drug resistance

The emerging threat of resistance to the current frontline drug artemisinin (ART), and its combination therapies (ACTs), is a cause of great concern. The mechanism of ART action, though generally agreed to generate free radical species which disrupt several essential pathways in the parasite, is highly debated. Immunoprecipitation studies with chemically tagged ART analogue (AP1) revealed that ART interacts with over a dozen proteins and is predominantly activated by free heme rather than free ferrous ions. *P. falciparum* Kelch 13 (PfK13) was identified as a key marker of ART resistance in several studies, most notably by Ariey et al., 2008 [38]. The studies have identified residues in the six Kelch propeller domains that are responsible for crucial protein-protein interactions, with the mutants failing to interact with its substrates *P. falciparum* phosphatidylinositol-3-phosphate (PfPI3P) [39]. PfPI3P has been shown to be involved in the unfolded protein response (UPR) pathway, thus helping the parasite cope with the free radical-induced stress (**Figure 3**). Localization studies indicated the PfK13 to co-localize with the *P. falciparum* erythrocyte membrane protein (PfEMP1) and majorly concentrated at various proteostasis system in the parasite including ER, cytoplasm, and the UPR. Specifically, PfK13 mutants were shown to elevate the PI3P-vesicle production and amplification, and their export throughout the parasite and into the infected erythrocyte [40].

Structural analysis and MD simulations of PfK13 indicated the presence of two evolutionarily highly conserved domains in the broad-complex, tramtrack, and bric à brac (BTB) domain and in the shallow binding pocket formed by the six propeller domain repeats. These domains displayed a different electrostatic surface potential unlike the rest of the bottom PfK13 face and are rich in highly conserved arginine and serine residues. While the BTB domain was shown to be involved in the recruitment of a scaffold protein Cullin, the propeller domain pocket binds to the substrate molecules for further ubiquitination. MD simulations showed that the validated PfK13 markers such as C580Y and R539T mutants induced a significant structural destabilization in the shallow pocket region as compared to wild type while maintaining the overall structural integrity. Specifically, the C580Y mutant disrupted a disulfide bridge (C532-C580) and additional H-bonds created with neighboring residues not present in wild type strains. In the case of R539T mutant, it was shown to have substantially less H-bond interactions along with a complete loss of a salt bridge interaction with E606 while also losing another inter-blade H-bond interaction [41]. Overall, these mutants lead to significantly diminished levels of functional protein which cause diminished substrate interaction, ultimately promoting the PfPI3P-mediated unfolded protein response pathway. Our own group, through Co-IP and mass spectrometric studies, has identified several novel proteins including Trx-like mero protein (PF3D7_1104400), pyridoxal kinase (PF3D7_0616000), trafficking protein particle complex subunit 3 (TRAPP), and

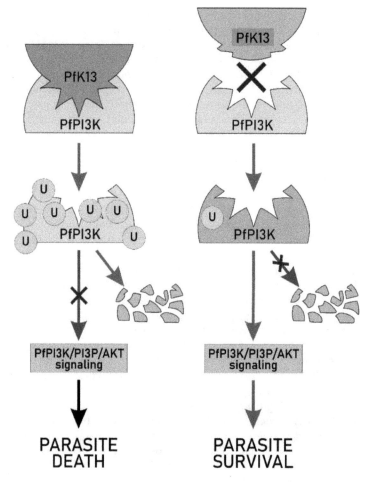

Figure 3.
Role of PfK13 in mediating ART resistance. In the presence of ART, wild PfK13 binds with PfPI3K, which results in PfPI3K ubiquitination and degradation, thus dysregulation of phosphoinositide signaling pathways ultimately leading to parasite death, while in ART-resistant strains, mutated PfK13 does not bind to PfPI3K initiating PI3P signaling thus promoting parasite survival. Adapted and modified from [39].

putative (PF3D7_0418500) that interact with PfK13 and could potentially have a role in stress-mediated response (Atul et al., 2019, unpublished).

4. PPI inhibition: peptidomimetics and design

While several strategies have been employed for PPI inhibition, bioinformatics-based drug design has been at the forefront to design specific PPI inhibitors. Structure-based drug design, where the solved structure of an enzyme in complex either with an inhibitor or a natural substrate was used to design inhibitors, was popularized in the 1990s. However, rational design for PPI inhibitors needs to overcome some common hurdles such as low proteolytic stability, analyzing extensive libraries of candidate molecules, and in some cases low ligand efficiency when compared to standard active site inhibitors. Thus, several strategies are employed in modern drug synthesis to overcome these problems. Short linear peptides tend to have lower conformational stability; thus cyclization of the peptide is preferred which rigidifies the structure in an active configuration. Certain modifications in the backbone of the peptide such as backbone extension, side-chain shifting to nitrogen atoms (peptoids), and altering the stereochemistry can also be applied. Peptoids can easily fold into helices or other structures as they consist of repeated nitrogen-substituted glycine units that give an added advantage of mimicking the peptide structure and function. Stereochemistry of a compound can be changed by using D-peptides instead of L-peptides as they are more susceptible to proteolytic degradation and are one of the most common strategies to develop potent bioactive compounds. Another modification involves using β-peptides; peptides with amino group bound at β-carbon instead of α-carbon for each amino acid, often called as foldamers, could confer additional proteolytic stability both in vitro and in vivo. A class of oligopeptides (<80 residues in length) called as miniproteins can also be utilized as they have a rigid, well-defined three-dimensional structure. The 19 kDa fragment of merozoite surface protein 1 (MSP1), the fragment that is finally displayed on the merozoite surface after several processing steps, was fused along with a glycosylphosphatidylinositol (GPI) tag used to create a miniprotein, which was successfully targeted by antibodies specific to the miniprotein and inhibited erythrocyte invasion [42]. Substantial effort has been made to develop rational strategies in designing PPI inhibitors for target proteins that have no well-defined binding site (so-called "hot-spot") and, thus, have previously been considered undruggable (**Figure 4**).

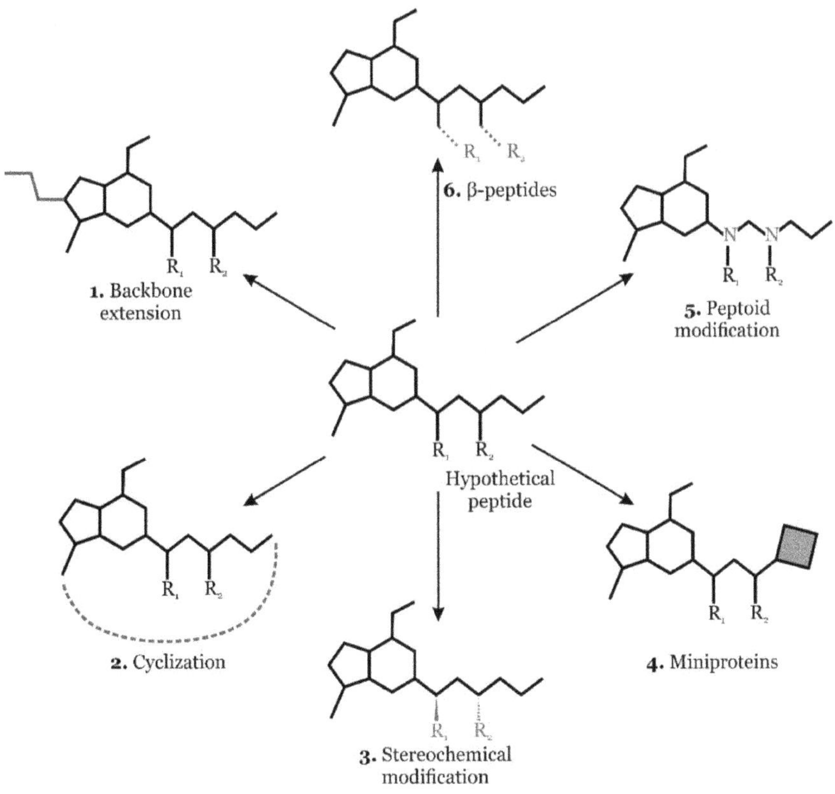

Figure 4.
Strategies for improving the potency of PPI inhibitors. Schematic showing the various ways peptides can be modified (highlighted in red) to achieve potency or improve bioavailability.

As described in the earlier section, Villa et al. designed and synthesized peptidomimetics belonging to 1,2,3-triazoles, specifically 1,4-disubstituted 1,2,3-triazoles. These compounds mimicked the contacts made by PfAtg3 template structure containing the residues W-L-L-P, as this template was shown to have the majority of interactions with PfAtg8. Of the four compounds synthesized, compound 2 (C2) exhibited prominent inhibition (IC$_{50}$–3.8 μM) in vitro, while C1 had better inhibitory effects in vivo [37].

Natural inhibitors of proteases are one of the best studies substrate groups in malaria as they are highly specific, stable, and reversible. *Plasmodium spp.* contain inhibitors of cysteine proteases (ICPs) and endogenous macromolecular inhibitors, which regulate the activity of cysteine proteases. Orthologs of ICPs are also observed in other apicomplexan groups such as *Trypanosoma cruzi*, whose ICP is called as chagasin [43]. Chagasin was shown to potently bind to the active site of both falcipains, FP2 and FP3. More importantly, three loop regions termed BC-, DE-, and FG loops

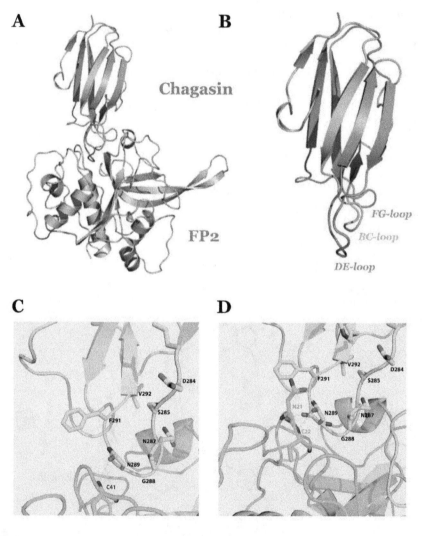

Figure 5.
Crucial interactions between falcipains and ICPs chagasin and falstatin. (A) Solved structure of FP2 and chagasin in that the ICP bound to the active site of falcipain and that (B) three loops BD, DE, and FG are involved in this interactions. (C, D) mutagenesis studies indicated that just the BC loop of falstatin was sufficient for inhibiting both FP2 (C) and FP3 (D), respectively. Adapted and modified from [44, 45].

were shown to be involved in active site inhibition (**Figure 5A,B**) [44]. However, further studies with the *P. falciparum* ICP, falstatin, indicated that unlike other ICPs, just the BC loop was sufficient for falcipain inhibition and that Asn289 of falstatin formed stabilizing hydrogen bonds and hydrophobic interactions (**Figure 5C,D**) [45].

5. Conclusion

Protein-protein interactions play roles of utmost importance in the growth and survival of any organism. Thus, focused targeting of such interactions specific to parasite can help produce robust and effective drugs. Recent research has indicated a renewed interest in targeting PPIs in the field of malaria. Various PPIs in pathways essential for parasite survival, erythrocyte invasion/egress, drug resistance, and others have been elucidated. These new classes of peptidomimetic compounds would form the future defense against an ever-increasing resistant parasite threat. Targeting PPIs offers several advantages over active site inhibition as 'hot-spots' are more flexible as compared to the active site and thus can be more selective in terms of drug interactions. In contrary to active site, the interactions at allosteric sites and exosites in an enzyme occur away from the active site; thus they tend to fall under less drug pressure and are less likely to develop resistance.

Acknowledgements

We thank NIMR, New Delhi, for providing basic infrastructure facilities. We also thank Indian Council of Medical Research for providing fellowship assistance to Mr. Rahul (45/16/2019-Bio/BMS).

Conflict of interest

The authors declare no conflict of interest.

Author details

Rahul Pasupureddy[1,2], Sriram Seshadri[2], Rajnikant Dixit[1] and Kailash C. Pandey[1*]

1 Host-Parasite Interaction Biology Group, ICMR-National Institute of Malaria Research, New Delhi, India

2 Institute of Science, Nirma University, Ahmedabad, Gujarat, India

*Address all correspondence to: pandey.kailash70@gmail.com; kailash.pandey@icmr.gov.in

IntechOpen

© 2019 The Author(s). Licensee IntechOpen. This chapter is distributed under the terms of the Creative Commons Attribution License (http://creativecommons.org/licenses/by/3.0), which permits unrestricted use, distribution, and reproduction in any medium, provided the original work is properly cited. [cc] BY

References

[1] World Health Organization. World Malaria Report 2018; 2018. ISBN 9789241564403

[2] Tilley L, Straimer J, Gnädig NF, et al. Artemisinin action and resistance in *Plasmodium falciparum*. Trends in Parasitology. 2016;**32**:682-696

[3] Davies DR, Cohen GH. Interactions of protein antigens with antibodies. Proceedings of the National Academy of Sciences of the United States of America. 1996;**93**:7-12

[4] Calejo AI, Taskén K. Targeting protein-protein interactions in complexes organized by a kinase anchoring proteins. Frontiers in Pharmacology. 2015;**6**:1-13

[5] Rao A, Bulusu G, Srinivasan R, et al. Protein-protein interactions and disease. Protein Interact. 2012;**8**:143-154. ISBN: 978-953-51-0244-1

[6] Liu K-QQ, Liu Z-PP, Hao J-KK, et al. Identifying dysregulated pathways in cancers from pathway interaction networks. BMC Bioinformatics. 2012;**13**:126

[7] Scott DE, Bayly AR, Abell C, et al. Small molecules, big targets: Drug discovery faces the protein-protein interaction challenge. Nature Reviews. Drug Discovery. 2016;**15**:533-550

[8] Snider J, Kittanakom S, Curak J, et al. Split-ubiquitin based membrane yeast two-hybrid (MYTH) system: A powerful tool for identifying protein-protein interactions. Journal of Visualized Experiments. 2010;(36):e1698

[9] Zhang X, Francis BF. New perspectives in predicting membrane protein-protein interactions. New Achievements in Evolutionary Computation. 2010;**7**:157-172. ISBN: 978-953-307-053-7

[10] Muangphrom P, Seki H, Fukushima EO, et al. Artemisinin-based antimalarial research: Application of biotechnology to the production of artemisinin, its mode of action, and the mechanism of resistance of plasmodium parasites. Journal of Natural Medicines. 2016;**70**:318-334

[11] Pasupureddy R, Atul SS, et al. Current scenario and future strategies to fight artemisinin resistance. Parasitology Research. 2019;**118**:29-42

[12] Dondorp AM, Nosten F, Yi P, et al. Artemisinin resistance in *Plasmodium falciparum* malaria. The New England Journal of Medicine. 2009;**361**:455-467

[13] Goldberg DE. Hemoglobin degradation. Malaria: Drugs, Disease and Post-genomic Biology. 2005;**295**:275-291

[14] Sundararaj S, Singh D, Saxena AK, et al. The ionic and hydrophobic interactions are required for the auto activation of cysteine proteases of *Plasmodium falciparum*. PLoS One. 2012;**7**:e47227

[15] Pant A, Kumar R, Wani NA, et al. Allosteric site inhibitor disrupting auto-processing of malarial cysteine proteases. Scientific Reports. 2018;**8**:e16193

[16] Salawu EO. In silico study reveals how E64 approaches, binds to, and inhibits falcipain-2 of *Plasmodium falciparum* that causes malaria in humans. Scientific Reports. 2018;**8**:1-13

[17] Bekono BD, Ntie-Kang F, Owono Owono LC, et al. Targeting cysteine proteases from *Plasmodium falciparum*: A general overview, rational drug design

and computational approaches for drug discovery. Current Drug Targets. 2018;**19**:501-526

[18] Nizi E, Sferrazza A, Fabbrini D, et al. Peptidomimetic nitrile inhibitors of malarial protease falcipain-2 with high selectivity against human cathepsins. Bioorganic & Medicinal Chemistry Letters. 2018;**28**:1540-1544

[19] Pandey KC, Wang SX, Sijwali PS, et al. The *Plasmodium falciparum* cysteine protease falcipain-2 captures its substrate, hemoglobin, via a unique motif. Proceedings of the National Academy of Sciences of the United States of America. 2005;**102**:9138 LP-9139143

[20] Pasupureddy R, Verma S, Pant A, et al. Crucial residues in falcipains that mediate hemoglobin hydrolysis. Experimental Parasitology. 2019;**197**:43-50

[21] Awasthi V, Chattopadhyay D, Das J. Potential hemoglobin A/F role in clinical malaria. Bioinformation. 2017;**13**:269-273

[22] Istvan ES, Dharia NV, Bopp SE, et al. Validation of isoleucine utilization targets in *Plasmodium falciparum*. Proceedings of the National Academy of Sciences. 2011;**108**:1627-1632

[23] Manickam Y, Chaturvedi R, Babbar P, et al. Drug targeting of one or more aminoacyl-tRNA synthetase in the malaria parasite *Plasmodium falciparum*. Drug Discovery Today. 2018;**23**:1233-1240

[24] Saint-Léger A, Sinadinos C, Ribas de Pouplana L. The growing pipeline of natural aminoacyl-tRNA synthetase inhibitors for malaria treatment. Bioengineered. 2016;7:60-64

[25] Burns AL, Dans MG, Balbin JM, et al. Targeting malaria parasite invasion of red blood cells as an antimalarial

strategy. FEMS Microbiology Reviews. 2019;**43**:223-238

[26] Bermúdez M, Arévalo-Pinzón G, Rubio L, et al. Receptor–ligand and parasite protein–protein interactions in *Plasmodium vivax*: Analysing rhoptry neck proteins 2 and 4. Cellular Microbiology. 2018;**20**:e12835

[27] Hossain ME, Dhawan S, Mohmmed A. The cysteine-rich regions of *Plasmodium falciparum* RON2 bind with host erythrocyte and AMA1 during merozoite invasion. Parasitology Research. 2012;**110**:1711-1721

[28] Nasamu AS, Glushakova S, Russo I, et al. Plasmepsins IX and X are essential and druggable mediators of malaria parasite egress and invasion. Science (80-). 2017;**358**:518-522

[29] Pino P, Mukherjee B, Klages N, et al. A multistage antimalarial targets the plasmepsins IX and X essential for invasion and egress. Science (80-). 2017;**358**:522-528

[30] Munsamy G, Agoni C, Soliman MES. A dual target of Plasmepsin IX and X: Unveiling the atomistic superiority of a core chemical scaffold in malaria therapy. Journal of Cellular Biochemistry. 2019;**120**:7876-7887

[31] Boucher LE, Hopp CS, Muthinja JM, et al. Discovery of plasmodium (M) TRAP-aldolase interaction stabilizers interfering with sporozoite motility and invasion. ACS Infectious Disease. 2018;**4**:620-634

[32] Chang HH, Falick AM, Carlton PM, et al. N-terminal processing of proteins exported by malaria parasites. Molecular and Biochemical Parasitology. 2008;**160**:107-115

[33] Gambini L, Rizzi L, Pedretti A, et al. Picomolar inhibition of plasmepsin V,

an essential malaria protease, achieved exploiting the prime region. PLoS One. 2015;**10**:e0142509

[34] Batinovic S, Mchugh E, Chisholm SA, et al. An exported protein-interacting complex involved in the trafficking of virulence determinants in plasmodium-infected erythrocytes. Nature Communications. 2017;**8**:1-14

[35] Marapana DS, Dagley LF, Sandow JJ, et al. Plasmepsin V cleaves malaria effector proteins in a distinct endoplasmic reticulum translocation interactome for export to the erythrocyte. Nature Microbiology. 2018;**3**:1010-1022

[36] Hain AUP, Weltzer RR, Hammond H, et al. Structural characterization and inhibition of the plasmodium Atg8-Atg3 interaction. Journal of Structural Biology. 2012;**180**:551-562

[37] Villa S, Legnani L, Colombo D, et al. Structure-based drug design, synthesis and biological assays of *P. falciparum* Atg3–Atg8 protein–protein interaction inhibitors. Journal of Computer-Aided Molecular Design. 2018;**32**:473-486

[38] Ariey F, Witkowski B, Amaratunga C, et al. A molecular marker of artemisinin-resistant *Plasmodium falciparum* malaria. Nature. 2014;**505**:50-55

[39] Mbengue A, Bhattacharjee S, Pandharkar T, et al. A molecular mechanism of artemisinin resistance in *Plasmodium falciparum* malaria. Nature. 2015;**520**:683

[40] Bhattacharjee S, Coppens I, Mbengue A, et al. Remodeling of the malaria parasite and host human red cell by vesicle amplification that induces artemisinin resistance. Blood. 2018;**131**:1234-1247

[41] Coppée R, Jeffares DC, Miteva MA, et al. Comparative structural and evolutionary analyses predict functional sites in the artemisinin resistance malaria protein K13. Scientific Reports. 2019;**9**:e10675

[42] Gilson PR, O'Donnell RA, Nebl T, et al. MSP119 miniproteins can serve as targets for invasion inhibitory antibodies in *Plasmodium falciparum* provided they contain the correct domains for cell surface trafficking. Molecular Microbiology. 2008;**68**:124-138

[43] Santos CC. Chagasin, the endogenous cysteine-protease inhibitor of *Trypanosoma cruzi*, modulates parasite differentiation and invasion of mammalian cells. Journal of Cell Science. 2005;**118**:901-915

[44] Wang SX, Pandey KC, Scharfstein J, et al. The structure of Chagasin in complex with a cysteine protease clarifies the binding mode and evolution of an inhibitor family. Structure. 2007;**15**:535-543

[45] Sundararaj S, Saxena AK, Sharma R, et al. Cross-talk between malarial cysteine proteases and falstatin: The BC loop as a hot-spot target. PLoS One. 2014;**9**:e93008

Chapter 6

Relationship of Parasitic Index and Cytokine Profile in Canine Visceral Leishmaniasis

José Nivaldo da Silva, Valéria Régia Franco Sousa,
Arleana do Bom Parto Ferreira de Almeida,
Adenilda Cristina Honorio-França and Eduardo Luzía França

Abstract

Visceral leishmaniasis (VL) is a zoonotic parasitic disease caused by *Leishmania infantum (L. chagasi)* that infects cells of the monocyte-phagocyte system. This work aims to describe the bone marrow parasitism in dogs naturally infected by *L. chagasi*, and to correlate with serum concentrations of cytokines and antibody level. It evaluated 42 dogs, 21 uninfected and 21 infected by *L. infantum*, of both sexes and of different ages; dogs were classified into three clinical stages: stage I, mild disease; stage II, moderate disease; and stage III, severe disease. Parasitic index was determined by real-time polymerase chain reaction (PCR) and cytokine serum concentration by flow cytometry. The average parasitic index of infected dogs was 4.59×10^{10} copies/μl. IL-4 and TNF-α concentrations were higher in infected dogs than in the control group. Antibody levels were positively correlated with IL-4 expression. There was a significant positive correlation of IL-6 cytokine levels with the evolution of stages I and III. Antibody levels were positively correlated with IL-4 expression. There was a significant positive correlation of IL-6 cytokine levels with the evolution of stages I and III. However, this cytokine can be used as a marker to distinguish between different clinical stages.

Keywords: *Leishmania infantum*, dogs, cytokines, parasitic index, cytometry

1. Introduction

Visceral leishmaniasis (VL) is a parasitic zoonotic disease caused by the protozoan *Leishmania infantum* (syn. *L. chagasi*), an intracellular parasite of the phagocytic mononuclear system [1, 2]. In Brazil, VL is transmitted by sandflies, *Lutzomyia longipalpis* [1, 3, 4].

In a global scenario, it is estimated that 300,000 new cases of VL occur with a rate of 20,000 deaths each year, with 94% new cases reported in Brazil, Ethiopia, India, Kenya, Somalia, South Sudan, and Sudan [5]. While in Latin America, LV spreads from Mexico to Argentina, with the largest number of cases concentrated in Brazil [6]. With the urbanization of VL in Brazil, annually, the country records approximately 3500 new cases, mainly in medium and large cities; probably, it is due to the disordered anthropic occupation of the geographic space [7].

IntechOpen

Despite scientific advances, cases of VL are expanding, which has a major impact on public health, as dogs are the main reservoirs in the urban environment and therefore play an important role in the transmission cycle [8, 9].

Canine visceral leishmaniasis (CVL) is characterized by a broad clinical spectrum, from mild and moderate to fatal clinical manifestations. Major clinical signs in dogs include hepatosplenomegaly, lymphadenopathy, exfoliative dermatitis, alopecia, onychogryphosis, keratoconjunctivitis, apathy, anorexia, and severe weight loss [10–13].

The clinical manifestation of CVL depends on the interaction of the parasite with the host immune response [2]. In susceptible dogs, clinicopathological abnormalities are preceded by an evident humoral response and depression of the cellular response, mediated by a non-protective Th2 immune response associated with cytokines IL-4, IL-5, IL-6, and IL-10 [14, 15]. Dogs that do not develop the disease have a protective cellular response (Th1) [16, 17], related to INF-γ, TNF-α, IL-2, and IL-12 cytokines.

Different procedures are used for the diagnosis of CVL [18]. The Brazilian Ministry of Health recommends serology in the investigation of canine disease by the Dual-Path Platform (DPP®) rapid method as a screening test and ELISA as confirmatory test [19]. Other tests are used to demonstrate infection, such as cytology, histopathology [20], and real-time PCR (RT-PCR) [21].

Similarly, determination of parasitic index has become important for early detection, but also evaluation of treatment efficacy and monitoring of relapses [22]. Thus, the aim of this study was to associate parasitic index to serum cytokine concentration in dogs naturally infected by *L. infantum* at different clinical stages of infection.

2. Methodological aspects

The procedures were previously approved by the Ethics Committee on the Use of Animals (ECUA)/UFMT, Brazil (n° 23108.019567/14-1), and collection of clinical samples was authorized by the dog owners by signing the informed consent form.

2.1 Animals

This study was conducted over a 16-month period, evaluating 42 male and female dogs of different ages and breeds from Barra do Garças, Mato Grosso State, Brazil (latitude, −15.893; longitude, 52.2599; south,15° 53′ 35″; west 52° 15′ 36″). Dogs with canine visceral leishmaniasis (n = 21) were classified into clinical stages at diagnosis as described by Solano et al. [23] and confirmed using the Dual-Path Platform Rapid Test (RT DPP®) and polymerase chain reaction (PCR). A control group (n = 21) was also formed, comprising dogs with no clinical changes and negative results for RT DPP® and conventional PCR.

2.2 Blood and bone marrow sample

Blood samples (5 mL) were collected by cephalic or jugular venipuncture, placed in tubes without anticoagulant to obtain serum. Serum was obtained by centrifuging the blood sample at $300 \times g$ for 5 minutes and was then transferred to 2 mL microtubes and stored at −80°C for cytokine dosing.

After dog restraint and local anesthesia with 2% lidocaine, bone marrow samples were obtained from the sternal manubrium, placed in microtubes with 0.5 mL 0.9% sterile NaCl solution, and stored at −20°C for subsequent molecular techniques.

2.3 Immunochromatographic rapid test: RT DPP® kit

The immunochromatographic rapid test for detection of anti-*Leishmania infantum* antibodies (DPP®—Canine Visceral Leishmaniasis-Bio-Manguinhos/ FIOCRUZ, Rio de Janeiro, Brazil) that uses the recombinant protein K39 (rK39) as an antigen, a cloned 39 amino acid sequence of the specific *L. infantum* kinase region, was performed according to the manufacturer's guidance.

2.4 DNA extraction, conventional PCR, and qPCR

DNA extraction from blood samples was performed by the phenol-chloroform method. The polymerase chain reaction assay was performed using the primers RV1 (sense) 5'-CTT TTC TGG TCC CGC GGG TAG G-3' and RV2 (antisense) 5'-CCA CCT GGC TAT TTT ACA CCA-3' [24], which amplifies the DNA fragment of a 145 bp region of conserved kDNA present in *L. infantum*. Amplification used 200 mM dNTP, 1 pM from each primer, a buffer solution (10 mM Tris–HCl and 50 mM KCl, pH 8.3), 2 mM MgCl2, 1.5 U Taq DNA polymerase, and 2 μl of the DNA sample in the final volume of 25 μl. Assays were performed for one cycle at 94°C for 4 minutes, followed by 30 cycles at 94°C for 30 seconds, 60°C for 30 seconds, and 72°C for 30 seconds, and final extension of one cycle at 72°C for 10 minutes. The amplification product was fractionated by 2.0% agarose gel electrophoresis, stained with red gel spot, and visualized on a transilluminator (UV, 300 nm).

Quantitative PCR (qPCR) was performed in triplicate using the StepOne™ Real-Time PCR System Sequence Detection System (Applied Biosystems) targeting RV1-5'-CTT TTC TGG TCC GGG TAG G-3' primers and RV2-5'-CCA CCT GGC TAT TTT ACA CCA-3' amplifying a 145 bp sequence of *L. infantum*-specific kDNA [24]. Reactions were prepared in a 25 μl final volume containing SYBR Green Master Mix, 0.3 μM of each primer, and 2 μl of target DNA. Amplification conditions included an initial incubation step at 94°C for 10 minutes, followed by 40 cycles of amplification, 94°C for 15 seconds, and 60°C for 60 seconds. The standard curve was established for each assay using known amounts of TOPO PCR 2.1 plasmid (Invitrogen Corp.) containing *L. infantum* kDNA gene. Serial (10×) dilutions of the recombinant plasmid containing 2.9×10^4–2.9×10^8 copies of the plasmid were performed and used on the standard curve.

2.5 Cytokine quantification by flow cytometry

Serum cytokine concentration (IL-2, IL-4, IL-6, IL-10, TNF-α, IFN-γ, and IL-17) was assessed using the Cytometric Bead Array (CBA) Kit (BD Bioscience, USA) and evaluated by a flow cytometer (FACSCalibur®, BD Bioscience, USA). The reading was done using the CellQuest. Data were analyzed in FCAP array software version 5.0.

2.6 Determination of serum immunoglobulins

Immunoglobulin concentrations (IgM and IgG) in the sera were determined by turbidimetric method. For 1:11 (v/v) IgM and 1:15 (v/v) IgG, antibody concentrations were determined using IgM (Bioclin®, Brazil, Ref K063) and IgG (Bioclin®, Brazil, Ref K062) antiserum diluted with 1:12 (v/v). The calibration curve obtained from the Multical calibrator (Bioclin®, Brazil, Ref K064) was used to determine the standard curve for each immunoglobulin. Positive and negative serum samples, standards, and controls were placed in 500 μl buffer solution (0.15 mol/L sodium chloride, Tris 50 mmol/L, 6.0000 PEG 50 g/L, and sodium azide 15.38 nmol/L). The suspensions were mixed and incubated at 37°C for 10 minutes. Reactions were read on a spectrophotometer at 340 nm.

2.7 Statistical analysis

For the analysis of the concentration of cytokines and immunoglobulins (IgG and IgM), the Student t-test independent samples were used. For the quantification of parasitic index of the bone marrow and cytokines when compared by clinical stage, Kruskal-Wallis analysis of variance was used. Parasite load correlation analysis of IgG in the presence of cytokines was also performed by calculating the Spearman correlation coefficient. Data were expressed as mean ± standard error. Values less than 0.05 ($p < 0.05$) were considered significant.

3. Results

Most of the 21 dogs in the control group were mongrel dog (15/71%), Labrador retriever (1/5%), dachshund (1/5%), pinscher (3/14%), and rottweiler (1/5%). Age ranged from 14 months to 8 years (average 3.4 years). Thirteen dogs were female (13/62%) and eight dogs were male (8/38%). Most of the 21 dogs with leishmaniasis were dogs from mongrel dog (12/57%), Labrador retriever (1/05%), American pit bull (1/05%), poodle (1/05%), and shih tzu (6/28%). Age ranged from 12 months to 11 years (mean 4.3 years). Six dogs were female (6/29%) and 15 dogs were male (15/72%).

At the time of clinical evaluation, all dogs diagnosed with VL had several clinicopathological findings typical of the disease. Clinical symptoms in seropositive animals (CVL) included lymphadenopathy (17/13%), skin ulcers (12/10%), onychogryphosis (11/09%), ear ulceration (11/09%), scaling (10/08%), weight loss (9/07%), dermatopathy (8/06%), ophthalmopathy (8/06%), muscle atrophy (4/03%), splenomegaly (7/06%), alopecia (6/05%), lethargy (5/04%), periocular alopecia (4/03%), skin nodules (3/02%), hepatomegaly (3/02%), cachexia (3/02%), and hyperkeratosis (2/01%).

Dogs were classified into three clinical stages: stage I, mild disease (n = 5/24%); stage II, moderate disease (n = 9/43%); and stage III, severe disease (n = 7/33%). Stage II dogs were not subclassified.

Leishmania infantum DNA was detected in all dogs of the group with CVL up to a concentration of 1 fg/µl. Real-time PCR of bone marrow samples was positive in all dogs in the CVL group (100%). There was no statistical difference in the distribution between clinical stages and parasitic index, as shown in **Table 1**.

The mean and standard error of concentrations (pg/ml) of IL-2, IL-4, IL-6, IL-10, TNF-α, IFN-γ, and IL-17 cytokines based on clinical staging in CVL-infected dogs are shown in **Table 1**. It was observed that IL-6 and TNF-α concentrations increased in serum of infected dogs with significant statistical difference between the clinical stages of CVL, although most infected dogs had moderate and severe clinical manifestations of the disease.

Among dogs with CVL and uninfected dogs, an increase of IL-4 and TNF-α concentrations in serum from dogs infected with CVL was observed. Similar serum concentrations of IL-2, IL-10, IL-17, and IFN-γ were observed between the groups studied (**Table 2**).

When comparing immunoglobulin means, IgG levels were elevated in the CVL group when compared to IgM levels. A significant difference (p = <0.0001) was observed. Similarly, IgG concentration between the control and CVL groups was evaluated. IgG levels were found to be higher in serum from dogs with CVL (2300.75 ± 678.463) when compared to control group IgG concentrations (636.94 ± 312.8 mg/dl), showing a significant difference between groups ($p = <0.0001$). Regarding the comparison of IgM concentration (mg/dl) in the CVL group (279.74 ± 37.755) compared to the control group (241.12 ± 59.835), there was no difference (**Table 3**).

Correlations of IL-6 and TNF-α concentrations were analyzed according to clinical staging with parasitic index according to stage I, IL-6 (rs = 0.400, p = 0.5046) and TNF-α (rs = 0.700, p = 0.1881); stage II, IL-6 (rs = 0.7000, p = 0.1881) and TNF-α (rs = −0.1590, p = 0.6828); and stage III, IL-6 (rs = −0.3571, p = 0.4316) and TNF-α (rs = −0.4643, p = 0.2939). There was no correlation between the other parameters evaluated.

The correlation between the parasitic index of dogs with CVL in the presence of cytokine IL-4 and TNF-α in the blood of dogs infected with CVL presented the IL-4 (rs = 0.0240, p = 0.9176) and TNF-α (rs = 0.0825, p = 0.7221). No additional significant correlations were found. Antibody levels were positively correlated with IL-4 expression (rs = 0.5997, p = 0.0040) (**Table 4**).

Cytokines/parasitemia	I	II	III	p-Value
IL-2	6.62 ± 1.18	12.01 ± 7.99	15.09 ± 6.34	0.152
IL-4	10.50 ± 2.05	11.38 ± 3.81	9.90 ± 2.73	0.9044
IL-6	2.14 ± 0.57	2.72 ± 0.66	3.12 ± 0.50	0.0350
IL-10	2.47 ± 0.97	2.85 ± 0.96	2.39 ± 0.84	0.8973
IL-17	2.22 ± 0.22	12.38 ± 9.63	13.27 ± 7.51	0.4345
TNF-α	4.52 ± 2.12	4.65 ± 2.31	6.14 ± 1.43	0.0462
IFN	3.07 ± 0.99	28.19 ± 23.21	2.58 ± 0.28	0.4648
Parasite copy number ($\times 10^7$)/ml	4.96 ± 1.00	4.63 ± 1.37	4.55 ± 1.49	0.9467

The results were expressed in mean and standard error.

Table 1.
Cytokine concentrations and parasite copy number ($\times 10^7$)/ml in dogs with visceral leishmaniasis in different clinical staging.

Cytokines	Control	CVL	p-Value
IL-2	9.18 ± 6.14	11.75 ± 6.89	0.3199
IL-4	7.43 ± 2.50	12.56 ± 5.37	0.0469
IL-6	2.87 ± 0.95	2.71 ± 0.67	0.3326
IL-10	2.98 ± 1.39	2.62 ± 0.87	0.2807
IL-17	11.12 ± 12.12	11.63 ± 9.66	0.4570
TNF-α	2.80 ± 0.52	5.12 ± 2.33	0.0009
IFN	13.26 ± 16.88	16.15 ± 19.01	0.3589

The results were expressed in mean and standard error.

Table 2.
Cytokine concentrations in dogs noninfected and dogs with canine visceral leishmaniasis.

Group	Control	CVL	p-Value
IgG	636.94 ± 255.52	2288.04 ± 610.08	<0.0001
IgM	241.12 ± 51.81	282.42 ± 33.99	0.0773

The results were expressed in mean and standard error.

Table 3.
Immunoglobulin concentrations (IgG and IgM) in serum from dogs with canine visceral leishmaniasis.

	IgG	
Parameters	rs	p-Value
IL-4	0.5997	0.0040
TNF-α	0.4164	0.0603
Parasitic index	−0.2243	0.3282

rs, correlation coefficient of Spearman.

Table 4.
Correlation between IgG concentrations with IL-4 and TNF-α and parasitic index of dogs infected with CVL.

Stage	I and II		I and III		II and III	
	rs	p	rs	p	rs	p
IL-6	0.6031	0.0855	0.8469	0.0162	0.5630	0.1144
TNF-α	0.0350	0.9288	0.3784	0.4026	0.0168	0.9658

rs, correlation coefficient of Spearman.

Table 5.
Correlation of IL-6 and TNF-α cytokine levels of dogs with canine visceral leishmaniasis by clinical staging of serum from dogs of the CVL group.

In this study, as shown in **Table 5**, the correlation of the evolution of clinical signs between the stages presented below was analyzed. There was a significant positive correlation of IL-6 cytokine levels between stage I and stage III.

4. Discussion

In this study the most dogs in the control group and CVL were mixed breed. The clinical symptoms of seropositive dogs (CVL) included lymphadenopathy, skin ulcers, onychogryphosis, ear ulceration, scaling, weight loss, and others. Dogs were classified into three clinical stages: stage I, mild disease; stage II, moderate disease; and stage III, severe disease. There was no statistical difference in the distribution between clinical stages and parasitic index. IL-6 and TNF-α concentrations increased in serum from infected dogs with a statistically significant difference between the clinical stages of CVL. Between the dogs with CVL and the control group, there was a statistical difference in the serum concentrations of cytokines IL-4 and TNF-α. IgG levels were elevated in the CVL group when compared to IgM levels. Antibody levels were positively correlated with IL-4 expression (rs = 0.5997; p = 0.0040). There was a significant positive correlation of IL-6 cytokine levels between stage I and stage III.

The clinical signs of CVL are important for the diagnosis. In the present study, the most prevalent clinical signs were lymphadenopathy, skin ulcers, onychogryphosis, ear ulceration, and scaling. However, prevalence is highly variable across studies, but generally these clinical signs are the most commonly reported in the literature. These results corroborate the findings of several authors [25, 26].

Regarding gender, there was a greater predominance of males in infected dogs and females in dogs in the control group. Regarding age, it did not present large variations. This fact seems to be associated with the higher risk of male exposure. However, the study shows no statistically significant differences for age and gender between healthy and sick dogs [27].

Bone marrow samples were taken from 21 dogs serologically positive for *L. infantum*. According to the clinical signs, dogs were classified as stages I, II, and III. Real-time PCR detected no parasite copies ($\times 10^{10}$)/µl *L. infantum* DNA in all animals of the CVL group, distributed as follows: stage I mean (4.964), stage II average (4.63), and stage III (4.55). No statistically significant difference was found in the average amount of DNA copy number between the different clinical stages (p = 0.9467). In bone marrow samples from dogs that are cytologically positive, a high parasitic index is detected [21].

Previous studies report that quantitative PCR on bone marrow samples from positive dogs in conventional tests contained a higher number of *Leishmania* kDNA copies than peripheral blood, although no significant differences were detected between symptomatic and asymptomatic dogs in terms of parasite load [28]. This literary quote converges with the findings of this study.

PCR can be used for detection of *Leishmania* in naturally infected dog samples, and PCR-RFLP (restriction fragment length polymorphism) is sensitive for identification of *Leishmania* species [28]. In addition, qPCR is effective in quantifying *Leishmania* DNA loading in clinical samples [29]. The blood sample from dogs infected by *L. infantum* was found by real-time PCR to have a sensitivity of 100% and specificity of 96.4% [30].

Most cytokines remain partially conserved between species; in this sense, the amino acid sequence of humans and canine cytokines shows 49–96% homology, suggesting a high probability of cross-reactivity between monoclonal antibodies; thus antibodies against human cytokines may be recommended as immunological biomarkers under pathological conditions by flow cytometry in human [31] and dogs [32] as used in this study.

In the present work, the serum concentration of cytokines (IL-2, IL-4, IL-6, IL-10, TNF-α, IFN-γ, and IL-17) was compared between the control groups and the group with CVL. In addition, cytokine levels were compared within the CVL group with clinical staging I, II, and III. When comparing the groups, IL-4 and TNF-α were higher in infected dogs than in the control group, showing significant difference between IL-4 (p = 0.0469) and TNF-α (p = 0.0009) groups. In the group with CVL there were differences between stages I and III with significant differences only for cytokines IL-6 (p = 0.0350) and TNF-α (p = 0.0462).

Elevated levels of IL-6 were found in serum from dogs with active leishmaniasis compared to healthy dogs [33]. These results corroborate the findings of this study. However, other authors reported that IL-6 production did not vary significantly between the groups studied [34]. On the other hand were described in the literature that elevated levels of IL-6 in dogs without clinical signs or symptoms in CVL dogs [35], and also highlights that, among other factors, it may indicate a balance between the parasite elimination effort and the active disease. Increased IL-6 levels suggest a restricted ability to control infection [36]. Even in the absence of clinical signs or symptoms, the animals showed granulomas on histopathological evaluation, suggesting chronicity and therefore a longtime course of infection [35]. Innate immune effector cells primarily neutrophils, monocytes, and macrophages produce and respond to IL-6, which may result in amplification of inflammation and a change from an acute inflammatory state to a chronic state [37].

IL-6 expression increases in dogs with active visceral leishmaniasis and may be a useful marker for active disease [33, 35]. Increased IL-6 production is not directly related to anti-*Leishmania* antibody titers, suggesting that other cytokines may be involved with hypergammaglobulinemia [33].

As shown in this work, it was observed that there was correlation of IL-6 expression between stages I and III of bone marrow aspirate of dogs infected with CVL. IL-6 production in dogs with active leishmaniasis appears to be associated with severe disease [33]. This statement converges with the findings in this study, as the dogs used in the control group were mostly stage II and III. IL-6 is essential for terminal B-cell differentiation and immunoglobulin production [38].

TNF-α concentration was higher in infected dogs than in the control group, as detected by de Lima et al. [33]. CVL susceptibility is closely associated with downregulation of key cytokines such as IFN-γ, TNF-α, and IL-17A, thus impairing iNOS activation and NO production and favoring parasite replication and disease development [39].

The increased activity of TNF-α in the liver of infected dogs compared to healthy canines has been reported [37, 40]. Higher TNF-α levels in infected dogs indicate that the presence of *L. infantum* induces an immune response with relevant TNF-α expression when the protozoan is present [40].

Studies suggest that decreased survival of L. *infantum* in canine macrophages is associated with increased TNF-α and IFN-γ production and decreased IL-10 production [41].

In dogs naturally infected with *L. infantum*, increased hepatic TNF-α may be associated with increased parasite load on this organ [42]. The cytokines IL-2, IL-4, IL-10, IFN-γ, TNF-α, and IL-12 may be used as markers in epidemiological studies conducted in endemic areas to distinguish between different clinical forms of VL [15]. However, Lima et al. [33] indicate that TNF-α is not considered a good marker of active disease in dogs with VL.

A study has reported a significant relationship between bone marrow IL-4 detection in naturally infected dogs with and without clinical signs and disease severity, suggesting that IL-4 production is associated with pathology [43]. Increased expression of IL-4 cytokine is associated with both severe clinical signs and a high parasitic index on skin lesions [44]. In bone marrow aspirates, IL-4 was elevated in naturally infected dogs with more severe symptoms [43].

The study points to evidence that IL-4 cytokine polymorphism may contribute to innate immunity to *L. infantum* infection [45].

Antibody levels were positively correlated with IL-4 expression (rs = 0.5997; p = 0.0040). IgG is also linked to chronic infection in patients with VL, where high levels of IgG are predictive of the disease. This finding is in line with the study by Lima et al. [33] suggesting that other cytokines, such as IL-10 or IL-4, may be associated with hypergammaglobulinemia observed in dogs with CVL. Previous studies have detected increased serum IgG levels in symptomatic dogs compared with healthy dogs and are related to pathophysiological disorders and active disease [33].

Response to natural infection of *L. infantum* is linked to the presence of IgG [43] and *Leishmania*-specific IgM antibodies that can be detected in infected dogs [46]. Some studies have reported that increased total protein is frequent in dogs infected with visceral leishmaniasis due to increased antibody production [47, 48].

5. Conclusion

These results may contribute to a better understanding of the immune response in dogs infected with *L. infantum*. Antibody levels were positively correlated with

IL-4 expression. There was a significant positive correlation of IL-6 cytokine levels with the evolution of stages I and III. However, this cytokine can be used as a marker to distinguish between different clinical stages.

Acknowledgements

This research received grants from the Mato Grosso Research Support Foundation (FAPEMAT No. 299032/2010) and from the National Council for Scientific and Technological Development (CNPq No. 447218/2014–0 and No. 305725/2018–1), in Brazil.

Conflict of interest

The authors declare that there is no conflict of interest and nonfinancial competitors.

Author details

José Nivaldo da Silva[1], Valéria Régia Franco Sousa[1],
Arleana do Bom Parto Ferreira de Almeida[1], Adenilda Cristina Honorio-França[2]
and Eduardo Luzía França[2*]

1 Faculty of Veterinary Medicine, Federal University of Mato Grosso, Cuiabá, Mato Grosso, Brazil

2 Institute of Biological and Health Sciences, Federal University of Mato Grosso, Barra do Garças, Mato Grosso, Brazil

*Address all correspondence to: elfranca@ufmt.br

IntechOpen

© 2019 The Author(s). Licensee IntechOpen. This chapter is distributed under the terms of the Creative Commons Attribution License (http://creativecommons.org/licenses/by/3.0), which permits unrestricted use, distribution, and reproduction in any medium, provided the original work is properly cited. (cc) BY

References

[1] Ferreira GE, dos Santos BN, Dorval ME, Ramos TP, Porrozzi R, Peixoto AA, et al. The genetic structure of *Leishmania infantum* populations in Brazil and its possible association with the transmission cycle of visceral leishmaniasis. PLoS One. 2012;7:e36242

[2] Saporito L, Giammanco GM, De Grazia S, Colomba C. Visceral leishmaniasis: Host-parasite interactions and clinical presentation in the immunocompetent and in the immunocompromised host. International Journal of Infectious Diseases. 2013;17:e572-e576

[3] Missawa NA, Lima GB. Spatial distribution of *Lutzomyia longipalpis* (Lutz & Neiva, 1912) and *Lutzomyia cruzi* (Mangabeira, 1938) in the state of Mato Grosso. Revista da Sociedade Brasileira de Medicina Tropical. 2006;39:337-340

[4] Missawa NA, Veloso MA, Maciel GB, Michalsky EM, Dias ES. Evidence of transmission of visceral leishmaniasis by *Lutzomyia cruzi* in the municipality of Jaciara, state of Mato Grosso, Brazil. Revista da Sociedade Brasileira de Medicina Tropical. 2011;44:76-78

[5] World Health Organization. 2019. Available from: http://www.who.ch [Accessed: November 18, 2019]

[6] Feitosa MM, Day MJ. Current status and management of canine leishmaniasis in Latin America. Research in Veterinary Science. 2019;123:261-272

[7] Carvalho AG, Luz JGG, Rodrigues LD, Dias JVL, Fontes CJF. Factors associated with *Leishmania* spp. infection in domestic dogs from an emerging area of high endemicity for visceral leishmaniasis in Central-Western Brazil. Research in Veterinary Science. 2019;125:205-211

[8] Reis AB, Martins-Filho OA, Teixeira-Carvalho A, Giunchetti RC, Carneiro CM, Mayrink W, et al. Systemic and compartmentalized immune response in canine visceral leishmaniasis. Veterinary Immunology and Immunopathology. 2009;128:87-95

[9] Travi BL, Cordeiro-da-Silva A, Dantas-Torres F, Miró G. Canine visceral leishmaniasis: Diagnosis and management of the reservoir living among us. PLoS Neglected Tropical Diseases. 2018;12:e0006082

[10] Reis AB, Teixeira-Carvalho A, Giunchetti RC, Guerra LL, Carvalho MG, Mayrink W, et al. Phenotypic features of circulating leucocytes as immunological markers for clinical status and bone marrow parasite density in dogs naturally infected by *Leishmania chagasi*. Clinical and Experimental Immunology. 2006;146:303-311

[11] Freitas JC, Nunes-Pinheiro DC, Lopes Neto BE, Santos GJ, Abreu CR, Braga RR, et al. Clinical and laboratory alterations in dogs naturally infected by *Leishmania chagasi*. Revista da Sociedade Brasileira de Medicina Tropical. 2012;45:24-29

[12] Nascimento MSL, Albuquerque TDR, Do-Valle-Matta MA, Caldas IS, Diniz LF, Talvani A, et al. Naturally *Leishmania infantum*-infected dogs display an overall impairment of chemokine and chemokine receptor expression during visceral leishmaniasis. Veterinary Immunology and Immunopathology. 2013;153:202-208

[13] Silva KL, de Andrade MM, Melo LM, Perosso J, Vasconcelos RO, Munari DP, et al. CD4+FOXP3+ cells produce IL-10 in the spleens of dogs with visceral leishmaniasis. Veterinary Parasitology. 2014;202:313-318

[14] Rogers KA, DeKrey GK, Mbow ML, Gillespie RD, Brodskyn CI, Titus RG. Type 1 and type 2 responses to *leishmania major*. FEMS Microbiology Letters. 2002;**209**:1-7

[15] Costa ASA, Costa GC, Aquino DMC, Mendonça VRR, Barral A, Barral-Netto M, et al. Cytokines and visceral leishmaniasis: A comparison of plasma cytokine profiles between the clinical forms of visceral leishmaniasis. Memórias do Instituto Oswaldo Cruz. 2012;**107**:735-739

[16] Ferrer L, Solano-Gallego L, Arboix M, Alberola J. Evaluation of the specific immune response in dogs infected by *Leishmania infantum*. Blackwell Science. 2002:92-99

[17] Baneth G, Koutinas AF, Solano-Gallego L, Bourdeau P, Ferrer L. Canine leishmaniosis—New concepts and insights on an expanding zoonosis: Part one. Trends in Parasitology. 2008;**24**:324-330

[18] Dantas-Torres F, Solano-Gallego L, Baneth G, Ribeiro VM, de Paiva-Cavalcanti M, Otranto D. Canine leishmaniosis in the old and new worlds: Unveiled similarities and differences. Trends in Parasitology. 2012;**28**:531-538

[19] MS. Secretaria de Vigilância em Saúde. Departamento de Análise de Situação de Saúde.Saúde Brasil 2011: uma análise da situação de saúde e a vigilância da saúde da mulher/Ministério da Saúde, Secretaria de Vigilância em Saúde, Departamento de Análise de Situação de Saúde. – Brasília: 444 p. il. Editora do Ministério da Saúde;2012

[20] Maia C, Campino L. Methods for diagnosis of canine leishmaniasis and immune response to infection. Veterinary Parasitology. 2008;**158**:274-287

[21] Ramos RA, Ramos CA, Santos EM, de Araújo FR, de Carvalho GA, Faustino MA, et al. Quantification of *Leishmania infantum* DNA in the bone marrow, lymph node and spleen of dogs. Revista Brasileira de Parasitologia Veterinária. 2013;**22**:346-350

[22] Paiva-Cavalcanti M, de Morais RC, Pessoa-E-Silva R, Trajano-Silva LA, Gonçalves-de-Albuquerque SAC, Tavares DEH, et al. Leishmaniases diagnosis: An update on the use of immunological and molecular tools. Cell and Bioscience. 2015;**5**:31

[23] Solano-Gallego L, Koutinas A, Miró G, Cardoso L, Pennisi MG, Ferrer L, et al. Directions for the diagnosis, clinical staging, treatment and prevention of canine leishmaniosis. Veterinary Parasitology. 2009;**165**:1-18

[24] Lachaud L, Marchergui-Hammami S, Chabbert E, Dereure J, Dedet JP, Bastien P. Comparison of six PCR methods using peripheral blood for detection of canine visceral leishmaniasis. Journal of Clinical Microbiology. 2002;**40**:210-215

[25] Noli C, Saridomichelakis MN. An update on the diagnosis and treatment of canine leishmaniosis caused by *Leishmania infantum* (syn. *L. chagasi*). Veterinary Journal. 2014;**202**:425-435

[26] Silva KR, Mendonça VR, Silva KM, Nascimento LF, Mendes-Sousa AF, Pinho FA, et al. Scoring clinical signs can help diagnose canine visceral leishmaniasis in a highly endemic area in Brazil. Memórias do Instituto Oswaldo Cruz. 2017;**112**:53-63

[27] Meléndez-Lazo A, Ordeix L, Planellas M, Pastor J, Solano-Gallego L. Clinicopathological findings in sick dogs naturally infected with *Leishmania infantum*: Comparison of five different clinical classification systems. Research in Veterinary Science. 2018;**117**:18-27

[28] Quaresma PF, Murta SMF, de Castro Ferreira E, da Rocha ACVM,

Xavier AAP, Gontijo CMF. Molecular diagnosis of canine visceral leishmaniasis: Identification of *Leishmania* species by PCR-RFLP and quantification of parasite DNA by real-time PCR. Acta Tropica. 2009;**111**:289-294

[29] Morais RCS, Costa Oliveira CN, Albuquerque SDCG, Silva LAMT, Pessoa-Silva R, Cruz HLA, et al. Real-time PCR for *Leishmania* species identification: Evaluation and comparison with classical techniques. Experimental Parasitology. 2016;**165**:43-50

[30] Mohammadiha A, Mohebali M, Haghighi A, Mahdian R, Abadi AR, Zarei Z, et al. Comparison of real-time PCR and conventional PCR with two DNA targets for detection of *Leishmania (Leishmania) infantum* infection in human and dog blood samples. Experimental Parasitology. 2013;**133**:89-94

[31] Scherer EF, Cantarini DG, Siqueira R, Ribeiro EB, Braga É, Honório-França AC, et al. Cytokine modulation of human blood viscosity from vivax malaria patients. Acta Tropica. 2016;**158**:139-147

[32] Moreira ML, Dorneles EM, Soares RP, Magalhães CP, Costa-Pereira C, Lage AP, et al. Cross-reactivity of commercially available anti-human monoclonal antibodies with canine cytokines: Establishment of a reliable panel to detect the functional profile of peripheral blood lymphocytes by intracytoplasmic staining. Acta Veterinaria Scandinavica. 2015;**57**:51

[33] de Lima VM, Peiro JR, de Oliveira Vasconcelos R. IL-6 and TNF-alpha production during active canine visceral leishmaniasis. Veterinary Immunology and Immunopathology. 2007;**115**:189-193

[34] Pinelli E, Killick-Kendrick R, Wagenaar J, Bernadina W, del

Real G, Ruitenberg J. Cellular and humoral immune responses in dogs experimentally and naturally infected with *Leishmania infantum*. Infection and Immunity. 1994;**62**:229-235

[35] De Vasconcelos TC, Doyen N, Cavaillon JM, Bruno SF, de Campos MP, de Miranda LH, et al. Cytokine and iNOS profiles in lymph nodes of dogs naturally infected with *Leishmania infantum* and their association with the parasitic DNA load and clinical and histopathological features. Veterinary Parasitology. 2016;**227**:8-14

[36] Solcà MS, Andrade BB, Abbehusen MM, Teixeira CR, Khouri R, Valenzuela JG, et al. Circulating biomarkers of immune activation, oxidative stress and inflammation characterize severe canine visceral leishmaniasis. Scientific Reports. 2016;**6**:32619

[37] Choy E, Rose-John S. Interleukin-6 as a multifunctional regulator: Inflammation, immune response, and fibrosis. Journal of Scleroderma and Related Disorders. 2017;**2**:S1-S5

[38] Le JM, Vilcek J. Interleukin 6: A multifunctional cytokine regulating immune reactions and the acute phase protein response. Laboratory Investigation. 1989;**61**:588-602

[39] Nascimento MS, Albuquerque TD, Nascimento AF, Caldas IS, Do-Valle-Matta MA, Souto JT, et al. Impairment of interleukin-17A expression in canine visceral leishmaniosis is correlated with reduced interferon-γ and inducible nitric oxide synthase expression. Journal of Comparative Pathology. 2015;**153**:197-205

[40] Michelin FA, Perri SH, De Lima VM. Evaluation of TNF-α, IL-4, and IL-10 and parasite density in spleen and liver of *L. chagasi* naturally infected

dogs. Annals of Tropical Medicine and Parasitology. 2011;**105**:373-383

[41] Turchetti AP, da Costa LF, Romão EEL, Fujiwara RT, da Paixão TA, Santos RL. Transcription of innate immunity genes and cytokine secretion by canine macrophages resistant or susceptible to intracellular survival of *Leishmania infantum*. Veterinary Immunology and Immunopathology. 2015;**163**:67-76

[42] Giunchetti RC, Mayrink W, Carneiro CM, Corrêa-Oliveira R, Martins-Filho OA, Marques MJ, et al. Histopathological and immuno-histochemical investigations of the hepatic compartment associated with parasitism and serum biochemical changes in canine visceral leishmaniasis. Research in Veterinary Science. 2008;**84**:269-277

[43] Quinnell RJ, Courtenay O, Shaw MA, Day MJ, Garcez LM, Dye C, et al. Tissue cytokine responses in canine visceral leishmaniasis. The Journal of Infectious Diseases. 2001;**183**:1421-1424

[44] Brachelente C, Müller N, Doherr MG, Sattler U, Welle M. Cutaneous leishmaniasis in naturally infected dogs is associated with a T helper-2-biased immune response. Veterinary Pathology. 2005;**42**:166-175

[45] Jeronimo SMB, Holst AKB, Jamieson SE, Francis R, Martins DRA, Bezerra FL, et al. Genes at human chromosome 5q31.1 regulate delayed-type hypersensitivity responses associated with *Leishmania chagasi* infection. Genetics of Immunity. 2007;**8**:539

[46] Rodríguez A, Solano-Gallego L, Ojeda A, Quintana J, Riera C, Gállego M, et al. Dynamics of *Leishmania*-specific immunoglobulin isotypes in dogs with clinical leishmaniasis before and after treatment. Journal of Veterinary Internal Medicine. 2006;**20**:495-498

[47] Ciaramella P, Oliva G, Luna RD, Gradoni L, Ambrosio R, Cortese L, et al. A retrospective clinical study of canine leishmaniasis in 150 dogs naturally infected by *Leishmania infantum*. The Veterinary Record. 1997;**141**:539-543

[48] Medeiros CMO, Melo AGC, Lima AKF, Silva ING, Oliveira LCO, Silva MC. Haematological profile of dogs with visceral leishmaniasis in the city of Fortaleza, Ceará. Ciência Animal. 2008;**18**:43-50

Chapter 7

Toxoplasma Immunomodulation Related to Neuropsychiatric Diseases

Mammari Nour and Halabi Mohamad Adnan

Abstract

Toxoplasma gondii (*T. gondii*) causes toxoplasmic encephalitis resulting from reactivation of latent toxoplasmosis. It is the most frequent clinical manifestation, characterized by multiple necrotizing brain lesions. Bradyzoite tissue cysts activate an immune response that has a major impact on controlling parasite persistence in the brain. The immune mechanisms stimulated in the brain cause a local inflammatory mediated by Th1 immune reaction cytokines. Several studies have linked this process to that active during different neuropsychiatric disorders, such as Schizophrenia. In addition to the immune reaction activated in the brain, this latter has the capacity to stimulate neurotransmitter production. *T. gondii* induces high concentrations of dopamine and tyrosine hydroxylase in the central nervous system and has also been shown to increase kynurenine/tryptophan ratio and elevated Kynurenic acid level, mainly in astrocyte cells. This imbalance plays a role in the pathophysiology of Schizophrenia. Results of different studies explain in this chapter support the idea that *Toxoplasma* is an etiological factor in Schizophrenia.

Keywords: *Toxoplasma gondii*, neuropsychiatric disorders, schizophrenia, immunity, neurotransmitter

1. Introduction

Toxoplasmosis is one of the most common parasitic zoonosis in the world. Its causative agent, *Toxoplasma gondii*, is an obligate intracellular protozoan, which has developed several potential pathways for the transmission between different host species. *T. gondii* is able to establish a persistent infection within the brain. In this case, the immunocompetent subject will harbor latent *Toxoplasma* cysts in his central nervous system (CNS). Chronic *Toxoplasma* infection is asymptomatic although studies suggest that it may be a factor associated with chronic neurological conditions (Schizophrenia, Parkinson, bipolar diseases, etc.) [1, 2]. When the infection occurs in a pregnant woman, contamination of the fetus is possible with varying consequences depending on the stage of embryogenesis and the degree of maturity of the immune system. The neurological disorders (hydrocephalus, microcephaly, mental retardation, intracranial calcification) or ocular (retino-choroiditis) of congenital toxoplasmosis reflect the neurological tropism of this parasite [3]. Similarly, during a progressive degradation of the immune system functions following infection with the human immunodeficiency virus (HIV) or immunosuppressive treatment, the brain is the preferred target for the reactivation

IntechOpen

of latent *Toxoplasma* cysts [4, 5]. Parasite multiplication in the CNS induces a local inflammatory reaction resulting in brain damage and a strong synthesis of neurotransmitters which are involved in necrotizing brain lesions and in neurological disorders. The relationship between *T. gondii* infection and the development of the bipolar disorder (BD) has long been investigated, Evidence studies suggest that this infection may be related to neuropsychiatric disorders, especially Schizophrenia. Immune response has a major role in the persistence of *T. gondii* cysts in the brain. The protective immune reaction against *Toxoplasma* is very complex. During primary infection, the components of the nonspecific immune response occur first. *T. gondii* tachyzoites reach the intestinal lumen, enter the intestinal cells, and multiply in the cells of the lamina propria [6]. At this stage, infected enterocytes activate an immune response to limit parasite multiplication [7]. This response mainly involves neutrophils, macrophages, monocytes and dendritic cells via the secretion of different chemoattractant proteins. Secondarily, cellular immune response is specifically activated against the parasite [8]. It is essentially an immune response Th1-type. This response is marked by interleukin (IL)-12 production by antigen presenting cells, and interferon-gamma (IFN-γ) production by CD4+ T cells, CD8+ T cells, and natural killer (NK) cells (**Figure 1**). The Th1-type reaction most often induces a local inflammatory reaction, hence the interest of activating a Th2-type immune reaction that inhibits the activation of the Th1 immune response. The Th2 response is mediated primarily by two interleukins IL-4 and IL-10 [6] (**Figure 1**). This immune regulation seems to be of great interest in reducing the inflammatory reactions responsible for most lesions, but it makes the soil favorable to parasite multiplication. Despite the immune responses against *T. gondii*, this parasite has the ability to escape and spread via the bloodstream to infect different organs. In the central nervous system, tachyzoites have the ability to cross the blood-brain barrier (BBB), infect different types of nerve cells, and become encysted bradyzoites that persist throughout the life of the host. Several studies have shown in the mouse model the importance of IFN-γ in this control [9]. Among the parasitic factors, the genotype also has a role in the influence of the evolution of *Toxoplasma* infection. Type I strains are associated with high virulence in mice, whereas type II or III strains are considered avirulent for mice. Type I tachyzoites have the ability to cross epithelial barriers and reach immune-privileged sites more rapidly than type II

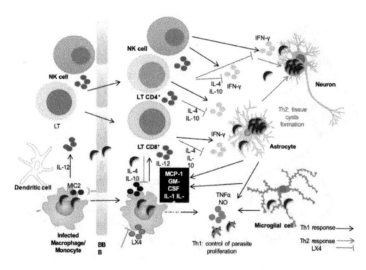

Figure 1.
Diagram showing the cerebral immune response during a cerebral toxoplasmosis infection in mice.

strains [10]. In human, several studies have reported severe acquired toxoplasmosis due to atypical strains in immunocompetent individuals. An overrepresentation of other atypical strains has been observed in patients with ocular toxoplasmosis [11]. The influence of the parasite strain on the development of the infection or the cerebral pathology remains however unknown.

2. The cerebral anti-*Toxoplasma* immune reaction

2.1 The central nervous system immunity

The central nervous system is closely linked to the immune system at several levels. The cerebral parenchyma is separated from the periphery by the BBB, the integrity of which is maintained by tight endothelial junctions. This barrier under normal conditions prevents the entry of mediators such as activated leukocytes, antibodies, complement factors, and cytokines. The myeloid cell line plays a crucial role in the development of immune responses at the central level, it includes two main subtypes: microglial cells, distributed in the cerebral parenchyma; perivascular macrophages located in the capillaries of the basal lamina brain and the choroid plexus. In addition, astrocytes, oligodendrocytes, endothelial cells, and neurons are also involved in the immune response in the CNS. By modulating synaptogenesis, microglial cells are more particularly involved in the restoration of neuronal connectivity following inflammation. These cells release immune mediators, such as cytokines, that modulate synaptic transmission and alter the morphology of dendritic spines during the inflammatory process after injury. Thus, the expression and release of immune mediators in the cerebral parenchyma are closely related to the plastic morphophysiological changes in the dendritic spines of neurons. Based on these data, it has been proposed that these immune mediators are also involved in the learning and memory processes. Microvasculature is a key element of brain damage. Endothelial cells are an important source of immune mediators such as a nitric oxide (NO), which are involved in the process of immune cell adhesion [12, 13]. A recent study shows that *T. gondii* invasion of neural tissue is mediated by epidermal growth factor receptor (EGFR), enhancing invasion likely by promoting survival of the parasite within endothelial cells [14]. Damage to the BBB can lead to increased permeability, which facilitates leucocyte access to the brain parenchyma. The release of mediators of endogenous inflammation and neurotoxins and the promotion of phagocytosis of cellular debris [6, 14]. Excessively activated microglial cells can cause major histocompatibility complex class II (MHCII) expression. This molecule facilitates the involvement of these cells in immune responses. Activation of microglial cells strongly influences the profile of cytokines released by two distinct mechanisms: recognition receptors and activation of the immune response [13, 15]. Activation of monocytes and macrophages is an important part of the innate immune response; it induces the production of pro-inflammatory cytokines and chemokines such as IL-8, monocyte chemoattractant protein1 (MCP-1), macrophage inflammatory proteins (MIP-1α and MIP-1β). Regulatory cytokines can also be activated within the CNS, such as IL-4 and IL-10 [8]. Expression of MHCII and adhesion molecules (CD11a, CD40, CD54, CD80, CD86) in activated microglial cells indicates that these cells can acquire antigen presenting activity and participate in the activation of T cells [16]. This suggests the existence of a network of complex interactions linking microglial cells, astrocytes and T cells; which creates a balance between the Th1/Th2 signals, which defines the immune response of the CNS. The role of astrocytes in the CNS is even more complex than that of microglial cells. Astrocytes are divided into two main subtypes: fibrous astrocytes located in the white matter; protoplasmic astrocytes located in the gray matter. These contribute to the formation of the BBB [6, 15]. Astrocytes also act as neuroprotectants by secreting neurotrophic and releasing potentially toxic pro-inflammatory molecules.

2.2 The mechanism of *T. gondii* invasion in the brain

In the brain, dendritic cells and monocytes are the most permissive cells for initial *Toxoplasma* infection [17]. These cell populations probably play an important role in the spread of the parasite, including in the brain. The CD11c$^+$ CD11b$^-$ dendritic cells infected promote the diffusion of *T. gondii* of the lamina propria to the mesenteric lymph nodes. Monocytes CD11c$^+$ CD11b$^-$ are the main cell population that contains tachyzoites in the blood [17]. *T. gondii* was detected in mononuclear cells + of infected mice 1 day after receiving an intravenous injection of CD11b$^+$ cells [18, 19].

The transepithelial migration capacity of tachyzoites is implicated in the passage of the parasite across the BBB. This could be done through the interaction of the intercellular adhesion molecule 1 (ICAM-1) of the BBB cells with the parasite MIC2 protein [20]. This interaction is important for transmigration of tachyzoites, as demonstrated *in vitro* in monolayers of several different cell lines [20] (**Figure 1**).

Macrophages are also responsible for the spread of *T. gondii* in the brain [21, 22]. The migration of infected macrophages into the CNS is mediated by the uPA/uPAR pathway and the expression of metalloproteinases 9 (MMP9) [23]. In the mouse brain during the acute phase of infection, *T. gondii* tachyzoites are able to infect all brain cells, mainly microglial cells, astrocytes and neurons. However, microglial cells tend to react against the parasite. These cells inhibit the growth of *T. gondii* and can, therefore, function as important inhibitors of *T. gondii* propagation in the CNS by mechanisms independent of NO and IFN-γ; but this does not prevent *T. gondii* from being able to encyst in these cells [15, 24]. Astrocytes and rat neurons are also suitable to host cells for the intracerebral proliferation of the PLK (type II) *T. gondii* strain [24]. These cells can harbor tachyzoites and cysts during the two respective phases of *Toxoplasma* infection [25]. Astrocytes also have the ability to control the proliferation of tachyzoites during the acute phase of infection for the local control of this opportunistic pathogen [26]. In neurons, the presence of tachyzoites or bradyzoites alters the functioning of infected neurons. These modifications will favor the persistence of the parasite [27, 28].

2.3 The regulation of the cerebral immune mechanism during *T. gondii* infection

After *T. gondii* has entered the CNS through the BBB, a cerebral immune response is triggered against the parasite. Experimental data on animal models show that the Th1-type immune response is activated against *T. gondii* to control the replication of the parasite in the brain. In the murine model, this immune response leads to the production of IFN-γ after infection with the ME49 (type II) strain [29–31]. This cytokine is the main mediator of parasite resistance in the murine model. IFN-γ produced by brain-resident cells is crucial for facilitating both the protective innate and T cell-mediated immune responses to control cerebral infection with *T. gondii*. Mice deficient for the IFN-γ receptor or those that are neutralized by an anti-IFN-γ antibody, are unable to control acute *Toxoplasma* infection [32]. During this host response, other cytokines and chemokines are produced. These may promote the infiltration of immune cells to the site of infection [33]. T cells and IFN-γ are essential for maintaining the latency of chronic infection in the brain and the prevention of reactivation of latent infection. The protective activity of T lymphocytes (CD4+, CD8+) results in the production of IFN-γ (**Figure 1**). The protective activity of these cells has been demonstrated in a transfer of immune cells T, which conferred protection against the reactivation of cerebral toxoplasmosis in an IFN-γ deficient mouse [34]. However, the presence of TCD4 and TCD8 cells appears to be critical for the long-term maintenance of the latency of chronic *Toxoplasma* infection in the brain. In addition, mRNA encoding IFN-γ was also detected in the brains of *T. gondii*-infected and NK-cell deficient mice. This suggests that IFN-γ could be produced by non-T cells and non-NK cells. This production is important for the maintenance of chronic toxoplasmosis in the brains of mice [35]. Microglial cells and macrophages are identified as the major non-T and non-NK cells that express IFN-γ in the brains of *T. gondii*-infected mice [36]. Therefore, it is possible that the production of IFN-γ by these cells plays an important role in the prevention of cerebral toxoplasmosis. Microglial cells play an important role on the one hand in the innate defense system that limits parasite proliferation and on the other hand by regulating the production of chemokines that facilitate the accumulation of T lymphocytes at the parasite multiplication site. Murine astrocytes have also been implicated in inhibiting the growth of type II *T. gondii* strain *in vitro*. Astrocytes infected with ME49 (type II) *Toxoplasma* strain, produce IL-1, IL-6 and Granulocyte-Macrophage Colony-Stimulating Factor (GM-CSF) [37]. During the innate immune response, dendritic cells, macrophages, and neutrophils produce IL-12 in response to *T. gondii* infection. This cytokine is essential for the production of IFN-γ. Neutralization of IL-12 with antibodies to this cytokine resulted in 100% mortality in mice infected with an avirulent strain of *T. gondii*, mortality was associated with decreased production of IFN-γ [38]. In addition, IL-12 is also important for maintaining IFN-γ production by T cells during chronic infection. The production of IL-12 is regulated by Lipoxin A4 (LXA4), in order to avoid pathogenic inflammatory reactions in the brain during the chronic phase of *T. gondii* infection. This has been demonstrated by the high production of LXA4 in the serum of mice during chronic *Toxoplasma* infection 5-Lipoxygenase (5-LO) is an essential enzyme in the production of LXA4, 5-LO deficient mice succumbed to infection during the chronic phase, thus presenting a cerebral inflammatory reaction [39]. LXA4 is important for the downregulation of pro-inflammatory responses during the chronic phase of *T. gondii* infection. Studies have shown that lipoxins activate two receptors (AhR and LXAR) in dendritic cells. This activation triggers the expression of the suppressor of cytokine signaling (SOCS)-2. SOCS-2 deficient mice succumb to chronic *T. gondii* infection. This is accompanied by a strong production of IL-12, IFN-γ, and reduction of cerebral cysts [40]. Although Th1 immune responses play a critical role in resistance to *T. gondii* infection, Th2-like immune responses are also implicated in protective immunity. IL-4 plays a major role in the development of the cellular immune response and in the differentiation of T cells into Th2 cells. During the chronic phase of *Toxoplasma* infection, IL-4 inhibits the production of pro-inflammatory mediators to prevent the development of local inflammations, promoting the persistence of cysts in the brain. Mice deficient in IL-4 die during the late phase of infection [41]. In these mice, a histological study reveals local areas of acute inflammation associated with the multiplication of tachyzoites in the brain. These results indicate that IL-4 is protective against the development of toxoplasmic encephalitis by preventing the formation of cysts and the proliferation of tachyzoites in the brain. The action of IL-4 during the chronic phase of infection is enhanced by the production of IL-10 by T cells [41]. IL-10 also exerts an immunomodulatory role in regulating the Th1-type inflammatory immune response [42]. Mice deficient in IL-10 and treated with sulfadiazine develop fatal inflammatory responses in the brain during the late stage of infection [43]. IL-10 is important for the survival of mice during the acute and chronic phases of infection. This is confirmed by the neutralization of this cytokine in *T. gondii*-infected mice [44] and following vaccination of the mice with *T. gondii* antigens (E/SA) [45].

3. The role of *T. gondii* in the etiopathogenetic of psychiatric diseases

Any infectious agent can affect neurons and brain structures after activation of the proinflammatory immune response and neurotransmitters, thus causing psychosis. Among the different infectious agents, *T. gondii* has received more attention for its location in the CNS. Many studies have suggested that toxoplasmosis is a risk factor for the development of behavioral changes and neuropsychiatric disorders such as depression, Schizophrenia, Alzheimer and Parkinson diseases. During an acute infection, the parasite is mainly present in peripheral tissues and blood, but also has access to the brain via immune circulating cells, as is explained in the part of *Regulation of the cerebral immune mechanism during T. gondii infection*. An early feature of *T. gondii* brain infection is the activation of glial cells, particularly astrocytes and microglia [24, 25, 46]. *Toxoplasma* cysts reside in the brain during latent infection. In individuals with acquired immune deficiencies, e.g., AIDS, or undergoing prolonged immunity, suppressive treatments, reactivation of the infection can lead to toxoplasmic encephalitis, also calling for cerebral toxoplasmosis. In recent years it has been shown that the latent toxoplasmosis, although often rejected as asymptomatic and clinically unimportant, can modify host behavior in human and rodents. This parasite has the capacity to be an etiological factor for some neuropsychiatric diseases [47].

A bunch of data hypothesizes that latent toxoplasmosis may be a risk factor for the depression. The low-grade inflammation caused by the chronic *Toxoplasma* infection it could be related to the development of behavioral symptoms, but the results have been varied multifactorial [48]. Regarding, the possible relationship between *Toxoplasma* infection and depression, study shows that specific *Toxoplasma* IgG titer levels correlated positively with depression [49]. One study found that this infection affected susceptibility to depression and severity of depressive symptoms in pregnant women [50]. Another study showed that male subjects infected with *Bartonella henselae* displayed more severe depressive symptoms when co-infected with *T. gondii* [51] but Pearce and collaborators, Sutterland and collaborators concluded that there is not any relationship between *T. gondii* infection and depression [52, 53]. Psychiatric patients with primarily severe or very severe depression are displaying more severe symptoms when are infected with *T. gondii*. In this recent study, results suggest that *Toxoplasma* infection can be related to anxiety, burnout and potentially to the severity of depression [48]. The possible link between *T. gondii* infection and Parkinson diseases is controversial. Tissue cysts of *T. gondii* reside especially in the amygdala, olfactory bulbs, hippocampus, cortical regions, and hypothalamus and could actively inhibit neuronal function in chronically infected mice [54]. Tachyzoite infection of neurons resulted in a dysregulated Ca^{2+} influx upon stimulation with glutamate, the major excitatory amino acid in the CNS leading either too hyper- or hypo-responsive neurons. Other experiments indicate that tachyzoites deplete Ca^{2+} stores in the endoplasmic reticulum that may contribute to the altered behavior of the host [54]. In addition, alteration of neurotransmitter pathways, degradation of dopamine-producing nerve cells and neurogenic inflammation induced by *T. gondii* infection are mentioned as etiology that could eventually lead to Parkinson disease [55]. Regarding the effect of *Toxoplasma* on the production of dopamine (DOPA) in the brain, studies have shown that this parasite-induced high concentrations of DOPA and tyrosine hydroxylase (TH) in CNS [56]. Parkinson disease is associated with lower levels of DOPA. So, the association between *Toxoplasma* infection and neuropsychiatric disorders could be strongly related to Schizophrenia but not Parkinson's disease [57]. Evidence suggests that *T. gondii* could be an etiological factor for Schizophrenia. Clinically, latent toxoplasmosis and Schizophrenia both induce similar alteration in brain morphology: gray matter atrophy, loss of brain parenchyma, ventricle system enlargement, CD4+ and CD8+ T cell influx, pro-inflammatory immune system infiltration, dendritic retraction in basolateral amygdala accompanied by reduced corticosterone secretion, which may deal with *T. gondii*-induced behavioral change [47, 58, 59]. Indeed, the relationship between chronic or acute *Toxoplasma* infection and Schizophrenia seems to exist. Researches in this field are increasing to determine the existence of this association by epidemiological, medical and biological studies. The following section presents an overview of the explanations published.

3.1 The cerebral immune response activated during schizophrenia and *T. gondii* infection

In cerebral toxoplasmosis, the balance between host immunity and defense mechanisms in the event of parasite escape is the basis of asymptomatic infection. Inflammation and immune deregulation have consistently been observed in both *Toxoplasma* infection and Schizophrenia. In the acute phase of infection, Th1 proinflammatory reaction is promoted by cytokines released in CNS to control parasite multiplication, this reaction was controlled by activation of Th2 immune reaction to minimize local cerebral inflammation. This immune response enhances the multiplication of parasite and promotes persistence of *Toxoplasma* tissue cysts in neuronal and glial cells. In Schizophrenia, an imbalance Th1 and Th2 reaction have shown with major activation of Th2 immune response and production of IL-6 and IL-10 [60]. IFN-γ, IL-12, TNF-α, IL-4 and IL-10, together with IL-1 and IL-1β, IL-2, IL-6, granulocytes (GM-CSF and GSF), IL-17 and IL-23 are variably expressed by astrocytes, microglial cells, neuron, TCD4+ and TCD8+ cells [9, 13, 31, 41–43] (**Figure 1**). All these immune mediators have shown to be markers for acute exacerbations of Schizophrenia [60]. This immune system can influence mood and behavior through their ability to modulate neurotransmission; therefore, the idea that latent infection is clinically asymptomatic may be associated with neuropsychiatric disorders. Since tachyzoites induce inflammatory tropism in host cells more than bradyzoites, the proliferation of tachyzoites in the brain after cyst rupture may be related to the onset of Schizophrenia and other mental illnesses [61]. In people with acute Schizophrenia, the display of symptoms has increased responses to cytokines. With regard to cytokine-induced effects, the role of IL-1β and IFN-γ in the activation of astrocytes have a major role. These immune proteins induce activation of astrocytes and microglia cells to inhibit tachyzoite replication by producing high levels of NO. In addition, experimental studies in rodents have shown that TCD8+ cells play a central role in long-term immunity to *Toxoplasma*. Depletion of CD8+ T cells may cause reactivation of latent disease in later phases of chronic toxoplasmosis. Interest in the potential correlation to this observation is the regulation of TCD8+ lymphocytes typically observed in schizophrenic patients [62]. After a short acute toxoplasmosis phase, the infection becomes latent and becomes encysted in the central nervous system and muscle tissue, probably throughout the life of the infected host. Evidence suggests that the parasite affects the synthesis of neurotransmitters, particularly DOPA, in infected individuals, which could lead to neurological and psychiatric disorders [63]. In addition to the studies that directly indicated the association between *Toxoplasma* infection and the increased incidence of Schizophrenia, some indirect evidence also highlighted the role of *T. gondii* in the etiology of Schizophrenia. More knowledge about the pathogenesis of the disorder would lead to more effective prevention and treatment strategies.

3.2 The neurobiological studies related to *T. gondii* infection to schizophrenia disease

There are differences in *T. gondii* infection; the acute phase and the chronic and phase. Cerebral cysts are formed in the cerebral hemispheres, hippocampus, amygdala, basal ganglia, cerebellum, cerebral cortex, brainstem, and olfactory bulb, and a variety of brain cells that may be infected, including neurons, microglia and mainly astrocytes [46] (**Figure 1**). Encysted *T. gondii* bradyzoites are capable of inhibiting apoptosis and modulates some signaling pathways such as nuclear factor (NF-κB), mitogen-activated protein kinase (MAPKinase), phosphoinositide 3 kinase (PI3K)/PKB/Akt and c-Jun N-terminal kinases (JNK); so that they can persist in host cells for long periods of time [64]. As cysts develop, the host cell degenerates and can break, releasing bradyzoites that can differentiate into tachyzoites, invade and kill surrounding cells, if uncontrolled by the immune system. Especially in immunocompromised patients, the infection is severe, sometimes with hydrocephalus, acute necrotizing encephalitis, and glial nodules formation. Lesions in the brain can manifest as behavioral symptoms by interfering with brain function in the area surrounding the lesion via mass effects or paracrine secretions. This explains the observation of high-concentration tissue cysts in the amygdala and nucleus accumbens, containing dopamine in limbic regions of the brain known to be an important control of motivation, pleasure, dependence, reward, and fear [47]. Other effects are more intriguing; Alteration of the neurotransmitter involves the production of homologous proteins to aromatic amino acid TH and dopamine (DOPA) 2 receptor (D2R) compounds with an increase in DOPA synthesis, tryptophan (TRP) degradation and the decrease in serotonin synthesis [56, 65].

The most likely mechanism of action in Schizophrenia affects neurotransmission in specific brain areas such as the thalamic-cortical limbic circuit of DOPA, 5-hydroxytryptamine (5-HT), gamma-aminobutyric acid (GABA), and glutamate. As a result, schizophrenic patients show abnormal levels of these neurotransmitters. Studies show an increase in DOPA release in the limbic system [47, 66]. In addition, *T. gondii* involves in the etiopathogenesis of Schizophrenia affecting neurotransmitters, especially DOPA [67]. The production *T. gondii* bradyzoites leads to induce liberation of TH, the enzyme that catalyzes the conversion of L-tyrosine (L-Tyr) to L-dihydroxyphenylalanine (L-DOPA) [68] and then L-DOPA is converted to DOPA by the enzyme DOPA decarboxylase. Dopamine is shown to be an essential product that stimulates proliferation and enhance infection and conversion of *T. gondii* in the brain [68]. After the synthesis of DOPA, it is transformed into phenylalanine (Phe) and tyrosine (Tyr) via the activity of phenylalanine hydroxylase (PAH). the elevation of the Phe/Tyr ratio and the alteration of PAH activity is related to the activation of the Th1-type immune response, which is activated during *T. gondii* infection. The increase in DOPA production was originally thought to be a product of inflammation of brain tissue (**Figure 2**). Blood levels of Phe and Tyr were increased in *T. gondii*-positive individuals with aggressive personality traits, and in particular those with overt history of aggression and suicidal behavior, so this mechanism could explain the link between Toxoplasmosis and Schizophrenia [69]. The increased concentration of DOPA in specific parts of the brain of patients is presumed to be responsible for the positive symptoms of this mental disorder. However, studies

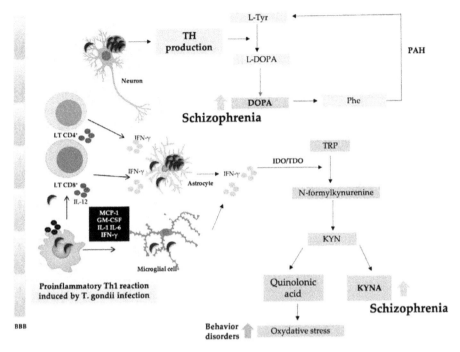

Figure 2.
Diagram showing the neurobiological pathway related to T. gondii *infection to schizophrenia disease.*

have identified two genes for limiting the TH synthesis in the genome of *T. gondii*; these genes expressed in the brain are responsible for DOPA overproduction in *T. gondii* tissue cysts that is responsible for the positive symptoms of some Schizophrenia patients [70].

In addition to DOPA, studies have also evaluated alterations of the kynurenine pathway (KYN) and involvement of TRP [71, 72]. In immunocompetent hosts, infection with *T. gondii* leads to the production of IFN-γ and production of indoleamine 2,3-dioxygenase (IDO), which converts the TRP to KYN and inhibits *T. gondii* growth. The metabolism of Tryptophan generates kynurenine and 3-hydroxykynurenine. The imbalance of these catabolites plays a role in the pathophysiology of Schizophrenia with positive and negative symptoms, which are reversible in response to antipsychotic treatment impact on such imbalance [71]. Additionally, alterations of the KYN pathway have also been shown with an increased KYN/TRP ratio and elevated kynurenic acid (KYNA) levels [73]. Activation of the KYN pathway following *T. gondii* infection may be part of a biological defense strategy against *T. gondii* infections. In the brain, this metabolism pathway takes place mainly in astrocytes that release newly produced KYNA into the extracellular environment, where it can influence surrounding neurons. KYNA synthesis is initiated also by tryptophan dioxygenase (TDO), this enzyme has shown that is elevated in the brains of Schizophrenia patients particularly in astrocytes and glial cells [74]. *T. gondii* infection in the CNS is accompanied, in response to parasite invasion or an inflammatory reaction, by strong activation of astrocytes and glial cells, resulting from high KYNA synthesis in these stimulated cells [75]. This reaction promotes high production of TDO or IDO in the brain and enhances proinflammatory cytokine expression in the site of *T. gondii* infection. These neurobiological data relating *Toxoplasma* infection to neuropsychiatric diseases.

4. Conclusion

The question that *Toxoplasma* infection could be the etiological cause psychological diseases and behavioral disorders is still under study. Recent studies try to prove this relationship. Study of Lindgren and collaborators demonstrated a significant association between *T. gondii* seropositivity and psychotic symptoms [76]. Vlatkovic and collaborators find an increased prevalence of *T. gondii* infection in a patient with Schizophrenia [77]. So, increased risk of developing toxoplasmosis infection prior to the onset of Schizophrenia was reported in several epidemiological, neurobiological and parasitological studies. One day this association will be a new method of diagnosis, treatment, and prevention of development of Schizophrenia. Therefore, health education on personal and nutritional hygiene given to patients and healthy people, especially early age, can help reduce the risk of contact with infectious agents and subsequently could decrease the incidence of behavior disorders.

Conflict of interest

The authors declare that there are no conflicts of interest regarding the publication of this chapter.

Author details

Mammari Nour* and Halabi Mohamad Adnan
Holy Family University, Batroun, Lebanon

*Address all correspondence to: nour.maamari@usf.edu.lb; nor-mammari@hotmail.fr

IntechOpen

© 2019 The Author(s). Licensee IntechOpen. This chapter is distributed under the terms of the Creative Commons Attribution License (http://creativecommons.org/licenses/by/3.0), which permits unrestricted use, distribution, and reproduction in any medium, provided the original work is properly cited. (cc) BY

References

[1] Dalimi A, Abdoli A. Latent toxoplasmosis and human. Iranian Journal of Parasitology. 2012;7:1-17

[2] Buoli M, Serati M, Caldiroli A, et al. Neurodevelopmental versus neurodegenerative model of schizophrenia and bipolar disorder: Comparison with physiological brain development and aging. Psychiatria Danubina. 2017;**29**:24-27

[3] Syn G, Anderson D, Blackwell JM, et al. Epigenetic dysregulation of host gene expression in *Toxoplasma* infection with specific reference to dopamine and amyloid pathways. Infection, Genetics and Evolution. 2018;**65**:159-162

[4] Soleymani E, Babamahmoodi F, Davoodi L, et al. Toxoplasmic encephalitis in an AIDS patient with normal CD4 count: A case report. Iranian Journal of Parasitology. 2018;**13**:317-322

[5] Marra CM. Central nervous system infection with *Toxoplasma gondii*. Handbook of Clinical Neurology. 2018;**152**:117-122

[6] Halonen SK, Weiss LM. Toxoplasmosis. Handbook of Clinical Neurology. 2013;**114**:125-145

[7] Długońska H. *Toxoplasma gondii* and the host cells. Annals of Parasitology. 2014;**60**:83-88

[8] Hunter CA, Sibley LD. Modulation of innate immunity by *Toxoplasma gondii* virulence effectors. Nature Reviews. Microbiology. 2012;**10**:766-778

[9] Mammari N, Vignoles P, Halabi MA, et al. Interferon gamma effect on immune mediator production in human nerve cells infected by two strains of *Toxoplasma gondii*. Parasite: Journal de la Société Française de Parasitologie. 2015;**22**:39

[10] Ajzenberg D. Type I strains in human toxoplasmosis: Myth or reality? Future Microbiology. 2010;**5**:841-843

[11] Delhaes L, Ajzenberg D, Sicot B, et al. Severe congenital toxoplasmosis due to a *Toxoplasma gondii* strain with an atypical genotype: Case report and review. Prenatal Diagnosis. 2010;**30**:902-905

[12] Konradt C, Ueno N, Christian DA, et al. Endothelial cells are a replicative niche for entry of *Toxoplasma gondii* to the central nervous system. Nature Microbiology. 2016;**1**:16001

[13] Mammari N, Vignoles P, Halabi MA, et al. In vitro infection of human nervous cells by two strains of *Toxoplasma gondii*: A kinetic analysis of immune mediators and parasite multiplication. PLoS ONE. 2014;**9**:e98491

[14] Corcino YL, Portillo J-AC, Subauste CS. Epidermal growth factor receptor promotes cerebral and retinal invasion by *Toxoplasma gondii*. Scientific Reports. 2019;**9**:669

[15] Schlüter D, Barragan A. Advances and challenges in understanding cerebral toxoplasmosis. Frontiers in Immunology. 14 February 2019;**10**. DOI: 10.3389/fimmu.2019.00242. [Epub ahead of print]

[16] Goverman J. Autoimmune T cell responses in the central nervous system. Nature Reviews. Immunology. 2009;**9**:393

[17] Tosh KW, Mittereder L, Bonne-Annee S, et al. The IL-12 response of primary human DC and monocytes to *Toxoplasma gondii* is stimulated by phagocytosis of live parasites rather than host cell invasion. Journal of Immunology (Baltimore, Md. : 1950). 2016;**196**:345-356

[18] Courret N, Darche S, Sonigo P, et al. CD11c- and CD11b-expressing mouse leukocytes transport single *Toxoplasma gondii* tachyzoites to the brain. Blood. 2006;**107**:309-316

[19] Lambert H, Hitziger N, Dellacasa I, et al. Induction of dendritic cell migration upon *Toxoplasma gondii* infection potentiates parasite dissemination. Cellular Microbiology. 2006;**8**:1611-1623

[20] Barragan A, Brossier F, Sibley LD. Transepithelial migration of *Toxoplasma gondii* involves an interaction of intercellular adhesion molecule 1 (ICAM-1) with the parasite adhesin MIC2. Cellular Microbiology. 2005;**7**:561-568

[21] Suzuki Y, Claflin J, Wang X, et al. Microglia and macrophages as innate producers of interferon-gamma in the brain following infection with *Toxoplasma gondii*. International Journal for Parasitology. 2005;**35**:83-90

[22] Ploix CC, Noor S, Crane J, et al. CNS-derived CCL21 is both sufficient to drive homeostatic CD4+ T cell proliferation and necessary for efficient CD4+ T cell migration into the CNS parenchyma following Toxoplasma gondii infection. Brain, Behavior, and Immunity. 2011;**25**:883-896

[23] Schuindt SHS, OBC d L, Pimentel PM de O, et al. Secretion of multi-protein migratory complex induced by *Toxoplasma gondii* infection in macrophages involves the uPA/uPAR activation system. Veterinary Parasitology. 2012;**186**:207-215

[24] Lüder CG, Giraldo-Velásquez M, Sendtner M, et al. *Toxoplasma gondii* in primary rat CNS cells: Differential contribution of neurons, astrocytes, and microglial cells for the intracerebral development and stage differentiation. Experimental Parasitology. 1999;**93**:23-32

[25] Contreras-Ochoa CO, Lagunas-Martínez A, Belkind-Gerson J, et al. *Toxoplasma gondii* invasion and replication within neonate mouse astrocytes and changes in apoptosis related molecules. Experimental Parasitology. 2013;**134**:256-265

[26] Hidano S, Randall LM, Dawson L, et al. STAT1 signaling in astrocytes is essential for control of infection in the central nervous system. MBio. 8 November 2016;**7**. DOI: 10.1128/mBio.01881-16. [Epub ahead of print]

[27] Song HB, Jung B-K, Kim JH, et al. Investigation of tissue cysts in the retina in a mouse model of ocular toxoplasmosis: Distribution and interaction with glial cells. Parasitology Research. 2018;**117**:2597-2605

[28] Halonen SK. Use of human neurons derived via cellular reprogramming methods to study host-parasite interactions of *Toxoplasma gondii* in neurons. Cell. 23 Sept 2017;**6**. DOI: 10.3390/cells6040032. [Epub ahead of print]

[29] Hwang YS, Shin J-H, Yang J-P, et al. Characteristics of infection immunity regulated by *Toxoplasma gondii* to maintain chronic infection in the brain. Frontiers in Immunology. 2018;**9**:158

[30] Lieberman LA, Hunter CA. Regulatory pathways involved in the infection-induced production of IFN-γ by NK cells. Microbes and Infection. 2002;**4**:1531-1538

[31] Sa Q, Ochiai E, Tiwari A, et al. Cutting edge: IFN-γ produced by brain-resident cells is crucial to control cerebral infection with *Toxoplasma gondii*. Journal of Immunology (Baltimore, Md. : 1950). 2015;**195**:796-800

[32] Scharton-Kersten T, Caspar P, Sher A, et al. *Toxoplasma gondii*: Evidence for interleukin-12-dependent

and-independent pathways of interferon-gamma production induced by an attenuated parasite strain. Experimental Parasitology. 1996;**84**:102-114

[33] Schlüter D, Deckert M, Hof H, et al. *Toxoplasma gondii* infection of neurons induces neuronal cytokine and chemokine production, but gamma interferon- and tumor necrosis factor-stimulated neurons fail to inhibit the invasion and growth of *T. gondii*. Infection and Immunity. 2001;**69**:7889-7893

[34] Kang H, Suzuki Y. Requirement of non-T cells that produce gamma interferon for prevention of reactivation of *Toxoplasma gondii* infection in the brain. Infection and Immunity. 2001;**69**:2920-2927

[35] Kang H, Suzuki Y. Requirement of Non-T cells That Produce Gamma Interferon for Prevention of Reactivation of *Toxoplasma gondii* infection in the brain. Infection and Immunity. 2001;**69**:2920-2927

[36] Wang X, Suzuki Y. Microglia produce IFN-γ independently from T cells during acute Toxoplasmosis in the brain. Journal of Interferon & Cytokine Research. 2007;**27**:599-605

[37] Halonen SK, Chiu F-C, Weiss LM. Effect of cytokines on growth of *Toxoplasma gondii* in murine astrocytes. Infection and Immunity. 1998;**66**:4989-4993

[38] Gazzinelli RT, Hieny S, Wynn TA, et al. Interleukin 12 is required for the T-lymphocyte-independent induction of interferon gamma by an intracellular parasite and induces resistance in T-cell-deficient hosts. Proceedings of the National Academy of Sciences of the United States of America. 1993;**90**:6115-6119

[39] Aliberti J, Serhan C, Sher A. Parasite-induced lipoxin A4 is an endogenous regulator of IL-12 production and immunopathology in *Toxoplasma gondii* infection. The Journal of Experimental Medicine. 2002;**196**:1253-1262

[40] Machado FS, Aliberti J. Impact of lipoxin-mediated regulation on immune response to infectious disease. Immunologic Research. 2006;**35**:209-218

[41] Suzuki Y, Yang Q, Yang S, et al. IL-4 is protective against development of toxoplasmic encephalitis. Journal of Immunology (Baltimore, Md. : 1950). 1996;**157**:2564-2569

[42] Ivanova DL, Denton SL, Fettel KD, et al. Innate lymphoid cells in protection, pathology, and adaptive immunity during apicomplexan infection. Frontiers in Immunology. 2019;**10**:196

[43] Wilson EH, Wille-Reece U, Dzierszinski F, et al. A critical role for IL-10 in limiting inflammation during toxoplasmic encephalitis. Journal of Neuroimmunology. 2005;**165**:63-74

[44] Jankovic D, Kullberg MC, Feng CG, et al. Conventional T-bet+Foxp3− Th1 cells are the major source of host-protective regulatory IL-10 during intracellular protozoan infection. The Journal of Experimental Medicine. 2007;**204**:273-283

[45] Abdollahi SH, Ayoobi F, Khorramdelazad H, et al. Interleukin-10 serum levels after vaccination with In vivo prepared *Toxoplasma gondii* excreted/secreted antigens. Oman Medical Journal. 2013;**28**:112-115

[46] Blanchard N, Dunay IR, Schlüter D. Persistence of *Toxoplasma gondii* in the central nervous system: A fine-tuned balance between the parasite, the brain and the immune system. Parasite Immunology. 2015;**37**:150-158

[47] Fabiani S, Pinto B, Bonuccelli U, et al. Neurobiological studies on the relationship between toxoplasmosis and neuropsychiatric diseases. Journal of the Neurological Sciences. 2015;**351**:3-8

[48] Bay-Richter C, Petersen E, Liebenberg N, et al. Latent toxoplasmosis aggravates anxiety- and depressive-like behaviour and suggest a role of gene-environment interactions in the behavioural response to the parasite. Behavioural Brain Research. 2019;**364**:133-139

[49] Suvisaari J, Torniainen-Holm M, Lindgren M, et al. *Toxoplasma gondii* infection and common mental disorders in the Finnish general population. Journal of Affective Disorders. 2017;**223**:20

[50] Nourollahpour Shiadeh M, Rostami A, Pearce BD, et al. The correlation between *Toxoplasma gondii* infection and prenatal depression in pregnant women. European Journal of Clinical Microbiology & Infectious Diseases. 2016;**35**:1829-1835

[51] Flegr J, Preiss M, Balátová P. Depressiveness and Neuroticism in bartonella seropositive and seronegative subjects-preregistered case-controls study. Frontiers in Psychiatry. 2018;**9**:314

[52] Pearce BD, Kruszon-Moran D, Jones JL. The relationship between *Toxoplasma gondii* infection and mood disorders in the NHANES III. Biological Psychiatry. 2012;**72**:290-295

[53] Sutterland AL, Fond G, Kuin A, et al. Beyond the association. *Toxoplasma gondii* in schizophrenia, bipolar disorder, and addiction: Systematic review and meta-analysis. Acta Psychiatrica Scandinavica. 2015;**132**:161-179

[54] Haroon F, Händel U, Angenstein F, et al. *Toxoplasma gondii* actively inhibits neuronal function in chronically infected mice. PLoS ONE. 2012;**7**:e35516

[55] Ramezani M, Shojaii M, Asadollahi M, et al. Seroprevalence of *Toxoplasma gondii* in Iranian patients with idiopathic Parkinson's disease. Clinical and Experimental Neuroimmunology. 2016;**7**:361-365

[56] Skallová A, Kodym P, Frynta D, et al. The role of dopamine in *Toxoplasma*-induced behavioural alterations in mice: An ethological and ethopharmacological study. Parasitology. 2006;**133**:525-535

[57] Fallahi S, Rostami A, Birjandi M, et al. Parkinson's disease and *Toxoplasma gondii* infection: Sero-molecular assess the possible link among patients. Acta Tropica. 2017;**173**:97-101

[58] Mitra R, Sapolsky RM, Vyas A. *Toxoplasma gondii* infection induces dendritic retraction in basolateral amygdala accompanied by reduced corticosterone secretion. Disease Models & Mechanisms. 2013;**6**:516-520

[59] Hermes G, Ajioka JW, Kelly KA, et al. Neurological and behavioral abnormalities, ventricular dilatation, altered cellular functions, inflammation, and neuronal injury in brains of mice due to common, persistent, parasitic infection. Journal of Neuroinflammation. 2008;**5**:48

[60] Miller BJ, Buckley P, Seabolt W, et al. Meta-analysis of cytokine alterations in schizophrenia: Clinical status and antipsychotic effects. Biological Psychiatry. 2011;**70**:663-671

[61] Tedford E, McConkey G. Neurophysiological changes induced by chronic *Toxoplasma gondii* infection. Pathogens (Basel, Switzerland). 17 May 2017;**6**. DOI: 10.3390/pathogens6020019. [Epub ahead of print]

[62] Bhadra R, Cobb DA, Weiss LM, et al. Psychiatric disorders in *Toxoplasma* seropositive patients—The CD8 connection. Schizophrenia Bulletin. 2013;**39**:485-489

[63] Del Grande C, Galli L, Schiavi E, et al. Is *Toxoplasma gondii* a trigger of bipolar disorder? Pathogens (Basel, Switzerland). 10 Jan 2017;**6**. DOI: 10.3390/pathogens6010003. [Epub ahead of print]

[64] Mammari N, Halabi MA, Yaacoub S, et al. *Toxoplasma gondii* modulates the host cell responses: An overview of apoptosis pathways. BioMed Research International. 2019:10

[65] Alsaady I, Tedford E, Alsaad M, et al. Downregulation of the central noradrenergic system by *Toxoplasma gondii* infection. Infection and Immunity. 2019;**87**:e00789-18

[66] Wang T, Sun X, Qin W, et al. From inflammatory reactions to neurotransmitter changes: Implications for understanding the neurobehavioral changes in mice chronically infected with *Toxoplasma gondii*. Behavioural Brain Research. 2019;**359**:737-748

[67] Xiao J, Prandovszky E, Kannan G, et al. *Toxoplasma gondii*: Biological parameters of the connection to schizophrenia. Schizophrenia Bulletin. 2018;**44**:983-992

[68] Gaskell EA, Smith JE, Pinney JW, Westhead DR, McConkey GA. A unique dual activity amino acid hydroxylase in *Toxoplasma gondii*. PLoS ONE 2009;**4**(3):e4801

[69] Mathai AJ, Lowry CA, Cook TB, et al. Reciprocal moderation by *Toxoplasma gondii* seropositivity and blood phenylalanine:tyrosine ratio of their associations with trait aggression. Pteridines. 2016;**27**:77-85

[70] Prandovszky E, Gaskell E, Martin H, et al. The neurotropic parasite *Toxoplasma gondii* increases dopamine metabolism. PLoS ONE. 2011;**6**(9):e23866. DOI: 10.1371/journal. pone.0023866

[71] Notarangelo FM, Wilson EH, Horning KJ, et al. Evaluation of kynurenine pathway metabolism in *Toxoplasma gondii*-infected mice: Implications for schizophrenia. Schizophrenia Research. 2014;**152**:261-267

[72] Bay-Richter C, Buttenschøn HN, Mors O, et al. Latent toxoplasmosis and psychiatric symptoms: A role of tryptophan metabolism? Journal of Psychiatric Research. 2019;**110**:45-50

[73] Schwarcz R, Hunter CA. *Toxoplasma gondii* and schizophrenia: Linkage through astrocyte-derived kynurenic acid? Schizophrenia Bulletin. 2007;**33**:652-653

[74] Miller CL, Llenos IC, Dulay JR, et al. Expression of the kynurenine pathway enzyme tryptophan 2,3-dioxygenase is increased in the frontal cortex of individuals with schizophrenia. Neurobiology of Disease. 2004;**15**:618-629

[75] Wurfel BE, Drevets WC, Bliss SA, et al. Serum kynurenic acid is reduced in affective psychosis. Translational Psychiatry. 2017;7:e1115

[76] Lindgren M, Torniainen-Holm M, Härkänen T, et al. The association between *Toxoplasma* and the psychosis continuum in a general population setting. Schizophrenia Research. 2018;**193**:329-335

[77] Vlatkovic S, Sagud M, Svob Strac D, et al. Increased prevalence of *Toxoplasma gondii* seropositivity in patients with treatment-resistant schizophrenia. Schizophrenia Research. 2018;**193**:480-481

Biology in Parasites and Microbes

Chapter 8

Sexual Processes in Microbial Eukaryotes

Harris Bernstein and Carol Bernstein

Abstract

Two principal ideas have been proposed to explain the primary adaptive function of the sexual process of meiosis: (1) meiosis, and particularly meiotic recombination, is a process for repairing DNA and (2) meiosis, by means of meiotic recombination, is a process for generating beneficial genetic variation among progeny. We review the sexual processes of a number of well-studied microbial eukaryotes: *Saccharomyces cerevisiae*, *Saccharomyces paradoxus*, *Schizosaccharomyces pombe*, *Candida albicans*, *Ustilago maydis*, *Paramecium tetraurelia*, *Volvox carteri*, *Trypanosoma brucei*, *Neurospora crassa*, and *Amoebozoa*. We indicate aspects of the sexual processes of these microbial eukaryotes, where they have been established, that support the idea that meiosis is primarily a process for repairing DNA. In addition, we review the likely origin of meiotic sex among the microbial eukaryotes. A prokaryotic archaeon is the likely ancestor of eukaryotes. Extant archaea are capable of a sexual process involving syngamy and recombinational repair of genome damage, suggesting that the precursor of eukaryotic meiotic sex may already have been present in the archaeal ancestor of eukaryotes. We believe that attainment of an understanding of the adaptive function of meiotic sex in microbial eukaryotes is of considerable importance since it will likely apply to meiotic sex in eukaryotes generally.

Keywords: meiosis, adaptive benefit, DNA repair, homologous recombination, genetic variation

1. Introduction

Different microbial eukaryotic species are capable of a variety of sexual processes. Basically, however, the different sexual processes have, as a central element, syngamy and meiosis. Syngamy is the fusion of two cells or two nuclei. Meiosis is ordinarily initiated in a diploid cell that contains a pair of homologs, which is two copies of each chromosome. In meiosis, generally, first the cell undergoes DNA replication, so each homolog now consists of two identical sister chromatids. Next, homologous chromosomes undergo intimate pairing with each other and exchange genetic information by homologous recombination. Recombination is succeeded by two cycles of cell division to yield four haploid daughter cells each having half the number of chromosomes as the original diploid cell. Some microbial eukaryotes, however, use a similar process, parasexual meiosis. This is where ploidy (the number of complete sets of chromosomes in a cell) is determined, both before and after homologous recombination, by processes other than those in standard meiosis. One of the microbial eukaryotes we discuss, below, *Candida albicans,* uses parasexual meiosis.

There appears to be broad agreement among geneticists that the key to under-standing why sex exists is to understand the adaptive benefit of meiotic homologous recombination, the molecular event that syngamy and meiosis seem designed to promote. The evidence reviewed here on microbial eukaryotes, we think, sup-ports the general view that the meiotic recombination mechanism is maintained by natural selection at each generation because of the benefit of DNA repair [1]. Recombinational repair is especially beneficial as an adaptation for responding to stressful conditions, such as starvation or oxidative stress, that cause DNA damage.

Meiotic sex appears to be very widespread among microbial eukaryotes. In 1999, Dacks and Roger [2] proposed, on the basis of phylogenetic evidence, that the common ancestor of all known eukaryotes was likely facultatively sexual. Since this proposal was presented, sex has been reported in several microbial eukaryotes that had previously been considered to be asexual. Examples of organisms recently recognized to be sexual are *Giardia intestinalis* (syn. *G. lamblia*) and *Trichomonas vaginalis*. These microbial eukaryotes were found to possess a core set of genes that function in meiosis, including genes that encode proteins that are specific to meiosis and act in homologous recombination [3, 4]. Both *G. intestinalis* and *T. vaginalis* are descended from ancient lineages that diverged from each other early in the evolu-tion of eukaryotes, thus indicating that core genes necessary for meiosis, and hence sex, were likely present in an early ancestor of both species. Parasitic protozoans of the genus *Leishmania* are another example of eukaryotic microbes once consid-ered to be asexual, but subsequently found upon further investigation, to have a sexual cycle [5]. Also, evidence for meiotic sex has recently been reported for the phylum *Amoebozoa*, another early diverging lineage in eukaryotic evolution (see Section 10). Fungi, a diverse group of eukaryotic microorganisms, also appear to be anciently sexual [6]. Recent findings on additional species, reviewed by Speijer et al. [7], also tend to substantiate the concept that sex is an ancient, ubiquitous and fundamental feature of eukaryotic life. Such varied reports have contributed to the current understanding that meiotic sex is likely a fundamental and primordial property of eukaryotes (e.g. [3, 4, 8]).

We describe here the typical stages of the sexual cycles of eukaryotic microbes, although the amount of time spent in each stage is variable among species. The stages are: (1) Haploid cells reproduce by mitosis (vegetative growth). (2) Haploid cell undergo cellular fusion (syngamy) to form a heterokaryon that may undergo further mitotic divisions (vegetative growth). (3) A diploid cell is formed when two haploid nuclei fuse. Diploid cells may also undergo additional mitotic divisions (vegetative growth). (4) The meiotic process is initiated in the nucleus of a diploid cell by undergoing a round of DNA replication without cell division, so that the nucleus has four copies of its genome. Conventionally, the nucleus at this stage is described as having two sets of homologous chromosomes where each chromo-some is composed of two sister chromatids (a chromatid being equivalent to a long DNA molecule bound with appropriate histone proteins). (5) Homologous chromatids undergo intimate pairing (synapsis) including pairing of non-sister homologous chromatids. (6) Genetic information is exchanged between the paired homologous chromatids by a process of recombination. Recombination may involve breakage and exchange between paired chromatids, but in most cases information is exchanged without breakage and exchange by a process referred to as synthesis dependent strand annealing [9]. (7) Meiosis is completed by two successive cell divisions whereby a cell nucleus, starting with four copies of the genome, produces four cell nuclei each having a single copy of the genome. During the first meiotic division chromosome segregation occurs so that after completion of the division there is one set of chromosomes (each with two chromatids) in each cell nucleus. During the second meiotic division there is only one set of chromatids (each

chromatid, now renamed as a chromosome, in each cell nucleus). That is, haploidy
is restored. In parasexual meiosis, control of ploidy both before and after homologous recombination may occur by processes other than those in "standard" meiosis
(see Section 5). The life cycle may now be repeated starting at stage (1).

2. *Saccharomyces cerevisiae* and *Saccharomyces paradoxus*

The budding yeast *S. cerevisiae* (**Figure 1A**) is a microbial fungus in the Division
Ascomycota. S. cerevisiae occurs in nature as haploid (n) or diploid (2n) cells
(**Figure 1B**). Haploid vegetative cells can reproduce by mitosis under favorable conditions. Diploid cells can also reproduce by mitosis when nutrients are abundant.
However, when quiescent *S. cerevisiae* are starved, they accumulate DNA damages
that include double-strand breaks and apurinic/apyrimidinic sites [10]. *S. cerevisiae*
cells maintained in a non-replicating quiescent state undergo chronological aging

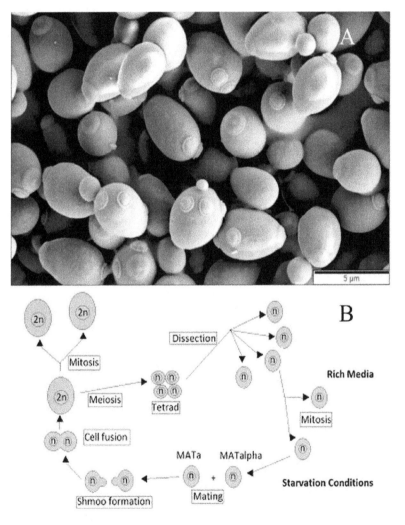

Figure 1.
(A) Budding yeast Saccharomyces cerevisiae *[13] and (B) cycle of sexual and vegetative reproduction*
S. cerevisiae *[14].*

during which they accumulate DNA double-strand breaks and their ability to repair such damages declines [11]. When starving (and accumulating DNA damages), haploid cells can mate to form diploid cells that can undergo meiosis to produce four haploid spores that are contained within a sac-like structure, the ascus (tetrad) [12] (**Figure 1B**). Such spores are resistant to stress, but under favorable conditions can germinate to produce haploid descendants by mitosis. When haploid cells of mating type MATa and MATalpha come into contact with each other they can fuse to form a diploid cell (syngamy) that may then either reproduce by mitosis or, if stressed, initiate another sexual cycle by undergoing meiosis. Recombination between homologous chromosomes is a central feature of meiosis and involves the systematic intimate pairing of homologous chromosomes. This process facilitates recombinational repair of DNA damages [9].

Increased sensitivity to killing by DNA damaging radiation or DNA damaging chemicals is a general characteristic of *S. cerevisiae* mutants that are defective in genes necessary for meiotic and mitotic recombination [15]. As an example, *Rad52* mutants of *S. cerevisiae* are deficient in meiotic and mitotic recombination and have increased susceptibility to killing by X-rays, methyl methanesulfonate and agents that introduce DNA crosslinks [15–17]. Homologous recombination is also necessary for recovery from oxidative DNA damage [18]. Such results demonstrate that DNA damages caused by diverse agents can be removed by recombinational repair.

A major effect of X-irradiation is the introduction of double-strand breaks in DNA. *S. cerevisiae* diploid cells in mitotic G1 phase are unable to repair such lethal X-ray induced damages [19]. However, *S. cerevisiae* cells in the G1 phase of meiosis are more resistant to the lethal effect of X-rays than cells in the mitotic G1 phase [19]. This suggests that X-ray induced lethal DNA damages are more efficiently repaired when occurring in meiotic G1 compared to mitotic G1. The increased resistance of cells undergoing meiosis may be explained by the intimate pairing of homologous chromosomes during meiosis which facilitates the replacement of damaged sequence information in one homolog by intact information from the other homolog.

Another proposed benefit of meiotic recombination, aside from DNA repair, is the production of progeny of varied genetic constitution, as occurs in outcross matings between unrelated individuals.

A study of the ancestry of natural *S. cerevisiae* strains indicated that outcrossing to an unrelated strain occurs only about once every 50,000 cell divisions [20]. That is, in nature, *S. cerevisiae* outcrossing is rare and mating is ordinarily between closely related cells. In nature, matings of *S. cerevisiae* tend to be between close relatives for two reasons [20]. First, the products of individual meiotic events are contained within the sac-like ascus, and each ascus contains a tetrad of ascospores, two ascospores of each mating type. Cells of different mating type from the same ascus tend to mate with each other because of their proximity, and such matings are between closely related individuals, which may not yield much, if any, genetic variation among the progeny. The second reason that mating tends to occur between genetically close relatives is mating type switching. Here, a cell of one mating type, upon mitotic cell division, produces two cells, usually one of the same mating types as the original cell and, often, a second cell of the opposite mating type. These two cells are physically adjacent and can mate with each other. Thus, in nature, the sexual cycle of *S. cerevisiae* can provide the benefit of recombinational repair, but only infrequently provides genetic variation.

In natural populations of the species *Saccharomyces paradoxus*, a sister species of *S. cerevisiae*, the frequency of matings between meiotic products from the same tetrad is estimated to be about 94% [21]. Also about 5% of matings are between clone-mates after switching of mating type. Only 1% of matings appear to be outcrossings. Outcrossing, in principal, may provide the adaptive benefit of generating beneficial genetic variants. Nevertheless, the low frequency of outcrossing in natural populations of *S. cerevisiae* and *S. paradoxus* indicates that the production of genetic variation is unlikely to be the principal selective force maintaining meiotic sex in these organisms. On the other hand, meiosis facilitates homologous recombinational repair of DNA damages and such repair is especially beneficial under stressful conditions that are likely to be common in nature. This proposed benefit is compatible with the hypothesis that, in general, the principal selective force maintaining meiotic sex is DNA repair [1, 22, 23].

3. *Schizosaccharomyces pombe*

S. pombe, also referred to as "fission yeast," is a unicellular rod-shaped eukaryotic microorganism in the Division *Ascomycota*. It grows vegetatively primarily as a haploid organism. *S. pombe* is facultatively sexual, so that when nutrients are limiting cells of opposite mating type tend to undergo syngamy (union of gametes) to form diploid zygotes [24]. The zygote can then enter meiosis leading to the production of four haploid products (spores) initially enclosed in a sac called an ascus.

Several different types of experiments have shown that DNA damages induce the sexual cycle and meiotic recombination in *S. pombe*. First, exposure of *S. pombe* cells to hydrogen peroxide, a reactive chemical that causes oxidative DNA damage, was observed to lead to an increase in sexual reproduction associated with a 4- to 18-fold increase in the formation of meiotic spores [25]. Second, DNA damages, in which the base cytosine is deaminated to uracil, forming the inappropriate base pair dU:dG, stimulate meiotic recombination [26]. Third, faulty processing of DNA replication intermediates (referred to as Okazaki fragments) produces DNA damages, including single-strand breaks or gaps, that stimulate meiotic recombination [27].

The fission yeast *S. pombe*, like the budding yeast *S. cerevisiae* (see above), switches mating type during vegetative growth, though they each use different mechanisms [28]. This provides *S. pombe* with increased mating opportunities with close relatives. The decreased opportunity for outcrossing in *S. pombe* indicates that the production of genetic variation is unlikely to be the principal selective force maintaining meiotic sex in these organisms. Overall, the findings with *S. pombe*, like those with the other yeasts, *S. cerevisiae* and *S. paradoxus,* suggest that meiotic recombination is primarily an adaptation for repairing DNA damage.

4. *Ustilago maydis*

U. maydis is a fungus in the Division *Basidiomycota*. It is a plant pathogen that causes corn smut. *U. maydis* teliospores are thick-walled rounded melanized cells with diploid nuclei that are capable of tolerating extreme temperatures and desiccation. Before teliospores mature in the infected corn plant, meiosis is initiated [29]. As teliospores germinate they complete meiosis to produce four haploid basidiospores [29].

Plants often defend themselves from pathogenic microbial invasion by releasing an oxidative burst that includes the production of reactive oxygen species [30]. *U. maydis* can protect against the host oxidative attack by an oxidative stress response [30]. In protecting against oxidative DNA damage, *U. maydis* employs a recombinational DNA repair system that includes the Rad51 protein (related to mammalian

Rad51), a Rec2 protein (more distantly related to mammalian Rad51), and the Brh2 protein [that is related to the mammalian Breast Cancer 2 (Brca2) protein)] [31]. When any of these proteins is inactive, *U. maydis* becomes more sensitive to DNA damaging agents, mitotic recombination is reduced, and there is failure to complete meiosis [31]. Recombinational repair occurring during meiosis as teliospores are formed by the pathogen likely contributes to the maintenance of its genome integrity by removing DNA damages incurred during infection.

5. *Candida albicans*

Candida albicans, a type of diploid yeast in the Division *Ascomycota*, is the most commonly encountered fungal pathogen in humans. The human infection candidiasis, resulting from overgrowth of *C. albicans*, often occurs in immunocompromised patients [32]. *C. albicans* can be induced to undergo a parasexual cycle that involves mating of diploids (syngamy) to form a tetraploid that subsequently appears to undergo a form of meiosis, followed by chromosome loss leading to approximately diploid cells with high levels of aneuploidy and homozygosity [33]. The *C. albicans* genome contains many genes that are homologous to genes in other species that function in meiosis [34]. One such gene, *Dmc1*, encodes a protein that has a central role in homologous recombination and is only known to express during meiosis [35]. Under appropriate conditions, *C. albicans* is capable of same sex mating and can undergo extensive genetic recombination between homologous chromosomes [36]. The two successive cell divisions that ordinarily occur subsequent to meiotic recombination in other organisms appear to be absent in *C. albicans* meiosis. Instead a reduction from four copies of the genome (tetraploidy) to two copies (diploidy) occurs by random chromosome loss during the mitotic cell division subsequent to meiotic recombination [37]. Although *C. albicans* populations are largely clonal, parasexual recombination can facilitate the evolution of resistance to the antifungal agent fluconazole upon exposure to the agent over successive generations [38].

The parasexual cycle appears to occur with greater frequency under environmental stress condition [33]. Glucose starvation and oxidative stress are environmental stresses that are commonly encountered by pathogenic *C. albicans*, and these stresses efficiently induce same-sex mating between cells from a single progenitor [39]. As suggested by Guan and collaborators [39], same sex mating in *C. albicans* may be an important mode of sexual reproduction that occurs often in nature. Oxidative stress, associated with an increase in reactive oxygen species, causes DNA damage and thus the induction of mating may reflect an adaptive DNA repair response.

Unlike *C. albicans*, several other *Candida* clade species have a sexual cycle that includes ordinary meiosis and formation of sexual spores [37]. It appears that *C. albicans* has retained meiotic homologous recombination, a principal feature of sexual reproduction that provides the adaptive benefit of DNA repair, while losing the ability to undergo successive cell divisions in an organized fashion to reduce ploidy.

6. *Paramecium tetraurelia*

P. tetraurelia is a unicellular eukaryotic ciliate in the Phylum *Ciliophora* (**Figure 2**). It has two diploid micronuclei and a polyploid macronucleus. The

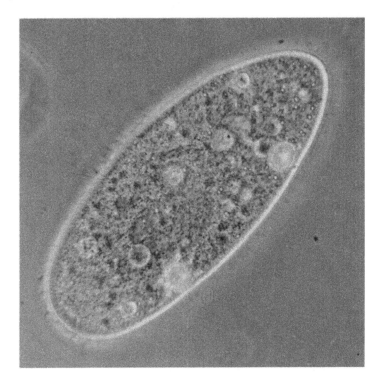

Figure 2.
Paramecium tetraurelia *[41].*

micronuclear chromosomal DNA contains the genetic information that is inherited from one generation to the next, whereas the macronucleus contains many chromosomal DNA copies that express cellular functions. *P. tetraurelia* is able to undergo both asexual and sexual reproduction. Asexual reproduction occurs by binary fission in which the micronuclei divide by mitosis and the macronucleus divides by amitotic division [40]. Sexual reproduction involves a meiotic process, either automixis or conjugation. Automixis is a kind of self-fertilization, whereas conjugation involves mating with another individual.

As *P. tetraurelia* undergoes asexual reproduction by binary fission over many successive generations, the vitality of the lineage declines (clonal aging) until the lineage reaches the end of its clonal lifespan at about 200 fissions [42]. However, if *P. tetraurelia* undergoes automixis or conjugation during clonal aging, vitality is restored. Several laboratories found that clonal aging is associated with a dramatic increase in DNA damage [42–44]. When clonally aged *P. tetraurelia* undergo automixis or conjugation, the micronuclei go through meiosis followed by pairwise nuclear fusion (syngamy) of haploid meiotic products either from the same individual (automixis) or from different individuals (conjugation) to form a new diploid micronucleus. Subsequent to the formation of a new diploid micronucleus, the old macronucleus disintegrates and the new micronucleus replicates to form a new macronucleus. The paramecia that undergo this process have their clonal lifespan restored and are rejuvenated. Clonal aging thus appears to be caused to a large extent by progressive accumulation of DNA damage and rejuvenation likely depends on the repair of such damages in the micronuclear DNA during meiosis followed by the reestablishment of macronuclear DNA by replication of the newly repaired micronuclear DNA.

7. *Volvox carteri*

Volvox carteri is in the Phylum *Chlorophyta*. It is a facultatively sexual species of colonial green algae. The *V. carteri* life cycle can include both a sexual and asexual phase. Under natural conditions, *V. carteri* reproduces asexually in temporary ponds during the spring. However, before the ponds dry up in the summer heat, it becomes sexual forming male and female gametes which can then undergo fertilization to form a desiccation resistant overwintering diploid zygospore. Germination of zygospores involves meiosis and takes place when environmental conditions become favorable, usually the next spring.

V. carteri can be induced by heat shock to undergo sexual reproduction [45]. Antioxidants can inhibit this induction, indicating that oxidative stress likely mediates the induction of sexual reproduction by heat shock [46]. Also implicating oxidative stress is the finding that an inhibitor of the mitochondrial electron transport chain, that causes an increase in reactive oxygen species, induces sex in *V. carteri* [47]. Thus the induction of facultative sex, even under natural conditions, may be due to oxidative stress, a condition that causes oxidative DNA damage [47].

8. *Trypanosoma brucei*

Human African trypanosomiasis (sleeping sickness) is caused by *T. brucei* infection (**Figure 3**). *T. brucei* undergoes meiosis within the salivary glands of its tsetse fly vector. Meiosis appears to be a normal part of the developmental cycle of *T. brucei* [49–51]. Three proteins that are only known to express during meiosis, Dmc1, Mad1 and Hop1, are found to be expressed in the nucleus of a small fraction of dividing epimastigote trypanosomes in the salivary glands and nowhere else [51, 52]. Haploid gametes produced by meiosis can subsequently undergo pairwise interaction leading to cell fusion [49].

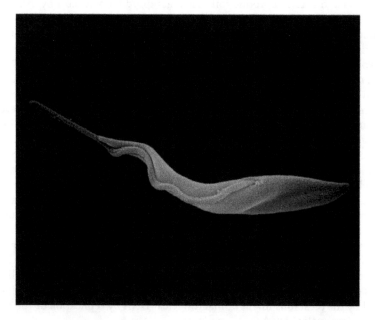

Figure 3.
Trypanosoma brucei *[48]*.

Tsetse flies are able to resist trypanosome infection by mounting immune defenses [50]. The flies' defenses include the ability to produce increased levels of reactive oxygen species (ROS) such as hydrogen peroxide [51, 53]. ROS can cause DNA damage, including double-strand breaks. *T. brucei* can carry out homologous recombinational repair of double-strand breaks [54]. Such a repair process is likely facilitated in *T. brucei* by homologous chromosome pairing during meiosis. This process may help protect *T. brucei* against the assault by ROS mounted by the tsetse fly host.

Trypanosomes are classified in the supergroup *Excavata* that are one of the earliest diverging eukaryotic lineages [55]. The discovery of a sexual stage in *T. brucei* supports the idea that meiotic sexual production is an ancestral characteristic of eukaryotes [49] (see Section 1).

9. *Neurospora crassa*

The *Ascomycete Neurospora crassa* grows vegetatively as a haploid filamentous fungus. **Figure 4A** illustrates a segment of haploid hyphae which form a mass of

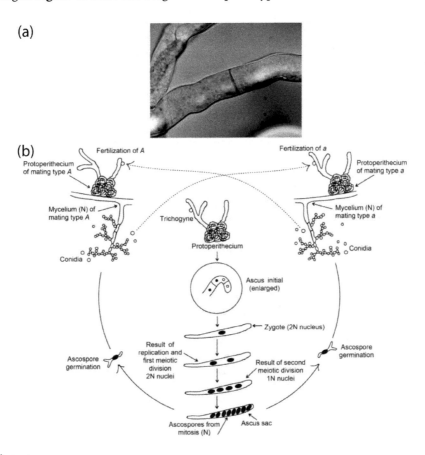

Figure 4.
(A) Neurospora crassa *hyphae [58], (B)* Neurospora crassa *life cycle. The haploid mycelium reproduces asexually by two processes: (1) simple proliferation of existing mycelium, and (2) formation of conidia (macro- and micro-) which can be dispersed and then germinate to produce new mycelium. In the sexual cycle, mating can only occur between individual strains of different mating type, A and a. Fertilization occurs by the passage of nuclei of conidia or mycelium of one mating type into the protoperithecia of the opposite mating type through the trichogyne. Fusion of the nuclei of opposite mating types occurs within the protoperithecium to form a zygote (2N) nucleus [59].*

thread-like filaments comprising the mycelium which is the vegetative part of the fungus. The life cycle of *N. crassa* is outlined in **Figure 4B** which indicates the structures and events of sexual reproduction. Like *S. cerevisiae*, *N. crassa* has two mating types. Sexual interaction in *N. crassa* can only occur between individuals of opposite mating type. The diploid stage is very brief, occurring just prior to entry into meiosis. However, the brief diploid stage of *N. crassa* involves considerable complexity. The haploid vegetative multicellular filamentous stage, although longer lasting and larger than the diploid stage, has a relatively simple modular structure. In natural populations, recessive mutations specifically affecting the diploid stage are quite frequent [56]. Such diplophase specific mutations, when homozygous, can cause barren fruiting bodies (perithecia) and failure to form asci. Homozygous mutations can also lead to an abnormal meiosis with faulty pachytene or diplotene stages, or defective chromosome pairing [57]. At least 435 genes were estimated to affect the diploid stage [56]. This is at least 4% of the total 9730 genes of *N. crassa*. Thus it appears that the requirement for union of opposite mating types provides the adaptive benefit, in the diploid stage, of allowing the masking of deleterious recessive mutations (complementation) while also promoting the recombinational repair benefits of meiosis.

Species of *Neurospora*, including *N. crassa*, have life cycles adapted to ecosystems arising as the result of fire [60]. *Neurospora* species are common primary colonizers of trees and shrubs that have been killed by fire in Western North America. Fire appears to provide heat and chemical byproducts necessary for germination of ascospores that have been produced by sexual reproduction. Also fire can create a sterile environment with an abundance of nutrients derived from dead plant tissues upon which *Neurospora* can grow. The distribution of *Neurospora* growing at natural sites suggests that initial colonization by heat resistant ascospores is followed by vegetative growth, the production of conidia and then the dispersal of the conidia.

10. *Amoebozoa*

The *Amoebozoa*, a phylum within the kingdom *Protozoa*, contains about 2400 described species. Amoebozoan species include a variety of lineages of polymorphic amoeboid forms that until recently were considered to be asexual. A recent study, however revealed that amoebozoans representing all major subclades possess most of the genes that function specifically in meiosis, as well as many of the genes involved in meiotic recombinational repair [61]. It was concluded that *Amoebozoa* is ancestrally sexual. Since the *Amoebozoa* diverged in eukaryotic evolution before 720 million years ago [62], these findings suggest that meiotic sex was present early in eukaryotic evolution.

Another analysis of the *Amoebozoa* also supported the probable occurrence of syngamy (cell fusion) and meiotic processes in all major amoebozoan lineages [63]. This study concluded that most amoebozoans are likely capable of a canonical meiotic process. As one example, wild populations of the social amoeba *Dictyostelium discoideum* undergo widespread mating and sexual reproduction including meiosis when food is scarce [64, 65]. The evidence for the occurrence of meiotic sex among the amoebozoa is consistent with the general idea (see Section 1) that meiotic sex is likely a primitive characteristic of eukaryotes.

11. Eukaryotic sexual processes likely arose in the archaea

From about 3.4 billion to 570 million years ago, microbes were the only forms of life. The last common ancestor of all eukaryotes arose before 1.5 billion years ago [66].

The eukaryotic common ancestor is considered to have arisen when an anaerobic host archaeal cell acquired an internalized aerobic bacterium [67]. The internalized aerobe eventually evolved into the mitochondrion, providing the capability for respiration. The ancestral archaeal genome appears to have contributed more important genes to the eukaryotic nuclear genome (such as those genes involved in transcription, translation and replication) than the internalized aerobe [68]. Meiotic sex appears to be a primordial characteristic of eukaryotes (see Section 1). This suggests that sexual processes may already have been present in the archaeal microbe from which eukaryotes arose. Extant archaeal species such as *Sulfolobus solfataricus* and *Sulfolobus acidocaldarius* as well as several other archaeal species undergo interactions that have key features similar to sexual processes in microbial eukaryotes [69].

For instance, the hyperthermophilic archaeon *S. solfataricus* expresses the RadA protein, a homolog of the eukaryotic proteins Rad51 and Dmc1 that catalyze DNA pairing and strand exchange, central steps in recombinational repair during meiosis [70]. Exposure of *S. solfataricus* to DNA damaging UV irradiation or agents that cause DNA double-strand breaks induces pilus formation leading to cellular aggregation [71]. UV-induced cellular aggregation mediates high frequency chromosomal marker exchange between cells [72]. The DNA damage inducible DNA transfer process and subsequent homologous recombination were hypothesized to represent an important mechanism for providing increased repair of damaged DNA via homologous recombination in order to maintain genome integrity [71–73]. Van Wolferan and collaborators [74, 75] also obtained evidence with *S. acidocaldarius* that led them to propose that DNA transfer occurs in order to repair DNA damages by homologous recombination. Thus it appears likely that key elements of eukaryotic meiosis, namely the coming together and intimate alignment of chromosomes from different cells followed by repair of DNA damage by homologous recombination, already existed in the archaeal ancestors of eukaryotes. To some extent, these key elements are also present in many extant eubacteria, particularly in those species capable of natural genetic transformation [1]. This suggests that sexual processes were even present in a common ancestor of both eubacteria and archaea.

12. Conclusions

Meiotic sex appears to be a primordial characteristic of microbial eukaryotes and has likely provided a continuous adaptive benefit for as long as 1.5 billion years in diverse lineages of microbial eukaryotes. Since eukaryotes appear to have evolved from an archaeal ancestor, the adaptive function of sexual processes, even in archaeal species, is relevant to understanding sexual processes in microbial eukaryotes. In the archaea, homologous recombinational repair of DNA damages appears to be the principal adaptive benefit of sexual processes. Conclusions bearing on the adaptive benefit of sexual processes (syngamy and meiosis) in microbial eukaryotes are summarized below.

The dikaryotic fungi (*Ascomycetes* and *Basidiomycetes*) include some of the most well-studied microbial eukaryotic species with respect to sexual reproduction. Wallen and Perlin [76] concluded in a 2018 review of the function and maintenance of sexual reproduction in the dikaryotic fungi that sexual reproduction, including its central feature of homologous recombination, evolved to repair DNA damages that arise particularly from environmental stresses. In the ascomycete yeast *S. cerevisiae*, DNA repair by homologous recombination during mitosis is well established. Recombinational repair during meiosis is stimulated under starvation conditions and appears to be even more efficient than during mitosis. In natural populations of *S. cerevisiae* and *S. paradoxus*, the great majority of matings that occur are between closely genetically related individuals. Thus sex in these species is unlikely to be primarily maintained by an adaptive benefit of producing genetic variation.

The ascomycete *S. pombe*, like *S. cerevisiae*, tends to mate when nutrients are scarce. Introduction of DNA damage by different DNA damaging conditions stimulates sexual reproduction and meiotic recombination, consistent with the idea that meiotic recombination is an adaptation for repair. Another ascomycete, *C. albicans* is regarded as a parasexual, rather than sexual, species since it appears to undergo a meiotic process that is not associated with the organized chromosome segregation that normally results in haploid meiotic products. Nevertheless *C. albicans* contains a set of genes homologous to genes that function in meiosis in other species including a key gene that only functions in meiosis. Same sex mating in *C. albicans* likely occurs frequently in nature especially under environmental stress conditions. *U. maydis* is a basidiomycete fungus. Upon infecting its plant host it can undergo meiosis. Recombinational repair occurring during meiosis likely helps protect the *U. maydis* genome from oxidative attack by the plant host's defensive system against invading fungal pathogens.

Paramecium tetraurelia, a unicellular ciliate, undergoes clonal aging over successive asexual generations leading eventually to extinction. However, if aging paramecia are allowed to undergo a sexual process, either conjugation (mating with another individual) or automixis (self-fertilization), the progeny have a lifespan characteristic of youthful paramecia. During clonal aging DNA damage dramatically increases. Presumably, during automixis or conjugation, age-related DNA damage is repaired by homologous recombination.

Volvox carteri is a facultatively sexual colonial green algae. Sex (syngamy and meiosis) can be induced by conditions that cause oxidative stress, suggesting that sex may be a response to oxidative DNA damage.

T. brucei is a trypanosome parasite that causes human sleeping sickness. The tsetse fly acts as a vector for transmitting the parasite. *T. brucei* after infecting the fly is able to undergo meiosis in the fly's salivary glands. The tsetse fly can defend itself against *T. brucei* infection, in part, by producing DNA damaging reactive oxygen species. When the trypanosomes within the fly's salivary glands undergo meiosis, the associated homologous recombination likely promotes repair of the oxidative damage in the trypanosome's genome.

The amoebozoa are a phylum of protozoans that diverged early in eukaryotic evolution. The amoebozoa include a large number of species that are classified into major subclades. Representative species from these subclades were recently found to have many genes that are related specifically to meiosis and to recombinational repair. This finding suggests that most amoebozoans are likely capable of meiosis, and contributes further to the idea that sex is a primitive character of eukaryotes.

Sexual processes in microbial eukaryotes are often induced by stress. In addition to the examples described above, sexual processes have also been demonstrated to be inducible by stress in other microbial eukaryotes. As an example, when *Chlamydomonas reinhardtii*, a unicellular green alga, is grown in a medium with limiting nitrogen, it differentiates to form gametes that are able to fuse together to produce a zygote capable of meiosis [77]. As another example, when the hyphae of the oomycete *Phytophthora cinnamomi* are exposed to hydrogen peroxide or mechanical damage, sexual reproduction is induced [78]. Also, meiotic processes can be induced in the human fungal pathogen *Cryptococcus neoformans* by desiccation or nitrogen starvation [79].

As noted in Section 1, the main focus of this review is to understand the principal adaptive function of meiotic sexual reproduction in microbial eukaryotes. The evidence reviewed in the preceding sections suggests that meiotic homologous recombination, the central process of meiosis, is an adaption for repairing DNA damages. The need for repair of DNA damages may be particularly critical in response to stress. The alternative possibility, that meiotic sex is primarily an adaptation for generating genetic variation seems less plausible because in well studied microbial eukaryotes, such as *S. cerevisiae* and *S. paradoxus,* all but a small percentage of matings in nature are between clonally related individuals. Nevertheless, the existence of mating types as in *S. cerevisiae, N. crassa* and other microbial eukaryotes suggests that some degree of out-crossing is adaptively beneficial. The benefit of out-crossing is that it promotes complementation, the masking of deleterious recessive mutations in diploid cells [80]. This masking benefit of out-crossing is generally recognized as underlying such concepts as heterosis, hybrid vigor or the avoidance of "inbreeding depression" [81]. Also, sexual processes can produce genetic variation that may be beneficial, as in the case of *C. albicans* populations where parasexual recombination can apparently facilitate, over successive generations, the evolution of resistance to the antifungal agent fluconazole [38].

Conflict of interest

Both authors declare that they have no conflict of interest.

Author details

Harris Bernstein and Carol Bernstein*
Department of Cellular and Molecular Medicine, University of Arizona, Tucson, AZ, USA

*Address all correspondence to: bernstein324@yahoo.com

IntechOpen

© 2019 The Author(s). Licensee IntechOpen. This chapter is distributed under the terms of the Creative Commons Attribution License (http://creativecommons.org/licenses/by/3.0), which permits unrestricted use, distribution, and reproduction in any medium, provided the original work is properly cited. [cc] BY

References

[1] Bernstein H, Bernstein C. Evolutionary origin and adaptive function of meiosis. In: Bernstein C, Bernstein H, editors. Meiosis. London: IntechOpen Limited; 2013. pp. 41-75. DOI: 5772/56557.ch3

[2] Dacks J, Roger AJ. The first sexual lineage and the relevance of facultative sex. Journal of Molecular Evolution. 1999;48(6):779-783

[3] Ramesh MA, Malik SB, Logsdon JM Jr. A phylogenomic inventory of meiotic genes; evidence for sex in Giardia and an early eukaryotic origin of meiosis. Current Biology. 2005;15(2):185-191. DOI: 10.1016/j.cub.2005.01.003

[4] Malik SB, Pightling AW, Stefaniak LM, Schurko AM, Logsdon JM Jr. An expanded inventory of conserved meiotic genes provides evidence for sex in *Trichomonas vaginalis*. PLoS One. 2007;3(8):e2879. DOI: 10.1371/journal.pone.0002879

[5] Akopyants NS, Kimblin N, Secundino N, Patrick R, Peters N, Lawyer P, et al. Demonstration of genetic exchange during cyclical development of *Leishmania* in the sand fly vector. Science. 2009;324(5924):265-268. DOI: 10.1126/science.1169464

[6] Nieuwenhuis BP, James TY. The frequency of sex in fungi. Philosophical Transactions of the Royal Society B: Biological Sciences. 2016;371(1706). pii: 20150540. DOI: 10.1098/rstb.2015.0540

[7] Speijer D, Lukeš J, Eliáš M. Sex is a ubiquitous, ancient, and inherent attribute of eukaryotic life. Proceedings of the National Academy of Sciences of the United States of America. 2015;112(29):8827-8834. DOI: 10.1073/pnas.1501725112

[8] Lahr DJ, Parfrey LW, Mitchell EA, Katz LA, Lara E. The chastity of amoebae: Re-evaluating evidence for sex in amoeboid organisms. Proceedings of the Biological Sciences. 2011;278(1715):2081-2090. DOI: 10.1098/rspb.2011.0289

[9] Bernstein H, Bernstein C, Michod RE. Meiosis as an evolutionary adaptation for DNA repair. In: Kruman I, editor. DNA Repair. London: InTech Open; 2011. p. 357-382 DOI:10.5772/25117.ch19

[10] Steinboeck F, Hubmann M, Bogusch A, Dorninger P, Lengheimer T, Heidenreich E. The relevance of oxidative stress and cytotoxic DNA lesions for spontaneous mutagenesis in non-replicating yeast cells. Mutation Research. 2010;688(1-2):47-52. DOI: 10.1016/j.mrfmmm.2010.03.006

[11] Pongpanich M, Patchsung M, Mutirangura A. Pathologic replication-independent endogenous DNA double-strand breaks repair defect in chronological aging yeast. Frontiers in Genetics. 2018;25(9):501. DOI: 10.3389/fgene.2018.00501

[12] Herskowitz I. Life cycle of the budding yeast *Saccharomyces cerevisiae*. Microbiological Reviews. 1988;52(4):536-553

[13] *Saccharomyces cereviciae* https://commons.wikimedia.org/wiki/File:Saccharomyces_cerevisiae_SEM.jpg by Mogana Das Murtey and Patchamuthu Ramasamy [CC BY-SA 3.0 (https://creativecommons.org/licenses/by-sa/3.0)]

[14] *Saccharomyces cereviciae* https://commons.wikimedia.org/wiki/File:YeastTetrad2.png by Wimblecf [CC BY-SA 3.0 (https://creativecommons.org/licenses/by-sa/3.0)]

[15] Haynes RH, Kunz BA. DNA repair and mutagenesis in yeast. In:

Strathern JN, Jones EW, Broach JR, editors. The Molecular Biology of the Yeast *Saccharomyces*: Life Cycle and Inheritance. Cold Spring Harbor, N.Y: Cold Spring Harbor Laboratory; 1981. pp. 371-414. DOI: 10.1101/87969139.11A.371

[16] Game JC, Zamb TJ, Braun RJ, Resnick M, Roth RM. The role of radiation (rad) genes in meiotic recombination in yeast. Genetics. 1980;**94**(1):51-68

[17] Henriques JAP, Moustacchi E. Sensitivity to photoaddition of mono- and bifunctional furocoumarins of X-ray sensitive mutants of *Saccharomyces cerevisiae*. Photochemistry and Photobiology. 1980;**31**(6):557-563. DOI: 10.1111/j.1751-1097.1980.tb03746.x

[18] Hayashi M, Umezu K. Homologous recombination is required for recovery from oxidative DNA damage. Genes & Genetic Systems. 2017;**92**(2):73-80. DOI: 10.1266/ggs.16-00066

[19] Kelly SL, Merrill C, Parry JM. Cyclic variations in sensitivity to X-irradiation during meiosis in *Saccharomyces cerevisiae*. Molecular & General Genetics. 1983;**191**(2):314-318

[20] Ruderfer DM, Pratt SC, Seidel HS, Kruglyak L. Population genomic analysis of outcrossing and recombination in yeast. Nature Genetics. 2006;**38**(9):1077-1081. DOI: 10.1038/ng1859

[21] Tsai IJ, Bensasson D, Burt A, Koufopanou V. Population genomics of the wild yeast *Saccharomyces paradoxus*: Quantifying the life cycle. Proceedings of the National Academy of Sciences of the United States of America. 2008;**105**(12):4957-4962. DOI: 10.1073/pnas.0707314105

[22] Birdsell JA, Wills C. The evolutionary origin and maintenance

of sexual recombination: A review of contemporary models. Evolutionary Biology. 2003;**33**:27-138. DOI: 10.1007/978-1-4757-5190-1_2

[23] Horandl E. Meiosis and the paradox of sex in nature. In: Bernstein C, Bernstein H, editors. Meiosis. London: IntechOpen Limited; 2013. pp. 17-39. DOI: 10.5772/56542.ch2

[24] Davey J. Fusion of a fission yeast. Yeast. 1998;**14**(16):1529-1566

[25] Bernstein C, Johns V. Sexual reproduction as a response to H_2O_2 damage in *Schizosaccharomyces pombe*. Journal of Bacteriology. 1989;**171**(4):1893-1897

[26] Pauklin S, Burkert JS, Martin J, Osman F, Weller S, Boulton SJ, et al. Alternative induction of meiotic recombination from single-base lesions of DNA deaminases. Genetics. 2009;**182**(1):41-54. DOI: 10.1534/genetics.109.101683

[27] Farah JA, Cromie G, Davis L, Steiner WW, Smith GR. Activation of an alternative, rec12 (spo11)-independent pathway of fission yeast meiotic recombination in the absence of a DNA flap endonuclease. Genetics. 2005;**171**(4):1499-1511. DOI: 10.1534/genetics.105.046821

[28] Thon G, Maki T, Haber JE, Iwasaki H. Mating-type switching by homology-directed recombinational repair: A matter of choice. Current Genetics. 2019;**65**(2):351-362. DOI: 10.1007/s00294-018-0900-2

[29] Kojic M, Sutherland JH, Pérez-MartínJ, HollomanWK. Initiation of meiotic recombination in *Ustilago maydis*. Genetics. 2013;**195**(4):1231-1240. DOI: 10.1534/genetics.113.156752

[30] Molina L, Kahmann R. An *Ustilago maydis* gene involved in H_2O_2

detoxification is required for virulence. The Plant Cell. 2007;**19**(7):2293-2309

[31] Kojic M, Zhou Q, Lisby M, Holloman WK. Rec2 interplay with both Brh2 and Rad51 balances recombinational repair in *Ustilago maydis*. Molecular and Cellular Biology. 2006;**26**(2):678-688

[32] Martins N, Ferreira IC, Barros L, Silva S, Henriques M. Candidiasis: Predisposing factors, prevention, diagnosis and alternative treatment. Mycopathologia. 2014;**177**(5-6):223-240. DOI: 10.1007/s11046-014-9749-1

[33] Berman J, Hadany L. Does stress induce (para)sex? Implications for *Candida albicans* evolution. Trends in Genetics. 2012;**28**(5):197-203. DOI: 10.1016/j.tig.2012.01.004

[34] Tzung KW, Williams RM, Scherer S, Federspiel N, Jones T, Hansen N, et al. Genomic evidence for a complete sexual cycle in *Candida albicans*. Proceedings of the National Academy of Sciences of the United States of America. 2001;**98**(6):3249-3253. DOI: 10.1073/pnas.061628798

[35] Diener AC, Fink GR. DLH1 is a functional *Candida albicans* homologue of the meiosis-specific gene DMC1. Genetics. 1996;**143**(2):769-776

[36] Forche A, Alby K, Schaefer D, Johnson AD, Berman J, Bennett RJ. The parasexual cycle in *Candida albicans* provides an alternative pathway to meiosis for the formation of recombinant strains. PLoS Biology. 2008;**6**(5):e110. DOI: 10.1371/journal.pbio.0060110

[37] Bennett RJ. The parasexual lifestyle of *Candida albicans*. Current Opinion in Microbiology. 2015;**28**:10-17. DOI: 10.1016/j.mib.2015.06.017

[38] Popp C, Ramírez-Zavala B, Schwanfelder S, Krüger I, Morschhäuser J. Evolution of fluconazole-resistant *Candida albicans* strains by drug-induced mating competence and parasexual recombination. MBio. 2019;**10**(1). pii: e02740-18. DOI: 10.1128/mBio.02740-18

[39] Guan G, Tao L, Yue H, Liang W, Gong J, Bing J, et al. Environment-induced same-sex mating in the yeast *Candida albicans* through the Hsf1-Hsp90 pathway. PLoS Biology. 2019;**17**(3):e2006966. DOI: 10.1371/journal.pbio.2006966

[40] Preer JR Jr. Whatever happened to paramecium genetics? Genetics. 1997;**145**(2):217-225

[41] *Paramecium tetrauralia* https://en.wikipedia.org/wiki/File:Paramecium.jpg#file by Barfooz at the English Wikipedia. CC BY-SA 3.0 (http://creativecommons.org/licenses/by-sa/3.0/) This file is licensed under the Creative Commons Attribution-Share Alike 3.0 Unported license.

[42] Gilley D, Blackburn EH. Lack of telomere shortening during senescence in *Paramecium*. Proceedings of the National Academy of Sciences of the United States of America. 1994;**91**(5):1955-1958

[43] Smith-Sonneborn J. DNA repair and longevity assurance in *Paramecium tetraurelia*. Science. 1979;**203**(4385):1115-1117

[44] Holmes GE, Holmes NR. Accumulation of DNA damages in aging *Paramecium tetraurelia*. Molecular & General Genetics. 1986;**204**(1):108-114

[45] Kirk DL, Kirk MM. Heat shock elicits production of sexual inducer in Volvox. Science. 1986;**231**(4733):51-54

[46] Nedelcu AM, Michod RE. Sex as a response to oxidative stress: The effect of antioxidants on sexual induction in a facultatively sexual lineage.

Proceedings of the Biological Sciences. 2003;**270**(Suppl 2):S136-S139. DOI: 10.1098/rsbl.2003.0062

[47] Nedelcu AM, Marcu O, Michod RE. Sex as a response to oxidative stress: A twofold increase in cellular reactive oxygen species activates sex genes. Proceedings of the Biological Sciences. 2004;**271**(1548):1591-1596. DOI: 10.1098/rspb.2004.2747

[48] Trypanosoma brucei https://commons.wikimedia.org/wiki/File:TrypanosomaBrucei_ProcyclicTrypomastigote_SEM.jpg by Zephyris. This file is licensed under the Creative Commons Attribution-Share Alike 3.0 Unported license

[49] Peacock L, Bailey M, Carrington M, Gibson W. Meiosis and haploid gametes in the pathogen *Trypanosoma brucei*. Current Biology. 2014;**24**(2):181-186. DOI: 10.1016/j.cub.2013.11.044

[50] Gibson W. Liaisons dangereuses: Sexual recombination among pathogenic trypanosomes. Research in Microbiology. 2015;**166**(6):459-466. DOI: 10.1016/j.resmic.2015.05.005

[51] Gibson W, Peacock L. Fluorescent proteins reveal what trypanosomes get up to inside the tsetse fly. Parasites & Vectors. 2019;**12**(1):6. DOI: 10.1186/s13071-018-3204-y

[52] Peacock L, Ferris V, Sharma R, Sunter J, Bailey M, Carrington M, et al. Identification of the meiotic life cycle stage of *Trypanosoma brucei* in the tsetse fly. Proceedings of the National Academy of Sciences of the United States of America. 2011;**108**(9):3671-3676. DOI: 10.1073/pnas.1019423108

[53] Hao Z, Kasumba I, Aksoy S. Proventriculus (cardia) plays a crucial role in immunity in tsetse fly (*Diptera: Glossinidiae*). Insect Biochemistry and Molecular Biology. 2003;**33**(11):1155-1164

[54] Marin PA, da Silva MS, Pavani RS, Machado CR, Elias MC. Recruitment kinetics of the homologous recombination pathway in procyclic forms of *Trypanosoma brucei* after ionizing radiation treatment. Scientific Reports. 2018;**8**(1):5405. DOI: 10.1038/s41598-018-23731-6

[55] Hampl V, Hug L, Leigh JW, Dacks JB, Lang BF, Simpson AG, et al. Phylogenomic analyses support the monophyly of Excavata and resolve relationships among eukaryotic "supergroups". Proceedings of the National Academy of Sciences of the United States of America. 2009;**106**(10):3859-3864. DOI: 10.1073/pnas.0807880106

[56] Leslie JF, Raju NB. Recessive mutations from natural populations of *Neurospora crassa* that are expressed in the sexual diplophase. Genetics. 1985;**111**(4):759-777

[57] Raju NB, Leslie JF. Cytology of recessive sexual-phase mutants from wild strains of *Neurospora crassa*. Genome. 1992;**35**(5):815-826

[58] *Neurospora crassa* hyphae. https://commons.wikimedia.org/wiki/File:Neurospora_crassahyphae.jpg by Roland Gromes. This file is licensed under the Creative Commons Attribution-Share Alike 3.0 Unported license

[59] *N. crassa* life cycle. https://en.wikipedia.org/wiki/Neurospora_crassa#/media/File:Neurospora_crassa_life_cycle.jpg by Chaya5260 [CC BY-SA 3.0] This file is licensed under the Creative Commons Attribution-Share Alike 3.0 Unported license.

[60] Jacobson DJ, Powell AJ, Dettman JR, Saenz GS, Barton MM, Hiltz MD, et al. *Neurospora* in temperate forests of

western North America. Mycologia. 2004;**96**(1):66-74

[61] Tekle YI, Wood FC, Katz LA, Cerón-Romero MA, Gorfu LA. Amoebozoans are secretly but ancestrally sexual: Evidence for sex genes and potential novel crossover pathways in diverse groups of amoebae. Genome Biology and Evolution. 2017;**9**(2):375-387. DOI: 10.1093/gbe/evx002

[62] Lahr DJG, Kosakyan A, Lara E, Mitchell EAD, Morais L, Porfirio-Sousa AL, et al. Phylogenomics and morphological reconstruction of *Arcellinida testate* amoebae highlight diversity of microbial eukaryotes in the Neoproterozoic. Current Biology. 2019;**29**(6):991-1001.e3. DOI: 10.1016/j.cub.2019.01.078

[63] Hofstatter PG, Brown MW, Lahr DJG. Comparative genomics supports sex and meiosis in diverse *Amoebozoa*. Genome Biology and Evolution. 2018;**10**(11):3118-3128. DOI: 10.1093/gbe/evy241

[64] Flowers JM, Li SI, Stathos A, Saxer G, Ostrowski EA, Queller DC, et al. Variation, sex, and social cooperation: Molecular population genetics of the social amoeba *Dictyostelium discoideum*. PLoS Genetics. 2010;**6**(7):e1001013. DOI: 10.1371/journal.pgen.1001013

[65] O'Day DH, Keszei A. Signalling and sex in the social amoebozoans. Biological Reviews of the Cambridge Philosophical Society. 2012;**87**(2):313-329. DOI: 10.1111/j.1469-185X.2011.00200.x

[66] Dacks JB, Field MC, Buick R, Eme L, Gribaldo S, Roger AJ, et al. The changing view of eukaryogenesis—Fossils, cells, lineages and how they all come together. Journal of Cell Science. 2016;**129**(20):3695-3703. DOI: 10.1242/jcs.178566

[67] Speijer D. Birth of the eukaryotes by a set of reactive innovations: New insights force us to relinquish gradual models. BioEssays. 2015;**37**(12):1268-1276. DOI: 10.1002/bies.201500107

[68] Cotton JA, McInerney JO. Eukaryotic genes of archaebacterial origin are more important than the more numerous eubacterial genes, irrespective of function. Proceedings of the National Academy of Sciences of the United States of America. 2010;**107**(40):17252-17255. DOI: 10.1073/pnas.1000265107

[69] Bernstein H, Bernstein C. Sexual communication in archaea, the precursor to eukaryotic meiosis. In: Witzany G, editor. Biocommunication of Archaea. Switzerland: Springer International Publisher; 2017. pp. 103-117. DOI: 10.007/978-3-319-65536-9-7

[70] Seitz EM, Brockman JP, Sandler SJ, Clark AJ, Kowalczykowski SC. RadA protein is an archaeal RecA protein homolog that catalyzes DNA strand exchange. Genes & Development. 1998;**12**(9):1248-1253. DOI: 10.1101/gad.12.9.1248

[71] Fröls S, Ajon M, Wagner M, Teichmann D, Zolghadr B, Folea M, et al. UV-inducible cellular aggregation of the hyperthermophilic archaeon *Sulfolobus solfataricus* is mediated by pili formation. Molecular Microbiology. 2008;**70**(4):938-952. DOI: 10.1111/j.1365-2958.2008.06459.x

[72] Ajon M, Fröls S, van Wolferen M, Stoecker K, Teichmann D, Driessen AJ, et al. UV-inducible DNA exchange in hyperthermophilic archaea mediated by type IV pili. Molecular Microbiology. 2011;**82**(4):807-817. DOI: 10.1111/j.1365-2958.2011.07861.x

[73] Fröls S, White MF, Schleper C. Reactions to UV damage in the model archaeon *Sulfolobus solfataricus*. Biochemical Society

Transactions. 2009;**37**(Pt 1):36-41. DOI:
10.1042/BST0370036

[74] van Wolferen M, Ma X,
Albers SV. DNA processing proteins
involved in the UV-induced stress
response of *Sulfolobales*. Journal of
Bacteriology. 2015;**197**(18):2941-2951.
DOI: 10.1128/JB.00344-15

[75] van Wolferen M, Wagner A, van
der Does C, Albers SV. The archaeal
Ced system imports DNA. Proceedings
of the National Academy of Sciences
of the United States of America.
2016;**113**(9):2496-2501. DOI: 10.1073/
pnas.1513740113

[76] Wallen RM, Perlin MH. An overview
of the function and maintenance of
sexual reproduction in dikaryotic fungi.
Frontiers in Microbiology. 2018;**9**:503.
DOI: 10.3389/fmicb.2018.00503

[77] Sager R, Granick S. Nutritional
control of sexuality in *Chlamydomonas
reinhardi*. The Journal of General
Physiology. 1954;**37**(6):729-742. DOI:
10.1085/jgp.37.6.729

[78] Reeves RJ, Jackson RM. Stimulation
of sexual reproduction in *Phytophthora*
by damage. Journal of General
Microbiology. 1974;**84**(2):303-310. DOI:
10.1099/00221287-84-2-303

[79] Lin X, Hull CM, Heitman J. Sexual
reproduction between partners
of the same mating type in
Cryptococcus neoformans. Nature.
2005;**434**(7036):1017-1021. DOI:
10.1038/nature03448

[80] Bernstein H, Byerly HC, Hopf FA,
Michod RE. Genetic damage, mutation,
and the evolution of sex. Science.
1985;**229**(4719):1277-1281

[81] Charlesworth D, Willis JH. The
genetics of inbreeding depression. Nature
Reviews. Genetics. 2009;**10**(11):783-796.
DOI: 10.1038/nrg2664

Chapter 9

An Insight into the Changing Scenario of Gut Microbiome during Type 2 Diabetes

Alpana Mukhuty, Chandrani Fouzder, Snehasis Das and Dipanjan Chattopadhyay

Abstract

The gut microbiome consists of bacteria, protozoans, viruses, and archaea collectively called as gut microbiota. Gut microbiome (GM) modulates a variety of physiological responses ranging from immune and inflammatory responses, neuronal signalling, gut barrier integrity and mobility, synthesis of vitamins, steroid hormones, neurotransmitters to metabolism of branched-chain aromatic amino acids, bile salts, and drugs. Type 2 diabetes mellitus (T2D) is a highly prevalent metabolic disorder that is featured by imbalance in blood glucose level, altered lipid profile, and their deleterious consequences. GM dysbiosis a major factor behind the incidence and progression of insulin resistance and is responsible for altering of intestinal barrier functions, host metabolic, and signaling pathways. The GM of type 2 diabetes (T2DM) patients is characterized by reduced levels of Firmicutes and Clostridia and an increased ratio of Bacteroidetes:Firmicutes. Endotoxemia stimulates a low-grade inflammatory response, which is known to trigger T2DM. Xenobiotics including dietary components, antibiotics, and nonsteroidal anti-inflammatory drugs strongly affect the gut microbial composition and can promote dysbiosis. However, the exact mechanisms behind the dynamics of gut microbes and their impact on host metabolism are yet to be deciphered. Interventions that can restore equilibrium in the GM have beneficial effects and can improve glycemic control.

Keywords: type 2 diabetes, inflammation, immune response, gut microbiome, xenobiotics

1. Introduction

Our quality of life and health status are modulated by our food habits and lifestyle. Hence several metabolic disorders and are the greatest global health issues are influenced by improper diet and lifestyle [1]. The other factors that are involved in the development of metabolic disorders and diseases are environmental factors, maternal health, and host genetic makeup. The resident microorganisms in our gastrointestinal tract are collectively collected as the gut microbiota (GM). GM consists of bacteria, fungi, Archaea, protozoa, and viruses. In case of mammals, GM comprises of four main phyla: Firmicutes (64%), Bacteroidetes (23%), Proteobacteria (8%), and Actinobacteria (3%). These phyla are important for the

IntechOpen

regulation of host metabolism and physiology [2]. The total number of both pro-karyotic cells and host eukaryotic cells in the gut is approximately 100 trillion, which is three times that of the total number of human body cells [3]. Hence, our unique gut environment is considered as a functional and measurable organ [4]. However, the composition of GM varies along the gastrointestinal tract, and differs within and between individuals depending on the gestational age, mode of delivery, breastfeeding, antibiotic exposure, dietary lifestyle and nutritional status of the individual status of [5, 6]. The colonization of GM is limited in stomach and small intestine, but quite dense and diverse in the colon owing to the absence of digestive secretions, slow peristalsis, and rich nutrient supply [7]. This variety in composition of GM and its function is influenced by the consumption of improper diet, which in turn affects the health condition of the host. GM regulates the energy homeostasis, intestinal integrity and immunity against invading pathogens by participating in the digestive process and energy production, hampering pathogen colonization, and modulating the immune system; hence GM can modulate the overall health status of the host. Gut microbiome also influences an individual's metabolic status such as calorie derived from indigestible dietary substances and storage of calories in adipose tissue, which regulates incidence of obesity in an individual. Studies from germ-free and wild type mice showed alteration in homeostasis in kidney, liver, and intestine in germ-free mice depicting the fact that GM influences whole body metabolism [8–13]. GM also plays a vital role in vitamin production, energy harvest and storage, fermentation and absorption of undigested carbohydrates. The distribution of GM is determined by diet to a large extent as evident from individuals who follow a diet high in animal fat have dominance of Bacteroides in GM, whereas those who follow a carbohydrate-rich diet have a *Prevotella* dominant GM (**Table 1**) [14–16]. According to conventional theories the relationship between genetic and environmental factors such as high-calorie diet and lack of physical activities was considered as the major main contributor to obesity but recently GM has attracted much attention in relation to human health and disease. Recent scientific investigations have shown that GM can be considered as an important endogenous factor controlling obesity [17, 18].

2. Host-gut microbiota metabolite interaction

Several reports have shown that the metabolites derived by GM from fermentation of food play a key role in maintenance of the host metabolism. Clostridium and Eubacterium from our GM break down bile acid in the intestine to its secondary metabolites like deoxycholic acid and lithocholic acid. These metabolites bind to Takeda G protein coupled receptor-5 TGR5 receptor (G-protein-coupled bile receptor) present in the endocrine glands, adipocytes, muscles, immune organs, spinal cord and enteric nervous system, and stimulates the secretion of incretin hormone GLP-1 and insulin. Hence these metabolites in turn promote energy expenditure (**Table 1**) [19]. Long chain fatty acids, for example linoleic acid produced by the GM regulates our lipid profile finally resulting in obesity [20]. Short chain fatty acids (SCFs) another secondary metabolite of gut microbial fermentation is formed by the digestion of indigestible polysaccharides and oligosaccharides that are neither digested nor absorbed in the proximal jejunum [21]. SCFs mainly acetate and propionate contributed by Bacteroidetes and butyrate produced by Firmicutes balance the host metabolism by influencing energy homeostasis, lipid accumulation and appetite [22]. SCF produced in the gastrointestinal tract are also known to control the pH of the lumen by increasing the absorption of nutrients. SCFs also act as a source of nutrition for GM due to high carbon content [23]. Butyrate is the main source of energy for colonocytes. It aids in the proliferation, maturation,

Gut microbiota	Facts and effects
Bifidobacteria	Population reduces in high fat-fed mice gut increasing endotoxemia [14]
Bacteroidetes	Population high in the gut of people consuming animal-based food rich diet [15]
Prevotella	Population high in the gut of people consuming plant-based food rich diet [16]
Clostridium and *Eubacterium*	Break down bile acid in the intestine to its secondary metabolites like deoxycholic acid and lithocholic acid. These metabolites bind to TGR5 receptor (G-protein-coupled receptor) present in the endocrine glands, adipocytes, muscles, immune organs, spinal cord and enteric nervous system, and stimulates the secretion of incretin hormone GLP-1 and insulin [19]
Lactobacillus reuteri GMNL-263	They are capable of reducing T2D markers like serum glucose, glycated hemoglobin and c-peptide in high-fructose-fed rats along with reduction in inflammatory cytokines IL-6 and TNF-α in adipose tissue and down-regulated forms of GLUT 4 and PPAR-γ [58]
Lactobacillus casei Shirota	They can increase lipopolysaccharide-binding protein expression in plasma and diminishes endotoxemia [63]
Bifidobacterium animalis subsp. lactis	They can restrict bacterial translocation in intestine alleviating bacteremia in early stages of T2D [64]
L. casei Zhang	Oral administration can ameliorate impaired glucose tolerance in hyperinsulinemic rats induced by high-fructose [65]
Lactobacillus	Oral administration is positively correlated with expression of CB2 receptor [76]
Clostridium	Oral administration is negatively correlated with CB2 expression probiotics control GM through CB2 receptor expression [76]
Bifidobacterium infantis	Impairs inflammation by altering the intestinal permeability [80, 81]
Bacteroidetes:Firmicutes ratio	Low in GM of obese patients [112, 113]
Butyrate-producing bacteria (*Roseburia* species and *Faecalibacterium prausnitzii*)	Low population in GM of T2DM patients [113]
Firmicutes (Gram-positive) and Bacteroidetes (Gram-negative)	90% of the bacterial species present in gut [15, 16]
Proteobacteria and particularly *Escherichia coli*	High in T2D patients [113, 121]
Enterobacteriaceae	Population elevated by T2D drugs [122]
Clostridium and *Eubacterium*	Population lowered by T2D drugs [122]
Akkermansia sp. *Akkermansia muciniphila*	Metformin increases the populations of *Akkermansia* sp. in high-fat diet-fed mice, hence improving glucose metabolism. Oral administration of *Akkermansia muciniphila* also improves metabolic dysfunctions like endotoxemia and adipose tissue inflammation [122]

Table 1.
Facts and effects of various types of bacteria present in GM

maintenance of colonocytes and also protects the colon by enhancing mucin expression and immune response [24]. Acetate and propionate can cross the liver epithelium, and propionate gets metabolized in the liver, whereas acetate stays in the peripheral circulation [25]. SCF also regulates epithelial barrier integrity by maintaining the tight junction proteins like claudin-1, occludin, and Zonula Occludens-1. Suppression of these proteins leads to invasion of bacteria and lipopolysaccharides (LPS) stimulating an inflammatory response [26]. Hence SCF acts as energy source and also regulates host biological responses including inflammation, oxidative stress, and immune response toward Crohn's disease, ulcerative colitis, and colorectal cancer [27, 28]. Host metabolism is activated by SCFs by direct stimulation of G-coupled receptors like free fatty acid receptors 2 and 3 (FFAR2/GPR41 and FFAR3/GPR41) occurring mainly in the gut epithelial cells. They also activate host metabolism by inhibiting nuclear class I histone deacetylases (HDACs) present in the epithelial cells [27]. FFAR2 acts as the receptor for acetate and FFAR3 is the receptor for butyrate and propionate. Activation of these receptors regulates the level of satiety hormones like ghrelin (orexigenic peptide), glucagon like peptide-1 (GLP-1), and peptide YY (PYY) (anorexigenic peptide) [29]. Ghrelin secretion occurs pre-meal, while GLP-1 and PYY are secreted post-meal, which in turn stimulates insulin production in the pancreatic β cells. GLP-1 and PYY also reduce food intake, normalizes weight loss and maintain the balance of energy intake. Increase in the production of SCFs enhances the secretion of PYY and GLP-1 but decreases secretion of ghrelin, which ultimately leads to increased satiety and reduction in food intake [30]. The other factors inducing reduced appetite is mediated by butyrate and propionate by (i) enhanced expression of leptin in adipocytes, direct regulation of body weight and energy homeostasis by decreased food intake and upregulated energy expenditure [31], (ii) promoting gluconeogenesis in the intestinal cells [32] and (iii) inhibition of histone acetyltransferase and deacetylases which exhibit anti-inflammatory responses, epigenetic modification necessary for proliferation and differentiation of immune cells, activated AMP-activated protein kinase (AMPK) pathway synchronised adiponectin secretion, induction of mitochondrial biogenesis and fatty acid oxidation [33]. In healthy subjects SCF regulates integrity of gut, secretion of hormones, and immune responses, while in metabolically unhealthy subjects SCF implements protection from diabetes, ulcerative colitis, colorectal cancer, and neurodegenerative disorders [24, 34].

2.1 Gut microbiota composition

Recent studies targeting metagenomics have disclosed that approximately 90% of the bacterial species in the GM of adult humans are Bacteroidetes (Gram-negative) and Firmicutes (Gram-positive) [35, 36]. A healthy person fosters 500–1000 bacterial species at a single time and almost 1012–1014 colony-forming units (CFU) with a total mass weight of about 1–2 kg in the total gut [37] with 109–1012 CFU/ml in the colon, 101–103 CFU/ml in jejunum and 104–108 CFU/ml in the ileum [38]. Transfer of microbiota from mother to embryo takes place in utero or during birth and attains strength by the 2 years. Composition of GM is shaped by host genetics, environmental factors and early exposure to microbes during birth. The other factors that regulate formation of a stale GM are exposure to vaginal microbiome during normal delivery, skin microbiota during cesarean sections, breast-feeding and antibiotics in neonatal or early childhood.

2.2 Role of gut microbiota in carbohydrate metabolism

Normal diet of a healthy human contains a considerable percentage of carbohydrates comprising of monosaccharides, disaccharides and complex polysaccharides. The difference lies in the absorption of the sugars, for example common sugars like cane sugar and fruit sugars are readily absorbed in the intestine, disaccharides like maltose, lactose and sucrose and complex polysaccharides like pectin, starch and hemicellulose are broken down into monosaccharides in the ileum with the help of bacterial enzymes like glycosidases before being absorbed [39]. After food intake consisting of carbohydrate-rich diet, glucose levels in the blood rise, and later are strongly regulated and kept at a homeostatic level by the help of two hormones, insulin and glucagon. Carbohydrate digestion and absorption occurs in the upper digestive tract via glucose transporters called GLUTs (glucose transporters) located on the epithelial cells [40]. GLUT proteins uptake glucose into the pancreatic β-cells. Metabolization of glucose stimulates insulin secretion due to increased ATP/ ADP ratio, membrane depolarization and closure of potassium channels, resulting in calcium dependant exocytosis of insulin [41].

The role of gut environment and gut associated lymphoid tissue plays a pivotal role in T2D [42]. T2D is a chronic metabolic disorder characterized by fasting serum hyperglycemia, non-responsiveness of insulin and insulin insufficiency [43]. Insulin resistance or non-responsiveness occurs in the liver and skeletal muscle cells when they undergo failure to sense insulin. Other factors in T2D are non-responsiveness or deficiency of incretins, amplified lipid catabolism, increased glucagon levels in circulation and increased salt and water renal retention [43, 44]. High-fat-diet-fed germ-free mice, wild type mice and standard diet fed mice exhibit different metabolic and immunological characters depending on diet and GM [45, 46]. Also mice belonging to same genotype and diet exhibit different metabolism of glucose depending on their GM [47].

2.3 Role of gut microbiota and its association with diet

In the earlier sections it has been discusses that our GM plays a key role in digestion and absorption of food. Increased population of Bacteroidetes lead to increase in energy production. The population of Bifidobacteria reduce in high fat-fed mice gut increasing endotoxemia. Prebiotic supplementation can restore Bifidobacteria levels in the mouse gut [48, 49]. Bacteroidetes are more widespread in the gut of people consuming animal-based food rich diet. *Prevotella* is prevalent in people consuming plant-based food rich diet. In case of people consuming plant-based foods, the GM produce more SCFAs and increased synthesis of amylase, glutamate and riboflavin [50, 51]. On the contrary, people consuming animal-based foods have GM modified for increased catabolic processes as for example degradation of glycans and amino acids [52]. SCFAs like butyrate, propionate and acetate along with some gases like hydrogen are produced by the breakdown of these polysaccharides, are further used in colonic fermentation and yield energy [53]. Butyrates can decrease calorie intake of an individual by inducing satiety via production of GLP-1 and gastric inhibitory peptide-1 [54]. Butyrates are also involved in maintenance of gut integrity by supplying energy for regulating the survival and proliferation of enterocytes.

Low-grade inflammation is a key pathophysiological factor behind the progression of type 2 diabetes (T2D), and incidence of hyperglycemia and insulin resistance [55]. Progression of T2D occurs along with reduced GM diversity and increased gut inflammation. Gut inflammation includes innate immune responses via toll-like receptors, (TLRs) secretion of proinflammatory cytokines and increased endotoxemia. Also during high-fat diet induced obesity, intestinal Gram-negative bacteria translocates in the circulatory system, adipose tissue and cause endotoxemia [56].

2.4 Role of probiotics upon gut microbiota

Probiotics enhance production of interleukin-10 (IL-10) an important regulatory and anti-inflammatory cytokine in diabetic mice. Increased IL-10 downregulates proinflammatory cytokines like interferon-γ (IFN-γ) and interleukin-2 (IL-2)/interleukin 1-β (IL-1β) preventing inflammation and incidence of diabetes [56, 57]. *Lactobacillus reuteri* GMNL-263 reduces T2D markers like serum glucose, glycated hemoglobin and c-peptide in high-fructose-fed rats along with reduction in inflammatory cytokines interleukin-6 (IL-6) and tumor necrosis factor-α (TNF-α) in adipose tissue and down-regulated forms of GLUT 4 and peroxisome proliferator activated receptor-γ (PPAR-γ) (**Figure 1** and **Table 1**) [58]. Methodical consumption of probiotic yoghurt reduces inflammatory markers such as high-sensitivity C-reactive protein levels in pregnant women and T2D [59, 60]. Probiotic strains decrease oxidative stress in pancreatic tissue, reducing inflammation and apoptosis of pancreatic cells [61]. Probiotic strains also lessen LDL cholesterol and total cholesterol in serum by regulating lipid metabolism, reducing the risk of T2D [62]. Consumption of *Lactobacillus casei* Shirota increase lipopolysaccharide-binding protein expression in plasma and diminishing endotoxemia (**Table 1**) [63]. *Bifidobacterium animalis* sub sp. lactis can restrict bacterial translocation in intestine alleviating bacteremia in early stages of T2D (**Table 1**) [64]. Oral administration of *L. casei* can also ameliorate impaired glucose tolerance in hyperinsulinemic rats induced by high-fructose (**Table 1**) [65].

2.5 Role of gut microbiota in maintaining intestinal integrity and metabolic conditions

Increased gut permeability provides the relation between high-fat diet and LPS by causing LPS entry into circulation via the portal system in T2D patients [66]. Animal model studies have provided evidence between increased intestinal permeability and progression of obesity and insulin resistance [67, 68]. Consumption of prebiotics increase gut microbiota, rectify intestinal permeability, diminish inflammation, alleviate endotoxemia and ameliorate glucose tolerance [68]. High-fat diet induce decrease in tight junction proteins regulating epithelial integrity of gut lining and gut permeability such as zonula occluden-1 (ZO-1) and occludin. Dietary fatty acids activate toll-like receptor 2 (TLR-2) and toll like receptor 4 (TLR-4) signaling pathways. TLR-4 leads to LPS translocation into intestinal capillaries and induces insulin resistance in mice [69–71]. Altered gut permeability and plasma LPS levels are related with distribution of ZO-1 and occluding and

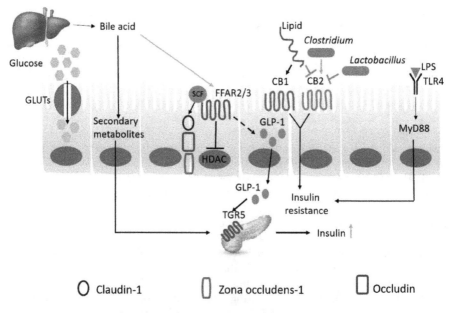

Figure 1.
Influence of gut microbiota in various physiological responses [80, 81, 83, 84, 110, 111].

endocannabinoid (eCB) system. Gut microbes selectively modify expression of the cannabinoid receptor 1 (CB1) in colon also affecting zona occluding ZO-1 and occludin [72]. Administration of probiotics changes the gut microbiota resulting in reduced gut permeability in obese mice. Antibiotic exposure induces metabolic endotoxemia in mice fed with high-fat diet, along with increased gut permeability, secretion of proinflammatory cytokines, and incidence of diabetes and obesity (**Figure 1**). Modulation of the eCB system is connected with inflammation and diabetes [72, 73]. Moderation of GM controls eCB expression in gut, thereby regulating gut permeability and plasma LPS levels through the CB1 receptor [72]. Changes in the gut microbiota due to prebiotic feeding reduce gut permeability in obese mice. Modulation of gut permeability occurs through the distribution of tight junction proteins through eCB systems [55]. Activation of cannabinoid CB2 receptor and blocking of CB1 receptor improves glucose tolerance [74, 75]. *Lactobacillus* administration is positively correlated with expression of CB2 receptor, and *Clostridium* spp. is negatively correlated with CB_2 expression (**Table 1**) [76]. Also probiotics control GM through CB2 receptor expression [77].

3. Gut microbiota and obesity mediated type 2 diabetes

GM has a close association with host obesity, since the increase in total body fat in wild type mice is high when compared to germ free mice consuming more food. Transplanting of cecum-derived microbiota induced an increase in body fat mass and insulin resistance, adipocyte hypertrophy, and increased level of circulating leptin and glucose [78]. Germ free mice when fed with a diet rich in fat and sugar content showed lean phenotype however wild type mice who were fed with the high sugar and high fat diet turned obese. Also the germ free mice showed enhanced insulin sensitivity, leading to improved glucose tolerance and altered cholesterol metabolism diminishing cholesterol storage and increasing cholesterol excretion via fecal route. GM alters intestinal permeability, causes endotoxemia, enhances calorie provision, stimulates endocannabinoid system (eCB), regulates lipid metabolism by increasing activity of lipoprotein lipase and lipogenesis resulting in host obesity. Lipopolysaccharides (LPS), present in the cell membrane of Gram-negative bacteria, stimulate low-grade inflammation and incidence of insulin resistance (IR). LPS reaches the circulation from gut by diffusion either by enhanced intestinal permeability or absorption after association with chylomicron [79]. LPS acts as a ligand for toll-like receptors TLR-4 occurring in immune cells, liver and adipose tissue. LPS activated TLR-4 prompts conformational changes recruiting adapter molecules like myeloid differentiation primary factor MyD88 protein, IL-1 receptor associated kinase IRAK, TNF receptor associated factor TRAF6, and NF-κB inducing kinase NIK, phosphorylating and degrading inhibitor of nuclear factor kappa B kinase IKKB, inhibitor of nuclear factor kappa light chain enhancer of activated B cells NF-κB. Activated NF-κB translocates to the nucleus triggering expression of inflammatory proteins and various pathways like janus kinase JNK, p38 microtubule associated protein kinase MAPK, and extracelluar signal regulated kinase ERK finally resulting in insulin resistance (**Figure 1**). Colonization of *Bifidobacterium infantis* can impair inflammation by altering the intestinal permeability. Excess of lipid in diet enhances exposure to free fatty acids and their derivatives, facilitates endotoxin absorption and increases plasma LPS level termed as "metabolic endotoxemia" (**Table 1**) [80, 81]. Interaction between endogenous lipid and cannabinoid receptor (CB1 and CB2) stimulates adenylate cyclase and MAPK, ERK, and NF-κB pathways, triggering inflammation, insulin resistance and obesity [82]. On the whole GM stimulates the eCB system, enhances intestinal permeability, triggering

LPS entry into circulatory system resulting in endotoxemia. Rise in LPS, modulates the integrity of the tight junctions of the intestinal membrane increasing LPS in circulation. Therefore, GM is a complex system having both advantageous and dangerous microbes, and understanding the GM and host integration system provides a generalized idea about the function of each unit of the GM-host system [83, 84].

3.1 Gut microbiota and carbohydrate metabolism during type 2 diabetes

Bile acids affect glucose homeostasis via activation of nuclear farnesoid X receptor (FXR) and the membrane-bound G protein coupled receptor, TGR5. These receptors are expressed in liver, ileum and pancreas [85]. Some bile acids act as agonists for FXR, and others are FXR antagonists [86–88]. Known FXR agonists are CDCA, lithocholic acid, deoxycholic acid, and cholic acid [89]. The antidiabetic effects exhibited by vertical sleeve gastrectomy, bariatric surgery, occurs through FXR [90]. Also, intestinal FXR agonist treatment can improve insulin sensitivity [91]. In the ileum, activation of FXR leads to the production of fibroblast growth factor-19, a hormone that affects glucose tolerance through mechanisms that are largely independent of insulin [92, 93]. Activation of TGR5 produces glucagon-like peptide-1 (GLP-1) from ileum improves both energy and glucose homeostasis [94]. Activation of FXR in pancreas regulates insulin transport and secretion [95], and protects the islets from lipotoxicity [96]. FXR activation in liver improves insulin sensitivity in T2D patients [97]. The GM can modulate the amount and type of secondary bile acids produced via FXR and TGR5 signaling. GM enzymes such as bile salt hydrolase for deconjugation, 7-alpha dehydroxylase for dihydroxylation and 7α-hydroxysteroid dehydrogenase for epimerization of bile acids are reduced in T2D patients compared to healthy controls [98]. Bile acid concentrations in the circulation show a diurnal pattern since they increase after food intake [99].

3.2 Gut microbiota and lipid metabolism during type 2 diabetes

Our body metabolism, inflammatory processes and innate immune system are regulated by dietary lipids [100]. The dietary lipids can also act as (proinflammatory) ligands which can bind to nuclear receptors [101]. The nuclear receptors are peroxisome-proliferator-activated receptors (PPAR) and liver X receptors (LXR) which regulate metabolic and inflammatory pathways. Hence the dietary lipids can improve insulin action and down-regulate secretion of pro-inflammatory cytokines [102, 103]. Lipids can also activate G-protein coupled receptors (Gpcr) such as Gpr43 when activated by dietary-metabolite acetate lipolysis in adipocytes is decreased leading to reduced plasma-free fatty acids. Gpr43 can be considered as a potential target for regulation of lipid metabolism [104]. Inflammation and lipid accumulation are characteristic features of atherosclerosis [105]. Recent evidences provide sufficient link between atherosclerosis and GM variety [106]. Short-term antibiotic administration can alter the composition of GM which can convert dietary choline and L-carnitine to trimethylamine (TMA). TMA is later oxidized into TMAO by the action of hepatic Flavin monooxygenases [107]. Dietary choline is highly available in foods rich in lipid phosphatidylcholine, lecithin, such as in eggs, red meat, milk, poultry, liver, and fish [108]. Bile acids are key modulators of lipid and cholesterol metabolism, and they facilitate intestinal absorption and transport of nutrients, vitamins, and lipids. Production of bile occurs in the liver and 95% of bile acids are reabsorbed in the ileum. Later the bile acids are re-absorbed in liver, entering the enterohepatic circulation. GM converts primary bile salts to secondary bile salts by bile acid de-hydroxylation [109]. Bile acids can also result in the release of GLP-1 from enteroendocrine L cells via activation of Takeda G protein coupled receptor-5

(TGR5) (**Figure 1**). This phenomenon affects insulin secretion sensitivity [110]. Bile acids have another receptor called farnesoid X receptor (FXR) present in liver, intestine, and pancreatic beta cells [111]. Hence, bile acids improve our metabolism in the long term after bariatric surgery by enhancing intestinal hormone secretion.

3.3 Gut microbiota composition during type 2 diabetes

The GM of T2D patients exhibit low population of Firmicutes and Clostridia and high ratio of Bacteroidetes:Firmicutes (**Table 1**) [112, 113]. However, the GM of T2DM and obese patients are not always identical because the GM of obese patients show decreased Bacteroidetes:Firmicutes ratio [113–115, 118]. GM of T2DM patients also show low population of butyrate-producing bacteria. Short-chain fatty acids (SCFAs) like butyrate, acetate, and propionate are fermented from dietary fiber in large intestine by GM. SCFAs regulate energy metabolism, immune responses and tumorigenesis in gut. Butyrate is the energy source for colonic epithelial cells. Butyrate perpetuates intestinal integrity and thereby avert translocation of Gram-negative intestinal bacteria across the lumen of the gut. This phenomenon ultimately leads to endotoxemia triggering a low-grade inflammation during T2D [15, 113, 115].

The major risk factors behind T2D are genetic predisposition, less physical activity, fetal programming, obesity and altered GM [114, 116]. Total weight of GM in the distal gut is about 1.5 kg and it is considered as a microbial organ. The GM consists of embers from Bacteria, Archaea, Eukarya and viruses, but a large part of the population includes anaerobic bacteria. 90% of the bacterial species present in gut are grouped into the two bacterial phyla Firmicutes (Gram-positive) and Bacteroidetes (Gram-negative) (**Table 1**) [15, 16]. An average adult fosters a minimum of 160 bacterial species and a set of genes in the GM is obligatory for proper functioning of the GM [15]. The GM gives protection from disease caus-ing pathogens and facilitates the immune system. GM also help in production of vitamin K and many B-vitamins like folate, vitamin B12. Metagenomic studies about sequencing of T2D patients exhibit dysbiotic GM and less butyrate-producing bacteria (*Roseburia* species and *Faecalibacterium prausnitzii*). Metabolic disorders like obesity and impaired glucose metabolism are related with an altered ratio of Firmicutes and Bacteroidetes [118–120]. Populations of Proteobacteria and particularly *Escherichia coli* are also high in T2D patients (**Table 1**) [113, 121]. Gram-negative bacteria contribute to inflammatory lipopolysaccharides (LPS) stimulating pro-inflammation, during T2D and obesity. Oral administration of metformin, a widely used drug for T2D elevates populations of Enterobacteriaceae and lowers populations of *Clostridium* and *Eubacterium*. Metformin also increases the populations of *Akkermansia* sp. in high-fat diet-fed mice, hence improving glucose metabolism [122]. Oral administration of *Akkermansia muciniphila* also improves metabolic dysfunctions like endotoxemia and adipose tissue inflammation (**Table 1**) [122, 123]. Hence metformin can be used as a potent drug in improvising the GM content in T2D patients, managing glucose tolerance and inflammation.

4. Modulation of gut microbiota to cure type 2 diabetes

4.1 Antibiotics

Antibiotics have become very popular for elimination of pathogenic bacte-ria. However, antibiotics are also harmful to the local population of beneficial GM. Hence excess use of antibiotics must be prevented for healthy maintenance of

GM. Bacterio-therapeutic use of antibiotics in farm animals has increased increase growth and food production, but has taken a toll of their metabolic pathways [115]. Excess of usage of antibiotics in early infancy show chronic effects on GM diversity, overweight in infants, obesity in adults. For example, excess of bacterio-therapy with vancomycin has increased the incidence of obesity in adults. Even, short-term treatment with vancomycin impeded peripheral insulin sensitivity and other related metabolic syndromes affecting GM (**Table 2**) [115]. Hence, even short-term treatment with oral antibiotics harness intense and chronic damage to GM diversity and function.

4.2 Prebiotics and probiotics

Recently prebiotics and probiotics have gained a lot of popularity among individuals as a healthy substitute for antibiotics. Prebiotics are actually indigestible carbohydrates that improve the growth and function of colonic bacteria boosting host health. Prebiotics include oligosaccharides which cannot be digested in the upper GI tract. These oligosaccharides are fermented, producing SCFAs in the colon and result in stimulation of growth of colonic. Prebiotics can be obtained from a large number of dietary elements like barley, garlic, asparagus, wheat bran and onions and both prebiotics and probiotics can be obtained from pickled and fermented foods like sauerkraut, kimchi, miso, yogurt [15, 16]. Probiotics obtained from food and supplements contain some very popular strains like bifidobacteria and lactobacilli. These bacteria alter the composition and function of GM as well as host system activity. The prebiotics and probiotics compete with pathogenic

Types of cure	Effects
Antibiotics	• Affect GM diversity
	• Overweight in infant
	• Obesity in adult
	• Vancomycin impede insulin sensitivity [115]
Prebiotics and probiotics	• Compete with pathogenic bacteria
	• Intensify intestinal barrier by secreting some antimicrobial substances
	• Enhances immune system [15, 16, 115]
Dietary modulation	• Increase GM ecosystem diversity
	• Enhances SCFA
	• Reduces fasting and postprandial glucose, A1C, serum cholesterol, insulin resistance, BMI, waist and hip circumferences [124]
Metformin	• Increases levels of butyrate-producing bacteria
	• Decreases levels of Lactobacillus [125]
Fecal microbiota transplant	• Allogenic infusion from lean donors lead to significant rise in GM diversity, enhanced levels of butyrate producing bacteria and improved insulin sensitivity [114, 115]
Bariatric surgery	• Proteobacteria rises and Firmicutes and Bacteroides lowers
	• BMI reduces by 15–32%
	• C-reactive protein decreases
	• T2DM is attenuated [112, 115]

Table 2.
Types of treatments for T2D involving modulation of GM and their effects.

bacteria, intensify the intestinal barrier by secreting some antimicrobial substances and enhances the immune system (**Table 2**) [15, 16, 115].

4.3 Dietary modulation

Changes in diet plan can modulate activity of GM and host metabolism. A fat and carbohydrate restricted diet increased the ratio of Bacteroidetes to Firmicutes in obese patients with T2D [118]. Also calorie deficient diet plans or diet plans rich in high-fiber macrobiotics like complex carbohydrates, legumes, fermented products, sea salt, and green tea and free of animal protein fat, and added sugar improved dysbiosis, increased GM ecosystem diversity, and enhanced SCFA producers in T2D patients. Macrobiotic diet can more efficiently reduce fasting and postprandial glucose, A1C, serum cholesterol, insulin resistance, BMI, waist and hip circumferences than the control diet. Also macrobiotic diet could effectively reduce pro-inflammatory bacterial strains (**Table 2**) [124].

4.4 Metformin

Metformin, already a well-established drug for T2D, has recently been known to have bacterio-therapeutic effects on microbial composition and production of SCFA. Several recent reports have shown that metformin affects GM of T2D patients like increasing the levels of butyrate-producing bacteria. Metformin can also decrease the levels of Lactobacillus which remains high in T2D patients (**Table 2**) [125].

4.5 Fecal microbiota transplant

Fecal microbiota transplant, or stool transplant also called bacteriotherapy, which is the process of replacing fecal bacteria from a healthy individual into a host individual has been quite effective in restoring GM composition. Fecal microbiota transplant is used in treating recurrent *Clostridium difficile colitis* recharging useful bacteria in the GI tract along with usage of antibiotics. Autologous infusion is reinfusion of one's collected feces and allogenic infusion is infusion with feces from a donor. Insulin resistant adults when autologously transplanted did not alter the GM composition but when transplanted with allogenic infusion from lean donors exhibited significant rise in GM diversity, enhanced levels of butyrate producing bacteria and improved sensitivity to insulin (**Table 2**) [114, 115].

4.6 Bariatric surgery

Bariatric surgery, or Roux-en-Y gastric bypass (RYGBP), is removal of a portion of stomach and re-routing the small intestine to a small stomach pouch. It is performed on people as an efficient tool to treat obesity. After bariatric surgery huge changes occur in the GM, Proteobacteria rises and Firmicutes and Bacteroides lowers, BMI reduces by 15–32%, C-reactive protein decreases and T2DM is attenuated. However, increase in some bacteria are highly significant than the normal levels in lean controls, which means these alterations are linked with GM modification, and not body weight (**Table 2**) [112, 117, 118].

5. Conclusion

The GM makes one of the largest organs in human body and remains the reason behind various metabolic disorders such as obesity, atherosclerosis, type 2 diabetes and so on. The alterations in GM is very susceptible to changes in our diet and environment which makes them vulnerable and ultimately ends in the incidence of diseases. Reversal of the GM alterations can restore the normal physiological functions and health. Hence further investigation is required in order to get a detailed scenario of the composition of various GM and their detailed function. Scrutiny of the composition of the GM and the change in their population in various metabolic disorders can create new avenues in finding out the treatment for those diseases. Deeper insights in the composition and function of GM can also provide more ideas for development of various techniques and drugs for the enhancement of the GM for better physiological responses and treatment of diseases.

Acknowledgements

AM is thankful to the Science & Engineering Research Board (SERB), Department of Science & Technology, Govt. of India, for her JRF fellowship (Grant No. ECR/2017/001028). DC thankful DBT for JRF. SD thanks UGC, New Delhi for SRF. The authors are thankful to Dr. Rakesh Kundu for technical assistance and constant encouragement.

Conflict of interest

The authors declare no conflict of interest.

Notes/thanks/other declarations

The authors thank to the Head of the Department of Zoology, for providing the assistance in their research work.

Author details

Alpana Mukhuty[1*], Chandrani Fouzder[1], Snehasis Das[2] and Dipanjan Chattopadhyay[2]

1 Cell Signaling Laboratory, Department of Zoology, Visva-Bharati University, Santiniketan, India

2 Molecular Endocrinology Laboratory, Department of Zoology, Visva-Bharati University, Santiniketan, India

*Address all correspondence to: alpanamukhuty@yahoo.com

IntechOpen

© 2019 The Author(s). Licensee IntechOpen. This chapter is distributed under the terms of the Creative Commons Attribution License (http://creativecommons.org/licenses/by/3.0), which permits unrestricted use, distribution, and reproduction in any medium, provided the original work is properly cited. [cc] BY

References

[1] Robson AA. Preventing diet induced disease: Bioavailable nutrient-rich, low-energy-dense diets. Nutrition and Health. 2009;**20**(2):135-166

[2] Qin J et al. A human gut microbial gene catalogue established by metagenomic sequencing. Nature. 2010;**464**:59-65

[3] Bianconi E et al. An estimation of the number of cells in the human body. Annals of Human Biology. 2013;**40**:463-471

[4] Fukuda S, Ohno H. Gut microbiome and metabolic diseases. Seminars in Immunopathology. 2014;**36**:103-114

[5] Collado MC et al. Factors influencing gastrointestinal tract and microbiota immune interaction in preterm infants. Pediatric Research. 2015;**77**(6):726-731

[6] Xu J et al. Evolution of symbiotic bacteria in the distal human intestine. PLoS Biology. 2007;**5**:1574-1586

[7] Sekirov I et al. Gut microbiota in health and disease. Physiological Reviews. 2010;**90**(3):859-904

[8] Zhao L, Shen J. Whole-body systems approaches for gut microbiota-targeted, preventive healthcare. Journal of Biotechnology. 2010;**149**(3):183-190

[9] Claus SP et al. Systemic multicompartmental effects of the gut microbiome on mouse metabolic phenotypes. Molecular Systems Biology. 2008;**4**:219

[10] Swann JR et al. Systemic gut microbial modulation of bile acid metabolism in host tissue compartments. Proceedings of the National Academy of Sciences of the United States of America. 2011;**108**(1):4523-4530

[11] Bäckhed F et al. The gut microbiota as an environmental factor that regulates fat storage. Proceedings of the National Academy of Sciences of the United States of America. 2004;**101**(44):15718-15723

[12] Bäckhed F et al. Host-bacterial mutualism in the human intestine. Science. 2005;**307**(5717):1915-1920

[13] Sonnenburg JL, Bäckhed F. Diet-microbiota interactions as moderators of human metabolism. Nature. 2016;**535**(7610):56-64

[14] Clemente JC et al. The impact of the gut microbiota on human health: An integrative view. Cell. 2012;**148**(6):1258-1270

[15] Barengolts E. Gut microbiota, prebiotics, probiotics and synbiotics in management of obesity and prediabetes: Review of randomized controlled trials. Endodontics: Principles and Practice. 2016;**22**(10):1224-1234

[16] Fujimura KE et al. Role of the gut microbiota in defining human health. Expert Review of Anti Infective Therapy. 2010;**8**(4):435-454

[17] Murphy EF et al. Composition and energy harvesting capacity of the gut microbiota: Relationship to diet, obesity and time in mouse models. Gut. 2010;**59**(12):1635-1642

[18] Lopez-Legarrea P et al. The influence of Mediterranean, carbohydrate and high protein diets on gut microbiota composition in the treatment of obesity and associated inflammatory state. Asia Pacific Journal of Clinical Nutrition. 2014;**23**(3):360-368

[19] Kishino S et al. Polyunsaturated fatty acid saturation by gut lactic acid bacteria affecting host lipid

composition. Proceedings of the National Academy of Sciences of the United States of America. 2013;**110**(44):17808-17813

[20] Miyamoto J et al. A gut microbial metabolite of linoleic acid, 10-hydroxy-cis-12-octadecenoic acid, ameliorates intestinal epithelial barrier impairment partially via GPR40-MEK-ERK pathway. E. Journal of Biological Chemistry. 2015;**290**(5):2902-2918

[21] Blachier F et al. Effects of amino acid-derived luminal metabolites on the colonic epithelium and physiopathological consequences. Amino Acids. 2007;**33**(4):547-562

[22] Postler TS, Ghosh S. Understanding the holobiont: How microbial metabolites affect human health and shape the immune system. Cell Metabolism. 2017;**26**(1):110-130

[23] Macfarlane GT, Macfarlane S. Bacteria, colonic fermentation, and gastrointestinal health. Journal of AOAC International. 2012;**95**(1):50-60

[24] van der Beek CM et al. Role of short-chain fatty acids in colonic inflammation, carcinogenesis, and mucosal protection and healing. Nutrition Reviews. 2017;**75**(4):286-305

[25] Koh A et al. From dietary fiber to host physiology: Short-chain fatty acids as key bacterialmetabolites. Cell. 2016;**165**(6):1332-1345

[26] Wang HB et al. Butyrate enhances intestinal epithelial barrier function via upregulation of tight junction protein claudin-1 transcription. Digestive Diseases and Sciences. 2012;**57**(12):3126-3135

[27] Tan J et al. The role of short-chain fatty acids in health and disease. Advances in Immunology. 2014;**121**:91-119

[28] Huang W et al. Short-chain fatty acids inhibit oxidative stress and inflammation in mesangial cells induced by high glucose and lipopolysaccharide. Experimental and Clinical Endocrinology & Diabetes. 2017;**125**(02):98-105

[29] Tolhurst G et al. Short-chain fatty acids stimulate glucagon-like peptide-1 secretion via the G-proteincoupled receptor FFAR2. Diabetes. 2012;**61**(2):364-371

[30] Li X et al. Gut microbial metabolite short-chain fatty acids and obesity. Bioscience of Microbiota, Food and Health. 2017;**36**(4):135-140

[31] Chambers ES et al. Effects of targeted delivery of propionate to the human colon on appetite regulation, body weight maintenance and adiposity in overweight adults. Gut. 2015;**64**(11):1744-1754

[32] de Vadder F et al. Microbiota-generated metabolites promote metabolic benefits via gut-brain neural circuits. Cell. 2014;**156**(1-2):84-96

[33] Jian H et al. Butyrate alleviates high fat diet-induced obesity through activation of adiponectinmediated pathway and stimulation of mitochondrial function in the skeletal muscle of mice. Oncotarget. 2016;**7**(35):56071-56082

[34] Bolognini D et al. The pharmacology and function of receptors for short-chain fatty acids. Molecular Pharmacology. 2016;**89**(3):388-398

[35] Human Microbiome Project C. A framework for human microbiome research. Nature. 2012;**486**:215-221

[36] Human Microbiome Project C. Structure, function and diversity of the healthy human microbiome. Nature. 2012;**486**:207-214

[37] Xu J et al. Does canine inflammatory bowel disease influence gut microbial profile and host metabolism? BMC Veterinary Research. 2016;**12**:114

[38] Blaut M, Clavel T. Metabolic diversity of the intestinal microbiota: Implications for health and disease. Journal of Nutrition. 2007;**137**:751S-755S

[39] Flint HJ et al. Microbial degradation of complex carbohydrates in the gut. Gut Microbes. 2012;**3**:289-306

[40] Arumugam M et al. Enterotypes of the human gut microbiome. Nature. 2011;**473**:174-180

[41] Hehemann JH et al. Transfer of carbohydrate-active enzymes from marine bacteria to Japanese gut microbiota. Nature. 2010;**464**:908-912

[42] Mason KL et al. Overview of gut immunology. Advances in Experimental Medicine and Biology. 2008;**635**:1-1

[43] Fonseca VA. Defining and characterizing the progression of type 2 diabetes. Diabetes Care. 2009;**32**(2):S151-S156

[44] Musso G et al. Interactions between gut microbiota and host metabolism predisposing to obesity and diabetes. Annual Review of Medicine. 2011;**62**:361-380

[45] Wen L, Duffy A. Factors influencing the gut microbiota, inflammation, and type 2 diabetes. Journal of Nutrition. 2017;**147**:1468S-1475S

[46] Caesar R et al. Gut derived lipopolysaccharide augments adipose macrophage accumulation but is not essential for impaired glucose or insulin tolerance in mice. Gut. 2012;**61**:1701-1707

[47] Backhed F et al. Mechanisms underlying the resistance to diet-induced obesity in germ-free mice.

Proceedings of the National Academy of Sciences of the United States of America. 2007;**104**:979-984

[48] Woting A et al. Alleviation of high fat diet-induced obesity by oligofructose in gnotobiotic mice is independent of presence of Bifidobacterium longum. Molecular Food and Nutrition Research. 2015;**59**:2267-2278

[49] Cani PD et al. Selective increases of bifidobacteria in gut microflora improve high-fat-diet-induced diabetes in mice through a mechanism associated with endotoxaemia. Diabetologia. 2007;**50**:2374-2383

[50] De Filippo C et al. Impact of diet in shaping gut microbiota revealed by a comparative study in children from Europe and rural Africa. Proceedings of the National Academy of Sciences of the United States of America. 2010;**107**:14691-14696

[51] Fan W et al. Impact of diet in shaping gut microbiota revealed by a comparative study in infants during the six months of life. Journal of Microbiology and Biotechnology. 2014;**24**:133-143

[52] Yatsunenko T et al. Human gut microbiome viewed across age and geography. Nature. 2012;**486**:222-227

[53] Nicholson JK et al. Host-gut microbiota metabolic interactions. Science. 2012;**336**:1262-1267

[54] den Besten G et al. The role of short-chain fatty acids in the interplay between diet, gut microbiota, and host energy metabolism. The Journal of Lipid Research. 2013;**54**:2325-2340

[55] Cani PD et al. Involvement of gut microbiota in the development of low-grade inflammation and type 2 diabetes associated with obesity. Gut Microbes. 2012;**3**:279-288

[56] Sanz Y et al. Understanding the role of gut microbes and probiotics in obesity: How far are we? Pharmacological Research. 2013;**69**:144-155

[57] Cano PG et al. Bifidobacterium CECT 7765 improves metabolic and immunological alterations associated with obesity in high-fat diet-fed mice. Obesity (Silver Spring). 2013;**21**:2310-2321

[58] Hsieh FC et al. Oral administration of *Lactobacillus reuteri* GMNL-263 improves insulin resistance and ameliorates hepatic steatosis in high fructose-fed rats. Nutrition and Metabolsim (London). 2013;**10**:35

[59] Asemi Z et al. Effects of daily consumption of probiotic yoghurt on inflammatory factors in pregnant women: A randomized controlled trial. Pakistan Journal of Biological Sciences. 2011;**14**:476-482

[60] Asemi Z et al. Effect of daily consumption of probiotic yoghurt on insulin resistance in pregnant women: A randomized controlled trial. European Journal of Clinical Nutrition. 2013;**67**:71-74

[61] Ejtahed HS et al. Probiotic yogurt improves antioxidant status in type 2 diabetic patients. Nutrition. 2012;**28**:539-543

[62] Ooi LG, Liong MT. Cholesterol-lowering effects of probiotics and prebiotics: A review of in vivo and in vitro findings. International Journal of Molecular Sciences. 2010;**11**:2499-2522

[63] Naito E et al. Beneficial effect of oral administration of *Lactobacillus casei* strain Shirota on insulin resistance in diet-induced obesity mice. Journal of Applied Microbiology. 2011;**110**:650-657

[64] Amar J et al. Intestinal mucosal adherence and translocation of commensal bacteria at the early onset of

type 2 diabetes: Molecular mechanisms and probiotic treatment. EMBO Molecular Medicine. 2011;**3**:559-572

[65] Zhang Y et al. Probiotic *Lactobacillus casei* Zhang ameliorates high-fructose-induced impaired glucose tolerance in hyperinsulinemia rats. European Journal of Nutrition. 2014;**53**:221-232

[66] Horton F et al. Increased intestinal permeability to oral chromium (51 Cr)-EDTA in human type 2 diabetes. Diabetic Medicine. 2014;**31**:559-563

[67] Ding S, Lund PK. Role of intestinal inflammation as an early event in obesity and insulin resistance. Current Opinion in Clinical Nutrition and Metabolic Care. 2011;**14**:328-333

[68] Xiao S et al. A gut microbiota-targeted dietary intervention for amelioration of chronic inflammation underlying metabolic syndrome. FEMS Microbiology Ecology. 2014;**87**:357-367

[69] Zhang X et al. Modulation of gut microbiota by berberine and metformin during the treatment of high-fat diet-induced obesity in rats. Scientific Reports. 2015;**5**:14405

[70] Saberi M et al. Hematopoietic cell-specific deletion of toll-like receptor 4 ameliorates hepatic and adipose tissue insulin resistance in high-fat-fed mice. Cell Metabolsim. 2009;**10**:419-429

[71] Poggi M et al. C3H/HeJ mice carrying a toll-like receptor 4 mutation are protected against the development of insulin resistance in white adipose tissue in response to a high-fat diet. Diabetologia. 2007;**50**:1267-1276

[72] Muccioli GG et al. The endocannabinoid system links gut microbiota to adipogenesis. Molecular Systems Biology. 2010;**6**:392

[73] Scherer T, Buettner C. The dysregulation of the endocannabinoid

system in diabesity—A tricky problem. Journal of Molecular Medicine (Berl). 2009;**87**:663-668

[74] Cani PD et al. Glucose metabolism: Focus on gut microbiota, the endocannabinoid system and beyond. Diabetes & Metabolism. 2014;**40**:246-257

[75] Bermudez-Silva FJ et al. Role of cannabinoid CB2 receptors in glucose homeostasis in rats. European Journal of Pharmacology. 2007;**565**:207-211

[76] Aguilera M et al. Stress and antibiotics alter luminal and wall adhered microbiota and enhance the local expression of visceral sensory-related systems in mice. Neurogastroenterology and Motility. 2013;**25**:e515-e529

[77] Rousseaux C et al. Lactobacillus acidophilus modulates intestinal pain and induces opioid and cannabinoid receptors. Nature Medicine. 2007;**13**:35-37

[78] Wostmann BS et al. Dietary intake, energy metabolism, and excretory losses of adult male germfree Wistar rats. Laboratory Animals. 1983;**33**(1):46-50

[79] Manco M et al. Gut microbiota, lipopolysaccharides, and innate immunity in the pathogenesis of obesity and cardiovascular risk. Endocrine Reviews. 2010;**31**(6):817-844

[80] Caesar R et al. Crosstalk between gut microbiota and dietary lipids aggravates WAT inflammation through TLR signalling. Cell Metabolism. 2015;**22**(4):658-668

[81] Moreira APB, Alfenas RCG. The influence of endotoxemia on the molecular mechanisms of insulin resistance. Nutricion Hospitalaria. 2012;**27**:382-390

[82] Muccioli GG et al. The endocannabinoid system links gut microbiota to adipogenesis. Molecular Systems Biology. 2010;**6**:392

[83] Nicholson JK, Lindon JC. Systems biology: Metabonomics. Nature. 2008;**455**(7216):1054-1056

[84] Knight R et al. The microbiome and human biology. Annual Review of Genomics and Human Genetics. 2017;**18**:65-86

[85] Kuipers F, Bloks VW, Groen AK. Beyond intestinal soap—bile acids in metabolic control. Nature Reviews Endocrinology. 2014;**10**:488-498

[86] Haeusler RA et al. Human insulin resistance is associated with increased plasma levels of 12alpha-hydroxylated bile acids. Diabetes. 2013;**62**: 4184-4191

[87] Wewalka M et al. Fasting serum taurine-conjugated bile acids are elevated in type 2 diabetes and do not change with intensification of insulin. Journal of Clinical Endocrinology and Metabolism. 2014;**99**:1442-1451

[88] Sayin SI et al. Gut microbiota regulates bile acid metabolism by reducing the levels of taurobeta-muricholic acid, a naturally occurring FXR antagonist. Cell Metabolism. 2013;**17**:225-235

[89] Ridlon JM et al. Bile acids and the gut microbiome. Current Opinion in Gastroenterology. 2014;**30**:332-338

[90] Ryan KK et al. FXR is a molecular target for the effects of vertical sleeve gastrectomy. Nature. 2014;**509**:183-188

[91] Fang S et al. Intestinal FXR agonism promotes adipose tissue browning and reduces obesity and insulin resistance. Nature Medicine. 2015;**21**:159-165

[92] Schaap FG. Role of fibroblast growth factor 19 in the control of glucose homeostasis. Current Opinion

in Clinical in Nutrition and Metabolic Care. 2012;**15**:386-391

[93] Morton GJ et al. FGF19 action in the brain induces insulin-independent glucose lowering. Journal of Clinical Investigation. 2013;**123**:4799-4808

[94] Sandoval DA, D'Alessio DA. Physiology of proglucagon peptides: Role of glucagon and GLP-1 in health and disease. Physiological Reviews. 2015;**95**:513-548

[95] Renga B et al. The bile acid sensor FXR regulates insulin transcription and secretion. Biochimica et Biophysica Acta. 1802;**2010**:363-372

[96] Popescu IR et al. The nuclear receptor FXR is expressed in pancreatic beta-cells and protects human islets from lipotoxicity. FEBS Letters. 2010;**584**:2845-2851

[97] Mudaliar S et al. Efficacy and safety of the farnesoid X receptor agonist obeticholic acid in patients with type 2 diabetes and nonalcoholic fatty liver disease. Gastroenterology. 2013;**145**:574-582

[98] Labbe A et al. Bacterial bile metabolising gene abundance in Crohn's, ulcerative colitis and type 2 diabetes metagenomes. PLoS One. 2014;**9**:e115175

[99] Steiner C et al. Bile acid metabolites in serum: Intraindividual variation and associations with coronary heart disease, metabolic syndrome and diabetes mellitus. PloS One. 2011;**6**:e25006

[100] Hotamisligil GS. Inflammation and metabolic disorders. Nature. 2006;**444**(7121):860-867

[101] Chawla A et al. Nuclear receptors and lipid physiology: Opening the X-files. Science. 2001;**294**(5548):1866-1870

[102] Glass CK, Ogawa S. Combinatorial roles of nuclear receptors in inflammation and immunity. Nature Reviews Immunology. 2006;**6**(1):44-55

[103] Wellen KE, Hotamisligil GS. Inflammation, stress, and diabetes. Journal of Clinical Investigation. 2005;**115**(5):1111-1119

[104] Ge H et al. Activation of G protein-coupled receptor 43 in adipocytes leads to inhibition of lipolysis and suppression of plasma free fatty acids. Endocrinology. 2008;**149**(9):4519-4526

[105] Semenkovich CF. Insulin resistance and atherosclerosis. Journal of Clinical Investigation. 2006;**116**(7):1813-1822

[106] Shapiro H et al. Personalized microbiome-based approaches to metabolic syndrome management and prevention. Journal of Diabetes. 2017;**9**(3):226-236

[107] Koeth RA et al. Intestinal microbiota metabolism of L-carnitine, a nutrient in red meat, promotes atherosclerosis. Nature Medicine. 2013;**19**(5):576-585

[108] Wang Z et al. Gut flora metabolism of phosphatidylcholine promotes cardiovascular disease. Nature. 2011;**472**(7341):57-63

[109] Chiang JY. Bile acids: Regulation of synthesis. Journal of Lipid Research. 2009;**50**(10):1955-1966

[110] Thomas C et al. TGR5-mediated bile acid sensing controls glucose homeostasis. Cell Metabolism. 2009;**10**(3):167-177

[111] Düfer M et al. Bile acids acutely stimulate insulin secretion of mouse b-cells via Farnesoid X receptor activation and KATP channel inhibition. Diabetes. 2012;**61**:1479-1489

[112] Graessler J et al. Metagenomic sequencing of the human gut microbiome before and after bariatric surgery in obese patients with type 2 diabetes: Correlation with inflammatory and metabolic parameters. The Pharmacogenomics Journal. 2013;**13**(6):514-522

[113] Larsen N et al. Gut microbiota in human adults with type 2 diabetes differs from non-diabetic adults. PLoS One. 2010;**5**(2):e9085

[114] Grarup N et al. Genetic susceptibility to type 2 diabetes and obesity: From genome-wide association studies to rare variants and beyond. Diabetologia. 2014;**57**:1528-1541

[115] Hartsra AV et al. Insights into the role of the microbiome in obesity and type 2 diabetes. Diabetes Care. 2015;**38**(1):159-165

[116] Gomes AC et al. The human gut microbiota: Metabolism and perspective in obesity. Gut Microbes. 2019;**9**:308-325

[117] Aron-Wisnewsky et al. Major microbiota dysbiosis in severe obesity: Fate after bariatric surgery. Gut. 2019;**68**:70-82

[118] Ley RE et al. Microbial ecology: Human gut microbes associated with obesity. Nature. 2006;**444**:1022-1023

[119] Heianza YD et al. Gut microbiota metabolites, amino acid metabolites and improvements in insulin sensitivity and glucose metabolism: The POUNDS lost trial. Gut. 2019;**68**:263-270

[120] Turnbaugh PJ et al. An obesity-associated gut microbiome with increased capacity for energy harvest. Nature. 2006;**444**:1027-1031

[121] Qin J et al. A metagenome-wide association study of gut microbiota in type 2 diabetes. Nature. 2012;**490**:55-60

[122] Shin NR et al. An increase in the Akkermansia spp. population induced by metformin treatment improves glucose homeostasis in diet-induced obese mice. Gut. 2014;**63**:727-735

[123] Everard A et al. Cross-talk between Akkermansia muciniphila and intestinal epithelium controls diet-induced obesity. Proceedings of the National Academy of Sciences of the United States of America. 2013;**110**:9066-9071

[124] Candela M et al. Modulation of gut microbiota dysbioses in type 2 diabetic patients by macrobiotic Ma-Pi 2 diet. British Journal of Nutrition. 2016;**116**(1):80-93

[125] Forslund K et al. Disentangling type 2 diabetes and metformin treatment signatures in the human gut microbiota. Nature. 2015;**528**(7581):262-266

Chapter 10

Gut Microbiome: A New Organ System in Body

Haseeb Anwar, Shahzad Irfan, Ghulam Hussain,
Muhammad Naeem Faisal, Humaira Muzaffar,
Imtiaz Mustafa, Imran Mukhtar, Saima Malik
and Muhammad Irfan Ullah

Abstract

The gut microbiome is comprised of various types of bacteria, fungi, protozoa, and viruses naturally occurring in humans and animals as normal microflora. Gut microorganisms are typically host specific, and their number and type vary according to different host species and environment. Gut microbes contribute directly and/or indirectly to various physiological processes including immune modulation, regulation of various neurotransmitter, and hormones, as well as production of many antioxidants and metabolites. They also play a role as antibiotic, anti-inflammatory, anti-diabetic, and anti-carcinogenic agents. Moreover, the ability of gut microbes to attenuate various systemic diseases like coronary heart disease, irritable bowel syndrome, metabolic diseases like diabetes mellitus, and infectious diseases like diarrhea has recently been reported. Current research findings have enough evidence to suggest that gut microbiome is a new organ system mainly due to the microorganisms' specific biochemical interaction with their hosts and their systemic integration into the host biology. Investigations into the potential ability of gut microbiome to influence metabolism inside their host via biochemical interaction with antibiotics and other drugs has recently been initiated. This chapter specifically focuses on the importance of gut microorganisms as a new organ system.

Keywords: gut microbiota, probiotics, metabolic disorders, gut health, drug metabolism

1. Introduction

Certain microorganisms have the unique ability to populate the human gastrointestinal tract and thus generally referred as gut microbiota. Gut microbiota is always non-pathological, and hence, the immune system is not triggered because of their presence. Humans co-evolved with a huge number of intestinal microbial species that offer to the host certain benefits by playing an important role in preventing them from pathogenic activities [1]. In addition to metabolic benefits, symbiotic bacteria benefit the host with various functions like boosting the immune homeostasis and inhibiting the colonization by other pathogenic microorganisms. The ability of symbiotic bacteria to inhibit pathogen colonization particularly in the gut is mediated

IntechOpen

via several mechanisms including direct killing of pathogen, competition for limited nutrients, and enhancement of immune responses [2]. The intestinal microorganisms also co-evolved and have strong affiliations and association towards each other. In this evolutionary process, the persistent and enduring members of this microflora become more competent during unsettling influences and thereby become essential for human health [3]. Definite composition of human microbiome varies between individuals [4] particularly among lean and obese people. The microbiome is also affected by the dietary modifications adapted for the weight loss [5]. Examination of metabolic profiles of human infant microbiota revealed that ingestion, storage and digestion of dietary lipids were explicitly regulated by the microbiome [6, 7].

The human gut microbial communities are a mixture of microorganisms. The classes of microbes that constitute the gut microbiome communities differ between hosts. The difference is attributed to factors such as, inability of a microorganism to migrate between different hosts, intense environmental conditions inside and outside host's gut and host inconsistency in terms of genotype, diet, and colonization history [8]. The co-evolution of humans and their symbiotic microorganism has created bilateral interactions which are important for the health of humans, and any genetic or ecological change in this bilateral interaction can result in pathological conditions like infection [8]. Gut microbial communities are important for diverse host functions, including metabolism, fertility, development, immunity, and even antioxidant activities which promote health and fitness of the host [9–12]. The gut microbiome has a much larger genetic variety compared to the genome of the host, e.g., human genome is comprised of 20-25,000 genes whereas microbiome inhabiting the body is estimated to be in trillions. Almost 10^{10} microorganisms enter the human body daily and with the progress of co-evolution of gut microbes in humans, the capability of microbes to exchange their genes and associated functions with the environment are some of the main factors leading to host adaptation. Therefore, the "hologenome" model appraises the host and its microbes genomes as one unit under assortment [13, 14]. It is acknowledged that host-symbiont co-evolution is accountable for basic biological aspects. In this chapter we aim to discuss the importance of gut microbiomes as a new organ system because of its association with the genetics and its role in the disease and health condition of the host. Moreover, the involvement of these microbiomes in shaping the overall health and constructing a symbiotic relationship with their host species is discussed as well as the co-evolution of gut microbes with the human body.

2. Inheritance of microbiome

2.1 Microbiome

A microbiome is the community of microbes dwelling collectively in a selected habitat. Humans, animals, vegetation, soils, oceans or even buildings have their own specific microbiome [15].

2.2 Host genetics and gut microbiome

The human gut environment is extremely complex with a unique ecology which comprises of trillion of microbiota with approximately 1.5 kg in mass. By using genetic techniques like 16S sequencing, 1000 microorganisms have been identified within the gut, with approx. 200 (0.5%) defining the core of the intestine microbiome [16]. These bacteria protect the gut epithelial cells against external pathogens. They also help the breakdown of indigestible dietary polysaccharides in the gut and

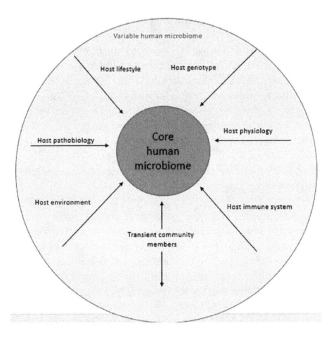

Figure 1.
Core human microbiome.

thus supply a quick chain of fatty acids, including acetate, butyrate, and propionate, which serve as vital metabolites for direct energy source of intestinal epithelial cells, prevention of insulin resistance and modulators of insulin secretion [17] (**Figure 1**).

The genetic makeup of humans is virtually identical, yet the small differences in DNA give rise to remarkable phenotypic assortment across the human population. The trillions of microbes inhabit our bodies and create complex, body-habitat-specific, adaptive ecosystems that are finely tuned to frequently changing host physiology [18]. A healthy "functional core" is actually a complement of metabolic and other molecular functions that are performed by the microbiome within a particular habitat but are not necessarily provided by the same organisms in different people [19].

2.3 Inherited microbiomes

The gastrointestinal tract (GIT) of humans is colonized by a vast variety of microbial population that can be understood as a complex and polygenetic trait which has been interacting and co-evolved with their host genetic environment [20–22]. It was previously considered that fetus lives in a germ free environment in the mother womb and the gut microbiota are transferred to the baby from mother's birth canal and body via horizontal transmission only [23]. But advanced researches have revealed that microbiota are also vertically transmitted to the infants from their mothers [24]. Presence of microbes in the meconium of the babies born by cesarean section clearly demonstrates that the gut microbes are not only derived after the birth [25, 26]. Moreover, presence of many microbes in the umbilical cord blood of the preterm babies and in the amniotic fluid substantiate the findings that the fetus in the mother womb is not totally sterile [27, 28]. Many gut bacterial genera are shared among the mammal species. The microbiomes of mice show strong fidelity throughout the generations and reiterate the intrinsic significance of these microorganisms in health.

2.4 Relationship of environment in shaping the microbiome

As mentioned above human intestinal microbiome composition is shaped by multiple factors like genetics, diet, environment and lifestyle. Several studies point towards stronger contribution by the environmental factors in shaping the gut microbial composition compared to the genetic factor [29]. It has also been speculated that gut microbial diversity affects the prediction accuracy for certain human traits including glucose and obesity problems, as compared to different animal models that use only host genetic and environmental factors [30].

2.5 Co-evolution and co-differentiation of host microbe interaction in exploring new drug targets

Horizontal gene transfer (HGT), genomic and metagenomics are possible approaches to identify drug targets that may also be considered as an evidence of co-evolution of hosts and their symbionts. Symbionts have the capacity to perform many metabolic activities including fermentation of dietary carbohydrates, drug metabolism, antimicrobial protection and immunomodulation, which is primarily due to the presence of genes in their genome which are missing in mammalian genomes. Therefore, horizontal gene transfer mechanisms are potential targets for drug discovery that become more evident with the use of gnotobiotics (germ free animal) in experimental trial to unveil the microbial function in the complex GIT microenvironment, and to investigate how orally administered drugs impact the gut microbial ecology in long term. HGT has gained immense interest in medical field as it contributes to the spreading of antibiotic resistance genes as well as it may cause closely related microbial strains to differ drastically in terms of clinical parameters [31]. Genetic variation in intestinal microbes may trigger the production of metabolites, but it may also generate changes in host's genome that may increase metabolite uptake or prevent their further synthesis. Co-evolution may lead to co-differentiation since permanent association of host and symbiont lineage can result in diversification [32]. The co-differentiation correlate resemblances in the microbial symbiont and the host [33, 34] which can be extended to an entire microbial community that passes vertically from host to offspring. Over the course of speciation, the microbial communities differentiate as a mirror to host phylogeny (such situation would be expected in hosts where parents immunize their offspring with microbial clique, e.g., Koala bear mother inoculate "pap" with dropping to shift young one from milk to eucalyptus leaves diet) [35]. Fecal microbiome from healthy humans is a mirror of distal gut microbiome which is highly rich in genes involved in the vitamin synthesis, breakdown of nutrients, and metabolism of xenobiotics as compared to already sequenced human genome and microbes genome [4]. The presence of conjugate transposons in gut microbiome is another important source of horizontal gene transfer in bacteria [36]. The HGT is involved not only in spreading antibiotic resistance genes, but also as a source of clinical response of closely related microbial strains of *Salmonella enterica* [37] such as the secretory system type III pathogenicity islands encoded by SPI-I and SPI-II (virulence genes are present in pathogenicity islands, and play a key role in the pathogenesis of *Salmonella* infections through invasion in host cell. Currently, 12 *Salmonella* pathogenicity islands have been investigated with common motifs) [38].

Novel strategies in drug discovery are being pursued by targeting horizontal gene transfer involved in the resistance to antibiotic [39] as well as virulence [40]. Targeting virulence factors with Salmonellosis inhibitors causes less damage to indigenous microbes compared to traditional antibiotic therapy, less selective pressure for evolution and transfer of resistance and may be more effective against divergent organisms that have acquired a particular virulence factor by HGT. Genomic islands which are a good source of genes and gene transfer systems are also being targeted with small molecule inhibitors that are co-administered with antibiotics to prevent resistance factors by targeted pathogenesis during the therapy [41].

2.5.1 Co-evolution of drug transporters in host and microbes

It has been established that the majority of molecules possessing physiological or pharmacological features are either transported into and or out of the cells by transporting proteins rather than by a passive transport mechanism where drug molecules cross cell membranes through solute transporters that are already involved in the movement of different metabolic intermediary molecules through channels. More than 1000 different types of transporting proteins (transporters) are present in humans [42] comprising solute carriers (SLC) and ATP binding cassettes (ABC) transporters involved in the transport of a broad range of substrates [43].

Human intestinal peptide transporter 1 (hPepT1) belonging to the proton-coupled oligopeptide transporter (POT) family which is also known as solute carrier 15A (SLC15A) is present in the enterocytes, the PepT2 (oligopeptide transporter 2, SLC15A2) in kidney, the PHT1 (peptide histidine transporter 1, SLC15A4) in brain and the PHT2 (peptide histidine transporter 2, SLC15A3) located in spleen, lungs and thymus. Both hPepT1 and PepT2 mediate the transport of di−/tri-peptides and a broad range of peptidomimetics in the organisms, whereas PHT1 and PHT2 mediate the translocation of histidine and with a few selected di- and tri-peptides [44]. The hPepT1, an oligopeptide transporter 1 located in the enterocystes of the small intestine, has low affinity and high capacity transporter protein to transport 400–800 different dipeptides and tripeptides and drugs like ACE'1 (Enalapril) and antiviral (acyclovir) [45]. The hPepT1 is also found in microbes like *Escherichia coli* residing the gut [46, 47] to uptake amino acids and on the microbial outer membrane channels (OmpC and OmpF) present in *E coli* [48] *S. typhi* [49] and *H. influenza* to uptake small and hydrophilic nutrients possessing a molecular weight lower than 600 kDa [50, 51].

Passive diffusion and secondary transport mechanisms in bacteria may involve uptake of drug into bacterial cytoplasm [52, 53]. In the inner membrane of *E. coli*, four protein transporters (PTR) namely YdgR or permease A (DtpA), YjdL, YhiP, and YbgH have been characterized as family members belonging to POT. Among these peptide transporters, the DtpA mediates the transport of dipeptides and tripeptides, thereby exhibiting peptide selectivity very similar to the human oligopeptide transporter (hPepT1) in gut enterocytes [54, 55]. These findings emphasize the potential of modifications of the human physiological state by indirectly modifying the microbiome through drugs [56].

3. Microbiome association with diseases

As described above microorganisms present in the gut of the living organisms contribute to health or cause disease of these organisms by interplay with their immune system. Microbiome is developed at birth according to host interaction but later it is evolved and modified by surrounding factors like environmental and diet. The variation in genetic expression of different individuals is thought to be linked with different microbial composition [57]. Genotype of the host affects the composition of gut microbes. Even mutation of a single gene can cause modification in the structure of gut microbiota. The exact mechanism of association between the gut microbes and the genotype of host is still unknown. Bifidobacteria are highly prevalent beneficial bacteria in gut microbiome and are associated with lactase non-persistent genotype. This genotype is responsible for the synthesis of lactase enzyme which helps to digest the lactose, present in the milk. Absence of this enzyme leads to lactose intolerance in different organisms. So it is important to investigate susceptibility of different underlying pathological conditions by studying microbiomes association with genotype and environmental factors that vary among different human populations [58].

Different studies showed that metabolic disorders are largely congenital and are associated with different microbiomes. For example, gut microbiomes have been linked to metabolic disorders and obesity [59].

3.1 Gut microbes and gastrointestinal tract (GIT) diseases

In gut microbiome, dysbiosis (imbalance of microbial flora) can be induced by host factors and/or external factors such as the intake of antibiotics, mental and physical stress, and nutrients in the diet. Dysbiosis is likely to impair the regular gut microbiota and the appearance of pathobionts and the production of metabolites which may be dangerous to the host or may deregulate beneficial microbial-derived metabolites. The microbial symbiosis has a significant role in the development of many diseases [60] such as the gastrointestinal diseases [61, 62], infections [63], metabolic disorders, liver diseases [64], autoimmune diseases [65], mental or psychological diseases [66] and respiratory diseases [67].

3.1.1 Inflammatory bowel disease

The inflammatory bowel disease (IBD), which includes Crohn's disease (CD) and ulcerative colitis (UC), has for quite some time been suspected to be a host reaction to its gut microbiota. CD represents the chronic inflammation of the GIT (involving any part from mouth to anus) with idiopathic etiology while UC is the chronic inflammation of the large bowel of the GIT with no known cause. Numerous aspects of the microbiota's association in IBD have been inspected in recent years. About 10–20% of adults and adolescents worldwide are affected by IBD [68]. The precise cause of IBD is unidentified, but it is believed to be a multifactorial disease. Inflammation, infection, visceral hypersensitivity, immunity, genetic factors, motor dysfunction of the GIT as well as psychopathological factors are suspected to play a role in its development [69]. Moreover, abnormal gut microbiota has been noticed in the IBD patients and in animals with intestinal inflammatory disease [70–73]. Some of the metabolically active anaerobic bacteria in the colon and terminal part of ileum interact with the immune system of epithelium and mucosal layer of the host intestine. Continuous stimulation of these microbial antigens promote pathogenic immune responses and may cause defects in the barrier functions of mucous layer by killing some beneficial bacteria or by immune dysregulation, consequently resulting in UC and CD. Moreover, disrupted microbiota structure and function in inflammatory bowel disease intensify the immune response of the host causing dysfunction of epithelium and increased permeability of the mucous layer of the intestine [74].

It is difficult to identify a single factor responsible of IBD; however, several observations have demonstrated a change in the gut microbial composition in IBD patients, both CD and UC [70]. Even though the gut microbiota has been recognized as responsible for the IBD establishment in non-predisposed hosts, numerous researches have revealed a high rate of pathogenic *E. coli* in ileal biopsies of CD patients [74]. *Mycobacterium avium* subspecies *paratuberculosis* is another bacterial species that has been commonly associated with the CD etiology [75]. Also, in IBD patients, large quantity of *Enterobacteriaceae* and a decline in *Faecalibacterium prausnitzii* was demonstrated to be related to the CD confined to the ileum [76]. However, it is not yet clear whether the IBD-related changes in the gut microbiota are the reason or the result of the disease.

3.1.2 Gastric cancer

For gastric cancer, *H. pylori*-associated chronic inflammation is considered as a risk factor and WHO has classified *H. pylori* as a class I carcinogen. In about 660,000 new cases every year of gastric cancer, *H. pylori* infection is identified as the major cause leading to the acid-producing parietal cells loss, and thereby prompting the gastric atrophy, metaplasia, dysplasia, and finally the formation of carcinoma [77]. The *H. pylori* elimination before the chronic atrophic gastritis may defend against gastric cancer [78]. The cancer-causing risk might be identified with the phylogenetic source of the *H. pylori* strain, host reaction, and host-microorganism communication [79, 80].

3.1.3 Colorectal cancer

Worldwide, the colorectal cancer (CRC) is the fourth most common cause of death associated with cancer [81]. Like other cancers, the CRC is a complex disease related to environmental and genetic factors. Ongoing research has proposed that gut microbiota assumes a role in the convergence of these factors, likely through forming a tumor-advancing environment.

In certain studies, by using a germ-free mice model of adenomatous polyposis coli (APC), a markedly reduced incidence of colonic tumor and a lower tumor load was revealed when compared to normally raised mice. Further other distinct CRC phenotypes such as bleeding from rectum and iron deficiency has also been shown with an invasion of inflammatory cells emerging from an intestinal epithelial barrier dysfunction. Therefore, it seems that the microbiome and host factors (for example, age and genetic predisposition) are important to the CRC growth and progression [82].

3.2 Role of gut microbiota in cardiovascular diseases

Cardiovascular and metabolic disorders are collectively known as cardiometabolic diseases and are associated with high morbidity and mortality along with significant health care expenditures [83]. The gut-derived and endogenously produced endotoxins including indoxyl sulfate, *para*-cresyl sulfate and lipopolysaccharides have been found to be involved in the development of pathological conditions ranging from atherosclerosis to cardio-renal failure or dysfunction [84, 85]. Furthermore, the development of some complex metabolic disorders including insulin resistance and obesity is also associated with differences in the composition of gut microbiota [86]. The metabolites L-carnitine, choline and phosphatidylcholine are metabolized by intestinal microbiota to generate TMA (trimethylamine) which then undergoes oxidation in liver to produce the proatherogenic metabolite known as TMAO (trimethylamine-N-oxide). Moreover, in atherosclerotic plaques was detected bacterial DNA of the intestinal microbiome indicating the direct involvement of intestinal microbiota in the development of atherosclerosis. Therefore, inhibition of intestinal microbiota-mediated TMAO production through dietary modulation has been suggested as a potential approach for treating atherosclerotic cardiovascular diseases [87].

In some earlier research studies, a significantly low synthetic capacity to produce TMA and TMAO from dietary L-carnitine as well as a subsequent lower plasma levels of TMAO have been observed in vegetarians as compared to omnivores. Likewise, significant variations in microbial communities have also been reported in vegetarians as compared to omnivores [88, 89] suggesting that chronic dietary exposure, i.e., omnivores vs. vegetarians, leads to shift of microbial composition with a selective advantage for bacterial species having potential for increased TMA production, and, thus, may interfere with treatment of atherosclerotic cardiovascular diseases.

3.3 Microbiota and integumentary system

The gastrointestinal (GI) system and skin are highly vascularized and densely innervated organs with crucial neuroendocrine and immune roles which are uniquely related to the normal function of skin [90]. Evidence of bidirectional and intimate connection between the gut and skin health as well as a close link between GI health to skin allostasis and homeostasis has been established [91]. GI disturbances resulted often in cutaneous manifestations and the GI system, especially the gut microbiota, appears to participate in the pathophysiology of many inflammatory diseases, i.e., acne, atopic dermatitis and psoriasis [92, 93].

3.3.1 Role of the gut microbiota in skin homeostasis

The mechanism by which GI flora exert their effect on skin homeostasis is still unknown; however it is postulated that probably such effect may be related to the modulatory influence of gut commensals on the systemic immunity [94]. Certain gut microbiota and their metabolites, i.e., polysaccharide A, retinoic acid from *Faecalibacterium prausnitzii, Bacteroides fragilis,* and bacteria belonging to the *Clostridium* cluster IV and XI potentiate the accumulation of the lymphocytes and regulatory T cells which assist in the anti-inflammatory responses [90]. In addition to this immunomodulatory effect there is recent evidence that the intestinal microbiota may influence cutaneous pathology, physiology and more directly the modification of the immune response by the metastasis of gut microbiome and their metabolic activity [95].

In cases of disturbance in intestinal barriers, it was found that intestinal bacteria and their metabolites may have the propensity to accumulate in the skin and have also access to the bloodstream which ultimately disrupts skin homeostasis. In fact, DNA of intestinal microbes has been separated from the plasma of psoriatic patients, thus showing a direct connection between the gut microbiota and skin homeostasis [90]. The short chain fatty acids (SCFAs), i.e., acetate, butyrate and propionate resulting from the fermentation of the fibers in GIT are believed to play an important role in the maintenance of certain skin microbiota which consequently affect cutaneous immune defense system. For example, propionic acid has an antimicrobial effect against the most common community-acquired methicillin-resistant *Staphylococcus aureus* (MRSA). Previous literature also demonstrates that SCFAs in skin play an important role in affecting the predominant residence of bacteria on normal human skin. It has been found that *P. acnes* and *S. epidermidis* have higher ability to tolerate the propionic acid than other pathogens. Thus, *P. acnes* and *S. epidermis* fermentation may have a low risk of disrupting the balance of skin microbiome. Altogether, these findings may provide supportive evidence for a functional interactive mechanistic approach between the skin and gut [96].

3.3.2 Dyshomeostasis due to dysbiosis

Intestinal dysbiosis may have the negative potential to affect the skin function since gut microbial flora has a huge potential to produce molecules, both harmful and beneficial, that could then reach the circulation and influence skin. Metabolic products of aromatic amino acids, i.e., *p*-cresol and free-phenols are considered biomarkers of a disturbed gut environment as their production is due to pathogenic bacteria such as *Clostridium difficile*. These metabolites may preferentially accumulate in the skin, enter the circulation blood and disrupt the epidermal differentiation and integrity of the skin barrier [90]. Indeed, high level of *p*-cresol and free-phenols is associated with impaired keratinization and decreased skin hydration [97]. Also, the intestinal dysbiosis is responsible for the increased permeability of epithelium which ultimately modulate the immune response by disrupting their balance with immunosuppressive regulatory T cells and thereby triggers the activation of T cells effectors. It has also been observed that epithelial permeability is further enhanced by the pro-inflammatory cytokines and result in chronic systemic inflammation [98].

3.4 Gut microbiome and pulmonary health

Infectious diseases of the respiratory tract including pneumonia and influenza result in deaths of approximately 3.25 million people annually [99]. The majority of the therapies being used currently are suboptimal because the problems of efficiency, toxicity and antibiotic resistance are difficult to overcome [100]. Most of the respiratory tract infections represent failure of host's immune defense. Recently, it was suggested that gut microbiota plays a crucial role in the initiation and adaptation of the immune response in other distal mucosal sites including lungs. Therefore, it is of interest to understand the underlying mechanisms that regulate the interplay between lung defense and gastrointestinal tract and how this interaction aids in achieving optimal lung health.

3.4.1 Asthma and allergies

An abnormal T-helper type 2 (Th2) cell responses is often associated with asthma and allergies. The Th2 cells are recognized by their ability to synthesize inflammatory cytokines including IL-13, IL-9, IL-5 and IL-4 [101] Evidence suggests that the development of allergic diseases in lung is directly affected by alteration in gut immune response [65]. In fact, a single oral dose of *Candida albicans* administered to antibiotic treated mice resulted in dysbiosis, i.e., an altered composition of the gut microbiome. These treated mice exhibited more CD4 cell mediated inflammation response in lung after aerosol administration of an allergen in comparison to those mice having normal intestinal flora [102], suggesting that an immunological predisposition to respiratory allergies can be facilitated by an altered gut microbiome. There is also an increasing interest in understanding the role of Th9 and Th17 cells in the development of asthma and allergies.

3.4.2 Viral and bacterial respiratory infections

Gut microbiota also plays a critical role in the immune response to respiratory tract viral infections like influenza. In infected mice, the CD8 and CD4 T cell subpopulations are directly influenced by the intestinal microbiota [103]. It has also been suggested that an intact intestinal microbiota is necessary for the expression of pro-inflammatory cytokines including pro-IL-18 and pro-IL-1β, which are essential for clearance of influenza [104]. This indicates that microbial signals are provided by gut microbiota which are crucial for the shaping and priming the immune response to viral pneumonia.

Similar findings regarding the role of gut microbiome in immune response to respiratory bacterial infections have also been observed in germ-free mice. These mice were found to be more susceptible to pulmonary infection caused by bacterial pathogen *Klebsiella pneumonia*, showing increased levels of IL-10 and suppressed recruitment of neutrophil that allows dissemination and growth of pathogens [105].

3.5 Gut microbiome and pregnancy

All systems of the body including maternal microbiome are affected by pregnancy. Changes in gut and vaginal microbiome during gestation are of particular significance because during vaginal delivery there is vertical transmission of microbes to the newborn [106–108]. During pregnancy the vaginal microbiota composition changes throughout the gestation period. In addition to vaginal microbiome, the maternal intestinal microbiome also undergoes change during pregnancy. It has been reported that bacterial diversity decreases in women as the pregnancy progresses [107]. Particularly, the ratio of pro-inflammatory *Proteobacteria*, which includes the *Streptococcus* genus and *Enterobacteriaceae* family, reduces during first and third trimester, while an increase in the anti-inflammatory *Faecalibacterium prausnitzii* occurs during these trimesters of pregnancy. These changes in microbiome are independent of body weight during pregnancy, diet, antibiotic use and gestational diabetes, suggesting the association of these changes with normal physiological pregnancy-related alteration in maternal immune and endocrine systems [109].

The consequences of changes in maternal vaginal and gut microbiota on mother health are not clear; however, the gestational changes in fecal and vaginal microbiota are considered to be important for the adaptive response necessary for protection as well as to promote the fetus health. These changes also help in providing a particular microbial inoculum to the newborn at birth before its exposure to other environmental microbes. Also the microbial communities' composition in maternal vagina and gut are not independent of each other. In fact, in pregnant women of 35–37 weeks of gestation most of bacteria, including species of *Bifidobacterium* and *Lactobacillus*, are common between vagina and rectum [110].

Some research studies reported that shift in gut microbiota of mother during pregnancy may be an adaptive response for the mother and newborn health. In mice, an increase in the gut bacteria associated with gestational age, promotes body weight gain indicating a co-evolution of these microbes with their hosts during pregnancy [107]. Moreover, during vaginal delivery, the vertical transmission of these maternal gut microbiomes to the neonate may help the newborn to get an immediate access to microbiota at birth [107, 111].

4. Role of gut-microbiome in brain physiology

Both extrinsic and intrinsic factors play an important role to regulate the development and maturation of the central nervous system (CNS) in humans. In germ-free and antibiotic-treated animals the physiology of the CNS can be affected by neurochemistry as well as by specific microbiota [112]. Evidences for interaction between neuropsychiatric and gastrointestinal pathology in humans have been reported in different psychiatric conditions including autism, depression and anxiety [113].

The role of gut-brain interaction in the nervous system development is also recognized. Gut-brain axis actually establishes a relationship between gut-microbiota and their interaction with brain leading to changes in the status of the CNS. The dysbiosis in microbial species of the gut may lead to induce imbalance in host homeostasis, atypical immune signaling and ultimately progression of CNS diseases [114].

The permeable blood brain barrier (BBB) and functional lymphatic vessels residing in dura meningeal membrane may serve as a gateway for transmission of signals [115]. The exposure to several environmental factors can affect the generation of neurons during the development of the CNS [113]. It has been suggested that maternal-fetal interface permeability permits regulatory factors from the gut microbiota to stimulate Toll-like receptor 2 (TLR2) that helps to promote neural development of fetus and also impart its effects on cognitive function during adulthood [116].

The combination of microbial strains (especially the probiotic) can actively counteract the deficient neurogenesis which further strengthen the developmental link of microbiome to the hippocampal neuronal generation [117]. The brain-blood barrier (BBB) is a highly selective and semipermeable barricade that permits the passage of neutral, low molecular weight and lipidic soluble molecules [118]. In the development of the structural components and growth of vasculature, BBB requires arachidonic acid (AA) and decohexaenoic acid (DHA) which are provided as polyunsaturated fatty acids (PUFA) by gut microbiome [119]. It has been demonstrated that the restoration of BBB is possible in germ-free mice by colonization of *Clostridium tyrobutyricum* that produce high level of butyrates [120].

5. Impact of different environmental conditions on gut microbiome

The most important environmental factors that may lead to dysbiosis include (i) Physical or psychological stress, (ii) use of antibiotics, and (iii) diet (**Figure 2**).

5.1 Physical or psychological stress

Stress is usually defined as homeostasis disruption due to physical, psychological or environmental stimuli known as stressors leading to adaptive behavioral and physiological response in order to restore homeostasis [121]. The effect of both psychological and physical stress on gut microbiome is widely recognized and has been observed in both humans as well as animals [122]. Some research conducted in mice has shown that the microbial composition in the cecum was altered in response to the exposure of a social stressor by placing an aggressive male mouse into the cages of non-aggressive mice. Furthermore, the plasma concentration of stress hormones such as adrenocorticotropic hormone (ACTH) and corticosterone was found to be significantly higher in germ-free mice as compared to specific pathogen-free mice. In addition, several stressors including acoustic stress, self-control conditions and food deprivation have a negative impact on the gut microbiome resulting in the impairment of the immune system [123, 124].

5.2 Use of antibiotics

It has been observed in both humans and animals that the treatment with antibiotics can result in a decreased population of beneficial bacteria including *Lactobacilli* and *Bifidobacteria* along with the increased population of potential pathogenic bacteria like *Clostridium difficile* and the pathogenic yeast *Candida albicans*. The GI symptoms for example diarrhea, abdominal pain, bloating as well as yeast infections may occur in response to microbial shifts or dysbiosis. However,

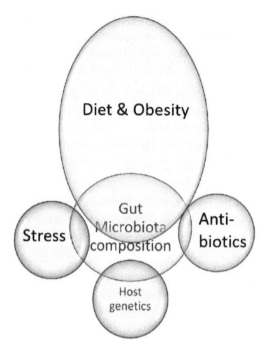

Figure 2.
Environmental factors influencing gut microbiota.

more serious and long-lasting consequences have been suggested. For example, it was reported that at the end of a 5-day treatment with the antibiotic ciprofloxacin, most of the gut bacteria was restored to the pre-treatment levels in 4 weeks, but some intestinal bacteria failed to recover even after 6-months. Moreover, a 7-day treatment with clindamycin, a drug of choice for treatment of *Bacteroides* infections, resulted in disrupted gut microbiome for up to 2 years [125].

5.3 Diet and obesity

Food is metabolized by the gut microbial species to extract nutrients, but some microbial species are more efficient in extracting nutrients from food as compared to other species. As different individuals have slightly different microbial populations, it is probable that more nutrients are harvested by some people's gut microbes making them perhaps more prone to become overweight. A high percentage of *Firmicutes* was found in the gut microbiome of genetically obese mice while a high percentage of *Bacteriodetes* were observed in lean mice. Similar observation was reported in lean and obese human volunteers. Moreover, it was also seen that the obese people who used a low-caloric diet to lose weight, their gut microbiota shifted to a similar bacterial population as observed in lean people [125].

6. Conclusions

The human body is a super-organism consisting of 10 times more microbial cells than our own body cells. The body's assortment of microorganisms is mainly in gastrointestinal tract, collectively called the gut microbiota. It can be comparable to an organ in because it performs functions necessary for our survival by contributing directly and/or indirectly in various physiological processes. For the past decade, human gut microbiota has been extensively studied as many scientists believe that human health mainly depends on microbes that are living on or in our body apart from our own genome. Recently, research findings have suggested that gut microbiome is evolving as a new organ system mainly due to its specific biochemical interaction with its host which affirm its systemic integration into the host physiology as gut bacteria are not only critical for regulating gut metabolism, but also important for other systems of host including immune system. The focus of this chapter was to highlight the importance of gut microorganisms as a new organ system and their possible involvement with host systems as well as the metabolism of different drugs and nutrients in the gut by these microbes. So, in this chapter, we have reviewed opinions of different researchers about the role of gut microbiota in maintaining health as well as its contributory role in different ailments. However, literature revealed that the involvement of gut microbiota in altering host genetics effecting disease progression needs further investigations.

Author details

Haseeb Anwar[1]*, Shahzad Irfan[1], Ghulam Hussain[1], Muhammad Naeem Faisal[2], Humaira Muzaffar[1], Imtiaz Mustafa[1], Imran Mukhtar[1], Saima Malik[1] and Muhammad Irfan Ullah[3]

1 Department of Physiology, Government College University, Faisalabad, Pakistan

2 Institute of Pharmacy, Physiology and Pharmacology, University of Agriculture, Faisalabad, Pakistan

3 Department of Pathobiology, Faculty of Veterinary Sciences, Bahauddin Zakariya University, Multan, Pakistan

*Address all correspondence to: drhaseebanwar@gcuf.edu.pk

IntechOpen

© 2019 The Author(s). Licensee IntechOpen. This chapter is distributed under the terms of the Creative Commons Attribution License (http://creativecommons.org/licenses/by/3.0), which permits unrestricted use, distribution, and reproduction in any medium, provided the original work is properly cited. (cc) BY

References

[1] Van den Abbeele P et al. The host selects mucosal and luminal associations of coevolved gut microorganisms: A novel concept. FEMS Microbiology Reviews. 2011;**35**(4):681-704

[2] Pickard JM et al. Gut microbiota: Role in pathogen colonization, immune responses, and inflammatory disease. Immunological Reviews. 2017;**279**(1):70-89

[3] Faust K et al. Microbial co-occurrence relationships in the human microbiome. PLoS Computational Biology. 2012;**8**(7):e1002606

[4] Gill SR et al. Metagenomic analysis of the human distal gut microbiome. Science. 2006;**312**(5778):1355-1359

[5] Ley RE et al. Microbial ecology: Human gut microbes associated with obesity. Nature. 2006;**444**(7122):1022

[6] Chen Z et al. Incorporation of therapeutically modified bacteria into gut microbiota inhibits obesity. The Journal of Clinical Investigation. 2014;**124**(8):3391-3406

[7] Martin FPJ et al. A top-down systems biology view of microbiome-mammalian metabolic interactions in a mouse model. Molecular Systems Biology. 2007;**3**(1):112

[8] Dethlefsen L, McFall-Ngai M, Relman DA. An ecological and evolutionary perspective on human–microbe mutualism and disease. Nature. 2007;**449**(7164):811

[9] Sison-Mangus MP, Mushegian AA, Ebert D. Water fleas require microbiota for survival, growth and reproduction. The ISME Journal. 2015;**9**(1):59

[10] Sampson TR, Mazmanian SK. Control of brain development, function, and behavior by the microbiome. Cell Host & Microbe. 2015;**17**(5):565-576

[11] McKenney PT, Pamer EG. From hype to hope: The gut microbiota in enteric infectious disease. Cell. 2015;**163**(6):1326-1332

[12] Nicholson JK et al. Host-gut microbiota metabolic interactions. Science. 2012;**336**(6086):1262-1267

[13] Zilber-Rosenberg I, Rosenberg E. Role of microorganisms in the evolution of animals and plants: The hologenome theory of evolution. FEMS Microbiology Reviews. 2008;**32**(5):723-735

[14] Rosenberg E, Zilber-Rosenberg I. The Hologenome Concept: Human, Animal and Plant Microbiota. Switzerland: Springer; 2014

[15] Blaser MJ, Cardon ZG, Cho MK, Dangl JL, Donohue TJ, Green JL et al. Toward a predictive understanding of Earth's microbiomes to address 21st century challenges. mBio. 2016;**7**(3):e00714-16.

[16] Izard J, Rivera M. Metagenomics for Microbiology. Academic Press Elsevier Science; 2014

[17] Macia L et al. Microbial influences on epithelial integrity and immune function as a basis for inflammatory diseases. Immunological Reviews. 2012;**245**(1):164-176

[18] Falony G et al. Population-level analysis of gut microbiome variation. Science. 2016;**352**(6285):560-564

[19] Heinken A, Thiele I. Systematic prediction of health-relevant human-microbial co-metabolism through a computational framework. Gut Microbes. 2015;**6**(2):120-130

[20] Ley RE, Peterson DA, Gordon JI. Ecological and evolutionary forces

shaping microbial diversity in the human intestine. Cell. 2006;**124**(4):837-848

[21] Sansonetti PJ, Medzhitov R. Learning tolerance while fighting ignorance. Cell. 2009;**138**(3):416-420

[22] Yang L et al. Gut microbiota co-microevolution with selection for host humoral immunity. Frontiers in Microbiology. 2017;**8**:1243

[23] Tissier H. Recherches sur la flore intestinale des nourrissons: (état normal et pathologique). G. Carre and C. Naud, Paris, France; 1900

[24] Blaser MJ. Who are we? Indigenous microbes and the ecology of human diseases. EMBO Reports. 2006;**7**(10):956-960

[25] Ardissone AN et al. Meconium microbiome analysis identifies bacteria correlated with premature birth. PLoS One. 2014;**9**(3):e90784

[26] Moles L et al. Bacterial diversity in meconium of preterm neonates and evolution of their fecal microbiota during the first month of life. PLoS One. 2013;**8**(6):e66986

[27] DiGiulio DB et al. Microbial prevalence, diversity and abundance in amniotic fluid during preterm labor: A molecular and culture-based investigation. PLoS One. 2008;**3**(8):e3056

[28] Moeller AH et al. Transmission modes of the mammalian gut microbiota. Science. 2018;**362**(6413):453-457

[29] Rothschild D et al. Environment dominates over host genetics in shaping human gut microbiota. Nature. 2018;**555**(7695):210

[30] Madupu R, Szpakowski S, Nelson KE. Microbiome in human

health and disease. Science Progress. 2013;**96**(2):153-170

[31] Zaneveld J et al. Host-bacterial coevolution and the search for new drug targets. Current Opinion in Chemical Biology. 2008;**12**(1):109-114

[32] Moran NA. Symbiosis as an adaptive process and source of phenotypic complexity. Proceedings of the National Academy of Sciences. 2007;**104** (Suppl. 1):8627-8633

[33] Charleston MA, Perkins SL. Traversing the tangle: Algorithms and applications for cophylogenetic studies. Journal of Biomedical Informatics. 2006;**39**(1):62-71

[34] Stevens J. Computational aspects of host–parasite phylogenies. Briefings in Bioinformatics. 2004;**5**(4):339-349

[35] Osawa R, Blanshard W, Ocallaghan P. Microbiological studies of the intestinal microflora of the koala, *Phascolarctos cinereus*. 2. Pap, a special maternal feces consumed by juvenile koalas. Australian Journal of Zoology. 1993;**41**(6):611-620

[36] Kurokawa K et al. Comparative metagenomics revealed commonly enriched gene sets in human gut microbiomes. DNA Research. 2007;**14**(4):169-181

[37] Hansen-Wester I, Stecher B, Hensel M. Analyses of the evolutionary distribution of *Salmonella* translocated effectors. Infection and Immunity. 2002;**70**(3):1619-1622

[38] Hensel M. Evolution of pathogenicity islands of *Salmonella enterica*. International Journal of Medical Microbiology. 2004;**294**(2-3):95-102

[39] Lujan SA et al. Disrupting antibiotic resistance propagation by inhibiting the conjugative DNA relaxase. Proceedings

of the National Academy of Sciences. 2007;**104**(30):12282-12287

[40] Dahlgren MK et al. Design, synthesis, and multivariate quantitative structure– activity relationship of Salicylanilides potent inhibitors of type III secretion in Yersinia. Journal of Medicinal Chemistry. 2007;**50**(24):6177-6188

[41] Hsiao WW et al. Evidence of a large novel gene pool associated with prokaryotic genomic islands. PLoS Genetics. 2005;**1**(5):e62

[42] Ekins S et al. Computational modeling to accelerate the identification of substrates and inhibitors for transporters that affect drug disposition. Clinical Pharmacology & Therapeutics. 2012;**92**(5):661-665

[43] Dobson PD, Kell DB. Carrier-mediated cellular uptake of pharmaceutical drugs: An exception or the rule? Nature Reviews Drug Discovery. 2008;**7**(3):205

[44] Rubio-Aliaga I, Daniel H. Peptide transporters and their roles in physiological processes and drug disposition. Xenobiotica. 2008;**38**(7-8):1022-1042

[45] Ma K, Hu Y, Smith DE. Peptide transporter 1 is responsible for intestinal uptake of the dipeptide glycylsarcosine: Studies in everted jejunal rings from wild-type and Pept1 null mice. Journal of Pharmaceutical Sciences. 2011;**100**(2):767-774

[46] Sussman A, Gilvarg C. Peptide transport and metabolism in bacteria. Annual Review of Biochemistry. 1971;**40**(1):397-408

[47] payne JW. Peptide Transport in Bacteria: Methods, Mutants and Energy Coupling. Biochemical Society Transactions. Portland Press Limited. 1983;**11**:794-798

[48] Mortimer PG, Piddok LJ. The accumulation of five antibacterial agents in porin-deficient mutants of Escherichia coli. Journal of Antimicrobial Chemotherapy. 1993;**32**(2):195-213

[49] Toro CS et al. Clinical isolate of a porinless *Salmonella typhi* resistant to high levels of chloramphenicol. Antimicrobial Agents and Chemotherapy. 1990;**34**(9):1715-1719

[50] Burns JL, Smith AL. A major outer-membrane protein functions as a porin in *Haemophilus influenzae*. Microbiology. 1987;**133**(5):1273-1277

[51] Srikumar R et al. Porins of *Haemophilus influenzae* type b mutated in loop 3 and in loop 4. Journal of Biological Chemistry. 1997;**272**(21):13614-13621

[52] Lewinson O et al. The *Escherichia coli* multidrug transporter MdfA catalyzes both electrogenic and electroneutral transport reactions. Proceedings of the National Academy of Sciences. 2003;**100**(4):1667-1672

[53] Abdel-Sayed S. Transport of chloramphenicol into sensitive strains of *Escherichia coli* and *Pseudomonas aeruginosa*. Journal of Antimicrobial Chemotherapy. 1987;**19**(1):7-20

[54] Harder D et al. DtpB (YhiP) and DtpA (TppB, YdgR) are prototypical proton-dependent peptide transporters of *Escherichia coli*. The FEBS Journal. 2008;**275**(13):3290-3298

[55] Casagrande F et al. Projection structure of DtpD (YbgH), a prokaryotic member of the peptide transporter family. Journal of Molecular Biology. 2009;**394**(4):708-717

[56] Garber K. Drugging the Gut Microbiome. Nature Publishing Group; 2015;**33**:228-231

[57] Pessione E. Lactic acid bacteria contribution to gut microbiota complexity: Lights and shadows. Frontiers in Cellular and Infection Microbiology. 2012;**2**:86

[58] Goodrich JK et al. The relationship between the human genome and microbiome comes into view. Annual Review of Genetics. 2017;**51**:413-433

[59] Snyder M. Genomics and Personalized Medicine: What Everyone Needs to Know. England: Oxford University Press; 2016

[60] Bassi C, Larvin M, Villatoro E. Antibiotic therapy for prophylaxis against infection of pancreatic necrosis in acute pancreatitis. The Cochrane Database of Systematic Reviews. 2003;**4**:CD002941

[61] Bik EM et al. Bacterial diversity in the oral cavity of 10 healthy individuals. The ISME Journal. 2010;**4**(8):962

[62] Bik EM et al. Molecular analysis of the bacterial microbiota in the human stomach. Proceedings of the National Academy of Sciences. 2006;**103**(3):732-737

[63] Bates JM et al. Intestinal alkaline phosphatase detoxifies lipopolysaccharide and prevents inflammation in zebrafish in response to the gut microbiota. Cell Host & Microbe. 2007;**2**(6):371-382

[64] Beutler B, Rietschel ET. Innate immune sensing and its roots: The story of endotoxin. Nature Reviews Immunology. 2003;**3**(2):169

[65] Björkstén B et al. Allergy development and the intestinal microflora during the first year of life. Journal of Allergy and Clinical Immunology. 2001;**108**(4):516-520

[66] Björkbacka H et al. Reduced atherosclerosis in MyD88-null mice links elevated serum cholesterol levels to activation of innate immunity signaling pathways. Nature Medicine. 2004;**10**(4):416

[67] Bingham S. Diet and Colorectal Cancer Prevention. Portland Press Limited; 2000

[68] Longstreth GF et al. Functional bowel disorders. Gastroenterology. 2006;**130**(5):1480-1491

[69] Ghoshal UC et al. The gut microbiota and irritable bowel syndrome: Friend or foe? International Journal of Inflammation. 2012:**151085**

[70] Peterson DA et al. Metagenomic approaches for defining the pathogenesis of inflammatory bowel diseases. Cell Host & Microbe. 2008;**3**(6):417-427

[71] Frank DN, Pace NR. Gastrointestinal microbiology enters the metagenomics era. Current Opinion in Gastroenterology. 2008;**24**(1):4-10

[72] Frank DN et al. Molecular-phylogenetic characterization of microbial community imbalances in human inflammatory bowel diseases. Proceedings of the National Academy of Sciences. 2007;**104**(34):13780-13785

[73] Lupp C et al. Host-mediated inflammation disrupts the intestinal microbiota and promotes the overgrowth of *Enterobacteriaceae*. Cell Host & Microbe. 2007;**2**(2):119-129

[74] Sartor RB. Microbial influences in inflammatory bowel diseases. Gastroenterology. 2008;**134**(2):577-594

[75] Packey CD, Sartor RB. Commensal bacteria, traditional and opportunistic pathogens, dysbiosis and bacterial killing in inflammatory bowel diseases. Current Opinion in Infectious Diseases. 2009;**22**(3):292

[76] Willing B et al. Twin studies reveal specific imbalances in the mucosaassociated microbiota of patients with ileal Crohn's disease. Inflammatory Bowel Diseases. 2008;**15**(5):653-660

[77] De Martel C et al. Global burden of cancers attributable to infections in 2008: A review and synthetic analysis. The Lancet Oncology. 2012;**13**(6):607-615

[78] Wong BC-Y et al. *Helicobacter pylori* eradication to prevent gastric cancer in a high-risk region of China: A randomized controlled trial. JAMA. 2004;**291**(2):187-194

[79] El-Omar EM et al. Interleukin-1 polymorphisms associated with increased risk of gastric cancer. Nature. 2000;**404**(6776):398

[80] de Sablet T et al. Phylogeographic origin of *Helicobacter pylori* is a determinant of gastric cancer risk. Gut. 2011;**60**(9):1189-1195

[81] Arnold M et al. Global patterns and trends in colorectal cancer incidence and mortality. Gut. 2017;**66**(4):683-691

[82] Li Y et al. Gut microbiota accelerate tumor growth via c-jun and STAT3 phosphorylation in APC Min/+ mice. Carcinogenesis. 2012;**33**(6):1231-1238

[83] Aron-Wisnewsky J, Clément K. The gut microbiome, diet, and links to cardiometabolic and chronic disorders. Nature Reviews Nephrology. 2016;**12**(3):169

[84] Buffie CG, Pamer EG. Microbiota-mediated colonization resistance against intestinal pathogens. Nature Reviews Immunology. 2013;**13**(11):790

[85] Collins SM. A role for the gut microbiota in IBS. Nature Reviews Gastroenterology & Hepatology. 2014;**11**(8):497

[86] Turnbaugh PJ et al. An obesity-associated gut microbiome with increased capacity for energy harvest. Nature. 2006;**444**(7122):1027

[87] Wang Z et al. Non-lethal inhibition of gut microbial trimethylamine production for the treatment of atherosclerosis. Cell. 2015;**163**(7):1585-1595

[88] Koeth RA et al. Intestinal microbiota metabolism of L-carnitine, a nutrient in red meat, promotes atherosclerosis. Nature Medicine. 2013;**19**(5):576

[89] Huijbers MM et al. Flavin dependent monooxygenases. Archives of Biochemistry and Biophysics. 2014;**544**:2-17

[90] O'Neill CA et al. The gut-skin axis in health and disease: A paradigm with therapeutic implications. BioEssays. 2016;**38**(11):1167-1176

[91] Levkovich T et al. Probiotic bacteria induce a 'glow of health'. PLoS One. 2013;**8**(1):e53867

[92] Shah KR et al. Cutaneous manifestations of gastrointestinal disease: Part I. Journal of the American Academy of Dermatology. 2013;**68**(2):189. e1-189. e21

[93] Salem I et al. The gut microbiome as a major regulator of the gut-skin axis. Frontiers in Microbiology. 2018;**9**:1459

[94] Forbes JD, Van Domselaar G, Bernstein CN. The gut microbiota in immune-mediated inflammatory diseases. Frontiers in Microbiology. 2016;**7**:1081

[95] Samuelson DR, Welsh DA, Shellito JE. Regulation of lung immunity and host defense by the intestinal microbiota. Frontiers in Microbiology. 2015;**6**:1085

[96] Schwarz A, Bruhs A, Schwarz T. The short-chain fatty acid sodium butyrate functions as a regulator of the skin immune system. Journal of Investigative Dermatology. 2017;**137**(4): 855-864

[97] Miyazaki K et al. Bifidobacterium fermented milk and galacto-oligosaccharides lead to improved skin health by decreasing phenols production by gut microbiota. Beneficial Microbes. 2013;**5**(2):121-128

[98] Kosiewicz MM et al. Relationship between gut microbiota and development of T cell associated disease. FEBS Letters. 2014;**588**(22):4195-4206

[99] Ruberto I et al. The availability and consistency of dengue surveillance data provided online by the World Health Organization. PLoS Neglected Tropical Diseases. 2015;**9**(4):e0003511

[100] Keely S, Talley NJ, Hansbro PM. Pulmonary-intestinal cross-talk in mucosal inflammatory disease. Mucosal Immunology. 2012;**5**(1):7

[101] McLoughlin RM, Mills KH. Influence of gastrointestinal commensal bacteria on the immune responses that mediate allergy and asthma. Journal of Allergy and Clinical Immunology. 2011;**127**(5):1097-1107

[102] Noverr MC et al. Role of antibiotics and fungal microbiota in driving pulmonary allergic responses. Infection and Immunity. 2004;**72**(9):4996-5003

[103] Ichinohe T et al. Microbiota regulates immune defense against respiratory tract influenza a virus infection. Proceedings of the National Academy of Sciences. 2011;**108**(13):5354-5359

[104] Ichinohe T, Pang IK, Iwasaki A. Influenza virus activates inflammasomes via its intracellular M2 ion channel. Nature Immunology. 2010;**11**(5):404

[105] Fagundes CT et al. Transient TLR activation restores inflammatory response and ability to control pulmonary bacterial infection in germfree mice. The Journal of Immunology. 2012;**188**(3):1411-1420

[106] Aagaard K et al. A metagenomic approach to characterization of the vaginal microbiome signature in pregnancy. PLoS One. 2012;**7**(6):e36466

[107] Koren O et al. Host remodeling of the gut microbiome and metabolic changes during pregnancy. Cell. 2012;**150**(3):470-480

[108] Romero R et al. The composition and stability of the vaginal microbiota of normal pregnant women is different from that of non-pregnant women. Microbiome. 2014;**2**(1):4

[109] Mueller NT et al. The infant microbiome development: Mom matters. Trends in Molecular Medicine. 2015;**21**(2):109-117

[110] El Aila NA et al. Identification and genotyping of bacteria from paired vaginal and rectal samples from pregnant women indicates similarity between vaginal and rectal microflora. BMC Infectious Diseases. 2009;**9**(1):167

[111] Pantoja-Feliciano IG et al. Biphasic assembly of the murine intestinal microbiota during early development. The ISME Journal. 2013;7(6):1112

[112] Smith PA. The tantalizing links between gut microbes and the brain. Nature News. 2015;**526**(7573):312

[113] Sharon G et al. The central nervous system and the gut microbiome. Cell. 2016;**167**(4):915-932

[114] Cussotto S et al. The neuroendocrinology of the

microbiota-gut-brain axis: A behavioural perspective. Frontiers in Neuroendocrinology. 2018;**51**:80-101

[115] Quail DF, Joyce JA. The microenvironmental landscape of brain tumors. Cancer Cell. 2017;**31**(3):326-341

[116] Humann J et al. Bacterial peptidoglycan traverses the placenta to induce fetal neuroproliferation and aberrant postnatal behavior. Cell Host & Microbe. 2016;**19**(3):388-399

[117] Möhle L et al. Ly6Chi monocytes provide a link between antibiotic-induced changes in gut microbiota and adult hippocampal neurogenesis. Cell Reports. 2016;**15**(9):1945-1956

[118] Wolak DJ, Thorne RG. Diffusion of macromolecules in the brain: Implications for drug delivery. Molecular Pharmaceutics. 2013;**10**(5):1492-1504

[119] Crawford M et al. The potential role for arachidonic and docosahexaenoic acids in protection against some central nervous system injuries in preterm infants. Lipids. 2003;**38**(4):303-315

[120] Braniste V et al. The gut microbiota influences blood-brain barrier permeability in mice. Science Translational Medicine. 2014;**6**(263):263ra158

[121] Glaser R, Kiecolt-Glaser JK. Stress-induced immune dysfunction: Implications for health. Nature Reviews Immunology. 2005;**5**(3):243

[122] Caso JR, Leza JC, Menchen L. The effects of physical and psychological stress on the gastrointestinal tract: Lessons from animal models. Current Molecular Medicine. 2008;**8**(4):299-312

[123] Bailey MT et al. Exposure to a social stressor alters the structure of the intestinal microbiota: Implications for stressor-induced immunomodulation. Brain, Behavior, and Immunity. 2011;**25**(3):397-407

[124] Sudo N et al. Postnatal microbial colonization programs the hypothalamic–pituitary–adrenal system for stress response in mice. The Journal of Physiology. 2004;**558**(1):263-275

[125] Phillips ML. Gut reaction: Environmental effects on the human microbiota. National Institute of Environmental Health Sciences. 2009;**117**(5):A198–A205

Chapter 11

Microscale Mechanics of Plug-and-Play In Vitro Cytoskeleton Networks

Shea N. Ricketts, Bekele Gurmessa
and Rae M. Robertson-Anderson

Abstract

This chapter describes recent techniques that have been developed to reconstitute and characterize well-controlled, tunable networks of actin and microtubules outside of cells. It describes optical tweezers microrheology techniques to characterize the linear and nonlinear mechanics of these plug-and-play in vitro networks from the molecular-level to mesoscopic scales. It also details fluorescence microscopy and single-molecule tracking methods to determine macromolecular transport properties and stress propagation through cytoskeleton networks. Throughout the chapter the intriguing results that this body of work has revealed are highlighted—including how the macromolecular constituents of cytoskeleton networks map to their signature responses to stress or strain; and the elegant couplings between network structure, macromolecular mobility, and stress response that cytoskeleton networks exhibit.

Keywords: cytoskeleton, actin, microtubules, microrheology, optical tweezers, fluorescence, microscopy, in vitro

1. Introduction

The cell cytoskeleton is a complex and dynamic network of filamentous proteins that provides cells with structural and mechanical integrity while enabling key dynamic features such as cell motility, cytokinesis, apoptosis, and division [1, 2]. The cytoskeleton is able to perform these diverse functions by exhibiting a wide range of mechanical and structural properties that are tuned by the properties of, and interactions between, its constituent filamentous proteins: actin, microtubules, and intermediate filaments.

Due to the critical importance of understanding cytoskeleton mechanics and structure, over the past several decades numerous researchers from diverse disciplines have performed in vitro, in vivo, in silico, and theoretical studies aimed at elucidating this open problem [1–17]. This collective body of work has made great strides in understanding the molecular structure and properties of individual actin filaments and microtubules, the viscoelastic properties of simple in vitro networks of cytoskeletal filaments, and the role that various crosslinking proteins play in the resulting architecture and mechanical properties of actin networks. Complementary in vivo studies have focused on identifying key motifs that arise in different cell types, in different regions of the cell, and during different phases in the cell cycle. These studies have demonstrated that the cytoskeleton can exhibit complex and nonlinear viscoelastic responses to strain; and that the lengths, concentrations and interactions between the comprising filaments play key roles in this response.

However, due to the diverse and complex mechanical responses and morphologies that cytoskeleton networks can exhibit, a connection between structure and mechanics in the cytoskeleton has proven elusive. The macromolecular properties and dynamics of the individual cytoskeleton filaments that give rise to the network stress response is also an open question. This chapter focuses on methods to overcome these issues including: the design of well-controlled in vitro cytoskeleton networks (Section 2), active microrheology methods to characterize the mechanical properties of these networks at the molecular and cellular scales (Section 3), and fluorescence microscopy techniques to measure network transport properties, mobility and structure (Section 4).

2. Preparation of tunable plug-and-play in vitro cytoskeleton networks

Over the past few decades, researchers have developed methods to create a range of cytoskeleton networks in vitro [3, 6, 11, 18–20]. Key issues that arise when creating and studying these networks are reproducibility and stability. There are also limited methods for creating networks comprised of multiple types of cytoskeleton filaments [6, 18]. Further, many of these systems exhibit structural and mechanical properties that vary from sample to sample, and exhibit aging and instability such that measurements are highly-dependent on the timescale of the measurement and age of the sample.

In vitro networks of semiflexible actin filaments have been most widely studied, spanning protein concentrations from the dilute to the nematic regimes, and incorporating numerous types of actin binding proteins (ABP) to create crosslinked and bundled networks [3, 13, 16, 19]. The motor protein, myosin II, has been used to create active and dynamic actin networks [4, 21, 22]. In vitro networks of rigid microtubules have also been studied, though less extensively [8, 14]. Far fewer studies have focused on composite networks of actin and microtubules, stemming from the incompatibility of established in vitro polymerization conditions for each protein. However, protocols have recently been developed to overcome this issue [18, 23].

Below are protocols to create highly stable, reproducible and tunable in vitro networks of actin and microtubules that mimic key biomimetic motifs and interactions. Further details regarding protocols can be found here [24]. These networks include actin networks with varying concentrations of crosslinkers, actin networks bundled by counterion condensation, and composite networks of sterically and chemically interacting actin filaments and microtubules. All networks are created by polymerization of actin monomers and/or tubulin dimers in an experimental sample chamber, rather than flowing in pre-formed filament networks, such that the native network structure and dynamics are preserved. To ensure reproducibility and stability, biotin-NeutrAvidin bonding and counterion condensation are used, rather than physiological ABPs, to create filament crosslinks and bundles.

2.1 Required buffers and reagents for networks described in Sections 2.2–2.4

PEM-100: 100 mM K-PIPES (pH 6.8), 2 mM EGTA, 2 mM MgCl$_2$. Store at room temperature (RT).

G-buffer: 2.0 mM Tris (pH 8), 0.2 mM ATP, 0.5 mM DTT, 0.1 mM CaCl$_2$. Store at −20°C.

10× F-buffer: 100 mM Imidazole (pH 7.0), 500 mM KCl, 10 mM MgCl$_2$, 10 mM EGTA, 2 mM ATP. Store at −20°C.

Oxygen scavenging system: 4.5 mg/mL glucose, 0.5% β-mercaptoethanol, 4.3 mg/mL glucose oxidase, 0.7 mg/mL catalase. Make fresh immediately prior to mixing into experimental sample. *Used to slow photobleaching during imaging when networks or microspheres have been fluorescent-labeled (see Section 4).*

1% (v/v) Tween: Used to prevent filaments from adsorbing to sample chamber surface. Dilute in working buffer.

100 mM GTP: Store at −20°C. Dilute to experimental concentration in PEM-100 and keep on ice.

100 mM ATP (pH to 7.0): Store at −20°C. Dilute to experimental concentration in working buffer (PEM-100 or G-buffer) and keep on ice.

2 mM Taxol: Suspend 1 mg Pacilitaxol (Sigma, T7402) in DMSO. Store at −20°C.

PEM-Taxol: 198 μL PEM-100, 2 μL 2 mM Taxol. Make fresh for every sample. Store at RT.

200 μM Taxol: 18 μL DMSO, 2 μL 2 mM Taxol. Make fresh for every sample. Store at RT.

Tubulin (*T*, Cytoskeleton #T240): Resuspend to 5 mg/mL in PEM-100. Store in 5 μL aliquots at −80°C.

Biotinylated Tubulin (*B-T*, Cytoskeleton #T333P): Resuspend to 5 mg/mL in PEM-100. Store in 2 μL aliquots at −80°C.

Rhodamine Tubulin (*R-T*, Cytoskeleton #TL590): Prepare 5 mg/mL solutions of 1:10 molar ratio [Rhodamine tubulin]:[tubulin]. Store in 5 μL aliquots at −80°C.

Example: bring 20 μg R-tubulin to 5 mg/mL by adding 4 μL PEM-100. Add 36 μL of 5 mg/mL tubulin (T) to 4 μL R-tubulin.

Actin (*A*, Cytoskeleton, #AKL99): Resuspend lyophilized protein to 2 mg/mL in G-buffer. Store in 25 μL aliquots at −80°C.

Biotinylated actin (*B-A*, Cytoskeleton #AB07): Resuspend lyophilized protein to 1 mg/mL in G-buffer. Store in 5 μL aliquots at −80°C.

Alexa-568-actin (*5-A*, ThermoFisher #A12374): Dilute to 1.5 mg/mL in G-buffer. Store in 5 μL aliquots at −80°C.

Alexa-488-actin (*4-A*, ThermoFisher #A12373): Dilute to 1.5 mg/mL in G-buffer. Store in 5 μL aliquots at −80°C.

Biotin (*B*, Sigma #B4501): Resuspend to 102 mM in deionized water (DI) and store at 4°C.

NeutrAvidin (*NA*, ThermoFisher #31000): Resuspend to 5 mg/mL in PEM-100. Store in 5 μL aliquots at −20°C.

Experimental sample preparation: For all cytoskeleton networks described below, a volume V_F = 20 μL of protein monomers, reagents, and buffers are mixed together and quickly pipetted into a sample chamber constructed from a glass slide and a microscope coverslip separated by two layers of double-sided tape. Sample chambers are sealed with epoxy and incubated (time and temperature depend on network) to form networks of filamentous proteins.

2.2 Entangled and crosslinked actin networks

2.2.1 Entangled actin at any concentration c (mg/mL) and final sample volume V_F

$$V_{PEM-100} = V_F - V_{Actin} - V_{ATP} - V_{Tween} - V_{OS}{}^*$$
$$V_{Actin} = (cV_F)/[A]$$
$$V_{ATP} = 0.1V_F \ 10 \text{ mM ATP}$$
$$V_{Tween} = 0.05V_F \ 1\% \text{ Tween}$$

$V_{OS} = 0.05V_F$ oxygen scavenging system*
If not imaging networks replace V_{OS} with PEM-100.
Incubate at RT for 60 min.

Actin concentrations should be c = 0.1–2.5 mg/mL for entangled networks.

2.2.2 Pre-assembled biotin-NeutrAvidin crosslinker assay

To reproducibly form stable networks of crosslinked actin filaments that are isotropically crosslinked and free of bundling, it is important to pre-assemble Biotin-NeutrAvidin crosslinker complexes before adding to actin monomers to initiate network formation. Each complex is comprised of 1 NeutrAvidin (NA), 2 biotins (B), and 2 biotin-actin monomers (B-A). The molar ratio R of crosslinker to total actin $[T$-$A]$ can be varied according to the following:
$[T$-$A] = [A] + [B$-$A]$; $R = [N$-$A]/([T$-$A])$; $R = \frac{1}{2} [B$-$A]/([T$-$A])$; $[NA] = \frac{1}{2} [B$-$A] = \frac{1}{2}[B]$
Recipe for preparing crosslinker complexes that are concentrated by a factor X in a volume V_{FC}. Prepared complexes are viable for ~24 h on ice.

	Equations for a given R	Ex. R = 0.07
Concentration factor, X	2–20	4 µL
G-buffer volume	$V_{G\text{-Buffer}} = V_{FC} - V_{NA} - V_{B\text{-}A} - V_B$	2.4 µL
NeutrAvidin volume	$V_{NA} = X(V_{FC}R[T\text{-}A]/[NA])$	0.8 µL
Biotinylated actin volume	$V_{BA} = X(V_{FC}2R[T\text{-}A]/[B\text{-}A])$	5.6 µL
Biotin volume	$V_B = X(V_{FC}2R[T\text{-}A]/[B])$	1.2 µL

Sonicate complex solution for 90 min at 4°C.
Add volume V_{CL} to solution below.

2.2.3 Crosslinked network with any given R and [T-A]

$V_{G\text{-buffer}} = V_F - V_{Actin} - V_{CL} - V_{10xF} - V_{OS}$
$V_{Actin} = ([T\text{-}A]V_F)/[A]$
$V_{CL} = V_F/X$
$V_{10\times F} = 0.1V_F$ 10× F-buffer
$V_{OS} = 0.05V_{Final}$ Oxygen scavenging system*
If not imaging networks replace V_{OS} with G-buffer.

2.3 Reversibly bundled actin networks

Bundled actin networks are formed via counterion condensation using high concentrations of $MgCl_2$ and KCl. $MgCl_2$ concentrations of c_M > 4 mM will bundle actin when paired with KCl at a concentration of $2c_M$ (**Figure 1**).

Bundled actin network with actin concentration c (mg/mL) and $MgCl_2$ concentration c_M (mg/mL) in a final volume V_F
$V_{PEM\text{-}100} = V_F - V_{Actin} - V_{ATP} - V_{Tween} - V_{MgCl2} - V_{KCl} - V_{OS}{}^*$
$V_{Actin} = cV_F/[A]$
$V_{ATP} = 0.1V_F$ 10 mM ATP
$V_{Tween} = 0.05V_F$ 1% Tween
$V_{MgCl2} = c_MV_F/[5\ M\ MgCl_2]$

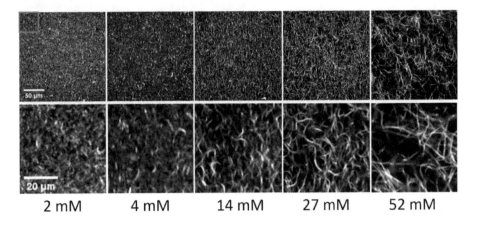

| 2 mM | 4 mM | 14 mM | 27 mM | 52 mM |

Figure 1.
Confocal micrographs of actin networks (c = 5.8 µM) with varying degrees of bundling determined by the MgCl$_2$ concentration (listed below each image). Images shown are average intensity projections from 60 s time-series (4 fps) taken on a Nikon A1R laser scanning confocal microscope with 60× objective.

$V_{KCl} = 2c_M V_F/[4 \text{ M KCl}]$
$V_{OS} = 0.05 V_{Final}$ oxygen scavenging system[*]
[*]*If not imaging networks replace V_{OS} with PEM-100.*

2.4 Composite networks of actin and microtubules

Co-entangled networks of actin and microtubules can be prepared with varying molar fractions of tubulin, $\phi_T = [tubulin]/([actin] + [tubulin])$, and total protein molarity, $[T\text{-}P] = [tubulin] + [actin]$. Composites are formed in PEM-100 with 1 mM ATP (for actin polymerization), 1 mM GTP (for tubulin polymerization) and 5 µM Taxol (for microtubule stabilization). To crosslink actin and/or microtubules within composites, biotin-NeutrAvidin complexes similar to those described in Section 2.2 can be prepared using either actin, tubulin, or both proteins (**Figure 2**).

2.4.1 Entangled actin-microtubule network with ϕ_T, [T-P] and final sample volume V_F

$V_{PEM-100} = V_F - V_{Tubulin} - V_{Actin} - V_{GTP} - V_{ATP} - V_{Tween} - V_{Taxol} - V_{OS}$[*]
$V_{Tubulin} = \phi_T[T\text{-}P]V_F/[T]$
$V_{Actin} = (1 - \phi_T)[T\text{-}P]V_F/[A]$
$V_{GTP} = 0.1V_F$ 10 mM GTP

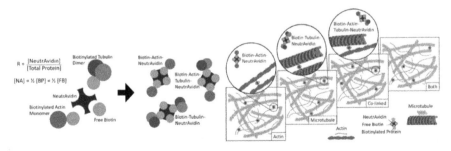

Figure 2.
(Left) Biotin-NeutrAvidin crosslinkers. (Right) Actin-microtubule networks in which: actin is crosslinked (Actin), microtubules are crosslinked (Microtubule), actin and microtubules are linked to each other (Co-linked), both the actin network and microtubule network are crosslinked (Both).

$V_{ATP} = 0.1V_F$ 10 mM ATP
$V_{Tween} = 0.025V_F$ 1% Tween
$V_{Taxol} = 0.025V_F$ 200 µM Taxol (in DMSO)
$V_{OS} = 0.05V_F$ oxygen scavenging system*
*If not imaging networks replace V_{OS} with PEM-100.
Incubate at 37°C for 60 min.

2.4.2 Recipe for preparing crosslinker complexes that are concentrated by a factor X in a volume V_{FC}

Prepared complexes are viable for ~24 h on ice. Biotinylated protein [B-P] used depends on the type of crosslinking as follows:
Actin: [B-P] = [B-A]
Microtubule: [B-P] = [B-T]
Co-linked: [B-P] = [B-A] + [B-T]; [B-A] = [B-T] = ½[B-P]
Both: Prepare Actin and Microtubule solutions. Add equal parts of each to final sample chamber.

	Equations for a given R	Ex. R = 0.02
Concentration factor, X	Number ranging from 2 to 20	4 µL
PEM-100 volume	$V_{PEM-100} = V_{FC} - V_{NA} - V_{B-P} - V_B$	5.28µL
NeutrAvidin volume	$V_{NA} = X(V_{FC}R[T-P]/[NA])$	2.79µL
Biotinylated protein volume	$V_{BP} = X(V_{FC}2R[T-P]/[B-P])$	1.02µL
Biotin volume	$V_B = X(V_{FC}2R[T-P]/[B])$	0.91µL

Sonicate complex solution for 90 min at 4°C.
Add volume V_{CL} to solution below.

2.4.3 Crosslinked network for any given R, ϕ_T and total protein concentration, [T-P]

$V_{PEM-100} = V_F - V_{Tubulin} - V_{Actin} - V_{CL} - V_{GTP} - V_{ATP} - V_{Tween} - V_{Taxol} - V_{OS}$*
$V_{Tubulin} = (\phi_T[T-P]V_F)/([T] - 2R[T-P])$
$V_{Actin} = ((1-\phi_T)[T-P]V_F)/([A] - 2R[T-P])$
$V_{CL} = V_F/X$
$V_{GTP} = 0.1V_F$ 10 mM GTP
$V_{ATP} = 0.1V_F$ 10 mM ATP
$V_{Tween} = 0.025V_F$ 1% Tween
$V_{Taxol} = 0.025V_F$ 200 µM Taxol (in DMSO)
$V_{OS} = 0.05V_F$ oxygen scavenging system*
*If not imaging networks replace V_{OS} with PEM-100.

3. Optical tweezers microrheology measurements

Given the importance of cytoskeleton mechanics to cell function, coupled with the complexity of mechanical properties that cells exhibit, understanding the response of cytoskeleton networks to stress and strain remains an important topic of research. Using standard bulk rheology techniques to measure the mechanical properties of cytoskeleton networks has been problematic due to the difficulty and expense in producing ~mL sample volumes often needed for these measurements.

Further, these measurements probe the macroscopic mechanical properties of the networks but are unable to probe mechanics at the molecular and cellular scales ($\sim\mu$m). Finally, these methods are ill-equipped to measure spatial heterogeneities in network response, and can irreversibly disrupt or damage the network.

Microrheology offers a complementary approach to characterizing the microscale mechanical and viscoelastic properties of cytoskeleton networks. While passive microrheology tracks freely diffusing microspheres embedded in networks to extract viscoelastic moduli, active microrheology uses optical tweezers to actively force embedded microspheres through networks and measure the force exerted to resist this strain. Active microrheology enables one to probe both molecular and mesoscopic scales and perturb networks far from equilibrium to access the nonlinear regime. Specifically, optical tweezers can be used to drag microspheres over distances that are large (5–30 μm) relative to the mesh size of the network (<μm) at speeds much faster than the molecular relaxation rates. The force exerted on the bead to resist the strain, as well as the subsequent relaxation of force following strain, is measured.

Reference [25] provides a thorough overview of the underlying principles and execution of optical tweezers microrheology to characterize the mechanics of bio-polymer networks. Here, the focus is on the key results obtained using the in vitro cytoskeleton networks described in Section 2 [18, 19, 26–28].

3.1 Entangled actin networks

Active microrheology experiments have been carried out on entangled actin networks (Section 2.1) to characterize the dependence of the viscoelastic response and stress relaxation on the rate of the applied microbead strain $\dot{\gamma}$ and actin concentration c (1 mg/mL = 23.2 μM) [26, 27]. The results are largely described within the framework of the tube model for entangled polymers, pioneered by de Gennes and Doi and Edwards [29, 30]. Comparisons to new theories and extensions of the tube model are also highlighted [31–33].

3.1.1 Strain rate dependence

Entangled actin networks (c = 0.5 mg/mL; mesh size ξ = 0.42 μm) subject to strain rates of $\dot{\gamma}$ = 1.4–9.4 s^{-1} (corresponding to speeds of v = 1.5–10 m/s) display a unique crossover to appreciable nonlinearity at a strain rate $\dot{\gamma}_c$ comparable to the theoretical rate of relaxation of individual entanglement segments τ_{ent}^{-1}. Above $\dot{\gamma}_c$, networks exhibit stress-stiffening, which, importantly, is not apparent at the macroscopic scale. This stiffening behavior occurs over very short time scales, comparable to the predicted timescale over which mesh size deformations relax τ_ξ, and has been shown to arise from suppressed filament bending. At times longer than τ_ξ, deformed entanglement segments are able to bend to release stress, and stress softening ensues until the network ultimately yields to an effectively viscous regime, over a timescale comparable to τ_{ent}. This terminal viscous regime exhibits shear thinning due to release of entanglements, with scaling $\eta \sim \dot{\gamma}^{-0.34}$, which is notably less pronounced than the thinning exhibited by flexible entangled polymers ($\eta \sim \dot{\gamma}^{-1}$). Surprisingly, the force relaxation following strain proceeds more quickly for increasing strain rates; and for rates greater than $\dot{\gamma}_c$, the relaxation displays a complex power-law dependence on time, as opposed to the expected exponential decay. This power-law relaxation is indicative of dynamic strain-induced entanglement tube dilation and healing, which corroborates recent theoretical predictions for rigid rods [31, 34].

3.1.2 Concentration dependence

These studies were extended to entangled actin networks of varying concentrations ($c = 0.2$–1.4 mg/mL) to reveal a previously unpredicted and unreported critical concentration $c_c = 0.4$ mg/mL for nonlinear response features to emerge. Beyond c_c, entangled actin stiffens for times below $\tau_{\bar{e}}$, with the degree of stiffening S and stiffening time scale t_{stiff} scaling inversely with the theoretical entanglement tube diameter d_t, i.e., $S \sim d_t^{-1} \sim c^{3/5}$. At longer times, the network yields to a viscous regime with the distance d_y and corresponding force f_y at which yielding occurs scaling inversely with the length between entanglements l_{ent} along each filament: $f_y \sim d_y \sim l_{ent}^{-1} \sim c^{2/5}$. Stiffening and yielding dynamics are consistent with recent predictions of nonlinear strain-induced breakdown of the cohesive entanglement force, which predicts the onset of yielding to occur when the induced force balances the cohesive elastic force provided by the entanglements [27, 32]. Following strain, the force relaxation displays distinct behaviors for $c > c_c$ versus $c < c_c$. For $c < c_c$, relaxation follows a single exponential decay with a decay time that scales according to tube model predictions for the disengagement time $\tau_D \sim c^{6/5}$. For $c > c_c$ relaxation proceeds via two distinct mechanisms: slow reptation out of dilated tubes with $\tau_{D'} \sim c^{1/5}$ coupled with $\sim 10\times$ faster lateral hopping. Tube dilation and the commensurate reduction in reptation time $\tau_{D'}/\tau_D$ scales as c^{-1}, in agreement with recent predictions for entangled rigid rods [34, 35]. This model also predicts faster lateral hopping out of constraining tubes due to temporary fluctuation-induced yielding. The coupled emergence of lateral hopping with concentration-dependent dilation indicates that hopping only plays a significant role when entanglement tubes are sufficiently dilated to allow for fluctuation-induced transient yielding of tube constraints.

3.2 Crosslinked actin networks

As detailed in Section 2.2, methods have been developed to produce highly stable and reproducible networks of randomly-oriented crosslinked actin filaments. With these methods, the crosslinker density can be systematically tuned while fixing the actin concentration and structural network properties (i.e., isotropic filament orientation, no bundling).

Nonlinear microrheological characterization of these networks have been carried out for crosslinking ratios of $R = 0$–0.07 ($c = 0.5$ mg/mL) [19]. For all R values, networks exhibit initial stiffening due to entropic stretching of filaments along the strain path, followed by stress softening and yielding to a steady-state regime. The maximum stiffness achieved K_{max} as well as the time to yield to the terminal regime scale exponentially with R. The critical decay constant associated with this scaling, $R^* \sim 0.014$, corresponds to a crosslinker length l_c equal to the theoretical entanglement length l_e. Networks with higher R values also exhibit more sustained elastic resistance in the terminal regime such that the terminal stiffness K_t scales exponentially with R with a similar critical ratio $R^* \sim 0.018$. These stress response characteristics suggest that softening and yielding arise from force-induced disentanglement and crosslinker unbinding while crosslinker rebinding events allow for the observed sustained terminal elasticity.

Following strain, all networks exhibit exponential force decay with two distinct timescales. Similar to the stress response characteristics, both fast and slow relaxation times scale exponentially with R with comparable R^* values of ~ 0.008, which likewise corresponds to $l_c \sim l_e$. For $R > R^*$ networks are able to maintain high levels of elastic stress following the strain, which is quantified by the terminal force value F_t at the end of the 30 s relaxation phase. Once again, $F_t \sim e^{R/R^*}$ with $R^* \sim 0.007$. As further discussed in Section 4.3, this long-lived post-strain stress is likely a result of the network distributing stress to a small fraction of highly strained connected filaments that span the network, allowing the rest of the network to relax [28].

These intriguing results, along with the corresponding actin filament deformations and stress propagation dynamics that lead to the force response, are further explored in Section 4.3.

3.3 Co-entangled composite networks of actin and microtubules

As described in Section 2.4, techniques have recently been developed to create randomly oriented, co-entangled networks of actin and microtubules by simultaneously co-polymerizing varying ratios of actin and tubulin in situ. The relative concentrations of actin and microtubules, quantified by the molar fraction of tubulin ϕ_T, as well as the overall protein concentration [T-P], can be systematically varied over a wide range of values while maintaining composite integrity and stability. Different crosslinking interactions and motifs can also be methodically introduced and tuned.

Seminal microrheology studies on these composites have been carried out for ϕ_T values of 0 to 1 with [T-P] held fixed at 11.6 µM [18, 23]. These studies show that composites comprised of mostly actin ($\phi_T < 0.5$) initially exert a $\sim$100× higher resistive force in response to strain, compared to networks comprised of mostly microtubules ($\phi_T > 0.5$). However, the rise in force with strain distance is steeper for $\phi_T > 0.5$ networks such that at $\sim$5 µm, the force became larger for $\phi_T > 0.5$ composites compared to $\phi_T < 0.5$. Actin-rich composites are also initially relatively stiff but quickly softened, whereas microtubule-rich composites display an initially soft/viscous response followed quickly by stiffening such that at the end of the strain the stiffness for $\phi_T > 0.5$ networks was $\sim$10× higher than their actin-rich counterparts. The initial force response can be understood in terms of poroelastic models, which consider the dynamics of the mesh as well as the pervading fluid [14, 36]. In these models, the faster the timescale for water to drain from the deformed mesh (τ_p), the faster the system can relax, such that it will exert a concomitantly smaller initial force on the bead. The poroelastic timescale, which depends both on the elastic modulus and mesh size of the network, is $\sim$40× longer for actin networks than for microtubule networks [18], resulting in a comparably higher initial force and stiffness for actin-rich composites versus microtubule-rich composites. The subsequent sharp transition from softening to stiffening when ϕ_T exceeds 0.5, arises from microtubules suppressing actin bending fluctuations.

The presence of a large fraction of microtubules ($\phi_T > 0.7$) result in large heterogeneities in force response as well as increased average resistive force. Heterogeneities arise from the increasing mesh size of the composite as ϕ_T increases, as well as more frequent microtubule buckling events. As ϕ_T increases the mesh size of the composite increases from $\xi_A \sim 0.42$ µm for $\phi_T = 0$ to $\xi_M \sim 0.89$ µm for $\phi_T = 1$. Thus, at the microscale, the system becomes increasingly more heterogeneous as ϕ_T increases. Further, for a composite with equal molar fractions of actin and microtubules ($\phi_T = 0.5$), the mesh size of the microtubule network is $\sim$2× that of the actin network ($\xi_A \sim 2\xi_M$), and the actin mesh remains smaller than the microtubule mesh until $\phi_T > 0.7$. Thus, actin network characteristics dominate the force response until relatively large fractions of microtubules are incorporated. This effect, combined with force-induced buckling of microtubules to alleviate stress, leads to a nonlinear increase in resistive force as ϕ_T increases.

Force relaxation following strain exhibits two-phase power-law decay with the first decay arising from actin bending modes while the long-time relaxation is indicative of filaments reptating out of deformed entanglement constraints.

Interestingly, the scaling exponents for the long-time relaxation exhibits a non-monotonic dependence on ϕ_T, reaching a maximum for equimolar composites (ϕ_T = 0.5), which suggests that filament diffusion (i.e., reptation) is fastest at ϕ_T = 0.5. This non-monotonic trend likely arises from a competition between increasing mesh size as ϕ_T increases, which increases filament mobility, versus increasing filament rigidity (replacing actin with microtubules), which suppresses filament mobility. See Section 4.2 for more discussion of this result.

4. Fluorescence imaging and characterization of network transport, mobility and structure

A key question regarding the cytoskeleton is how the mechanical force response couples to both network structure as well as the mobility and deformations of the comprising filaments. To address this problem, a range of fluorescence labeling schemes can be incorporated into in vitro networks, and various microscopy methods can be employed to image networks and quantify mobility and structure. This section describes different in vitro labeling and imaging methods as well as key results and parameters that can be obtained with the described methods.

4.1 Fluorescence labeling of proteins for varied measurement methods

Below are protocols for three different labeling schemes optimized for different network characterizations and imaging methods: (1) doping networks with pre-formed labeled filaments [18, 27], (2) in situ network labeling [23], and (3) labeling discrete filament segments for particle-tracking [19, 28].

4.1.1 Doping networks with pre-formed labeled filaments

This method is ideal for measuring filament length distributions and resolving single-filament fluctuations and mobility (**Figure 3**).

Figure 3.
Two-color laser scanning confocal imaging of fluorescent-labeled equimolar actin-microtubule composite ([T-P] = 11.6 μM). (A) The actin (green) channel, (B) microtubule (red) channel and (C) both channels show actin filaments and microtubules within composites form networks that overlap with each other forming a homogeneous network with no phase separation or clustering. The scale bar is 50 μm and applies to all images. The 512 × 512 image is taken on a Nikon A1R laser scanning confocal microscope with a 60× objective and QImaging CCD camera.

4.1.1.1 Labeled actin filaments for actin networks (Sections 2.2 and 2.3)

Prepare 10 μL of a 5 μM solution of 1:1 [5-A]:[A] to polymerize prior to adding to actin network:
7.75 μL G-buffer

0.72 µL 5-A

0.54 µL A

1 µL 10× F-buffer

Incubate for 60 min at RT.

Prepare a 1:2 dilution in PEM-100 or F-buffer (depending on desired final buffer).

Add 1 µL of dilution to final sample chamber solution from Section 2.2 or 2.3, replacing the equivalent volume of PEM-100 or G-buffer (depending on network).

4.1.1.2 Labeled filaments for actin-microtubule composites (Section 2.4)

Alexa-488-actin filaments

Prepare 10 µL of a 5 µM solution of 1:1 [4-A]:[A] to polymerize prior to adding to composite:

6.74 µL PEM-100

0.72 µL 4-A

0.54 µL A

2.00 µL 10 mM ATP

Incubate for 60 min at RT.

Immediately prior to imaging prepare a 1:2 dilution in PEM-100 + 2 mM ATP.

Add 1 µL to final sample chamber solution from Section 2.4, replacing the equivalent volume of PEM-100.

Rhodamine-labeled microtubules

Prepare 5 µL of a 37 µM solution of R-T to polymerize prior to adding to composite as follows:

Thaw R-T aliquot in hand.

Add 0.55 µL 10 mM GTP.

Incubate at 37°C for 30 min.

Add 0.6 µL of 200 µM Taxol.

Incubate at 37°C for 30 min.

Immediately prior to imaging prepare a 1:10 dilution in PEM-Taxol.

Add 1 µL to final sample chamber solution from Section 2.4, replacing the equivalent volume of PEM-100.

Labeled filaments can be stored at RT for up to 1 week. After day 1, shear microtubules with a sterile hamilton syringe before adding to the sample chamber.

4.1.2 In situ network labeling

In this method labeled monomers are added to solution prior to in situ network formation, rather than adding pre-formed filaments [23]. This method, demonstrated in **Figures 1** and **4** provides the most accurate depiction of network architecture and enables evaluation of network formation during polymerization. The drawback is that rarely are discrete single filaments visible, preventing filament length measurements. The ratio of labeled (*4-A, 5-A* or *R-T*) to unlabeled (*A* or *T*) monomers can range from 1:50 to 1:5 depending on the overall protein concentration and type of fluorescent dye used. Below are recipes for optimized samples of entangled actin and actin-microtubule composites.

4.1.2.1 Example of in situ labeled actin network

$c = 1$ mg/mL, [5-A]:[A] = 1:9.6, $V_F = 20$ µL

6.3 µL PEM-100

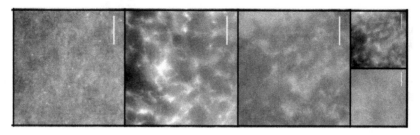

Figure 4.
Epifluorescence imaging of in situ labeling of an actin network (left), microtubule network (middle), and equimolar actin-microtubule composite (right). Images are sum projections of 400-frame time series (40 fps) taken using an Olympus IX73 microscope with 60× objective. The composite image also shows the separate channels for microtubules (top, far right) and actin (bottom, far right). All scale bars represent 10 μm.

1.2 μL 5-A
9.1 μL A
0.4 μL 100 μM ATP
1 μL 1% Tween
2 μL oxygen scavenging system.

4.1.2.2 Example of in situ labeled actin-microtubule composite

$[T\text{-}P] = 11.6$ μM, $\phi_T = 0.5$, $[4\text{-}A]:[A] = 1:4.8$, $[R\text{-}T]:[T] = 1:35.7$, $V_F = 20$ μL

3.43 μL PEM-100
0.29 μL 4-A
1.03 μL A
0.83 μL R-T
0.87 μL T
1 μL 10 mM ATP
1 μL 10 mM GTP
0.5 μL 200 μM Taxol
0.5 μL 1% Tween
1 μL oxygen scavenging system

4.1.3 Labeling discrete filament segments for particle-tracking

Because actin and microtubules are extended filaments, standard particle-tracking methods, optimized for punctile objects, cannot be used. To overcome this limitation, one can generate actin filaments with discrete, well-separated labeled segments (**Figure 5**) through a multi-stage polymerization process that includes shearing and annealing of labeled actin segments. Below is the protocol to create discrete-labeled actin filaments.

Follow protocol in Section 4.1.1.1 to prepare pre-formed Alexa-568-labeled actin filaments.

Shear filaments with a 26 gauge Hamilton syringe 15 times.

Quickly add 1 μL of 2 mg/mL actin (*A*) and mix by pipetting 5 times. Incubate at RT for 20 min to allow labeled and unlabeled segments to anneal.

Prepare a 1:20 dilution in F-buffer. Mix by pipetting 5 times.

Add to final sample solution from Section 2.2 at a volume of $0.05V_F$, replacing the equivalent volume of PEM-100.

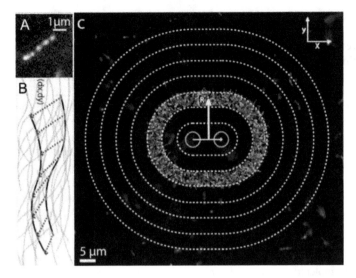

Figure 5.
Discrete labeling of actin filament segments for particle-tracking. (A) Microscope image of filament with interspersed ~0.45 μm labeled segments that can be centroid-tracked during experiments. (B) Cartoon of tracking labeled segments along an actin filament. (C) Tracking discrete segments at varying distances R from strain path during microrheology experiments described in Section 3. Orange circles represent bead position before/after strain and yellow line represents strain path. Dotted lines outline annuli positioned every 4.5 μm from strain path (R = 6.75, 11.25, ..., 29.25 μm). All tracks within each annulus are used to determine R dependence of strain-induced actin mobility.

4.2 Fluorescence confocal microscopy methods

Two-color fluorescence confocal microscopy allows for characterization of the 3D structure and mobility of networks comprised of multiple species (i.e., actin and microtubules). Use labeling method (1), the lengths, orientations, and mobility of single filaments within cytoskeleton composites can be resolved.

This method has been used to quantify the mobility of actin and microtubules within composites as described in Ref. [18]. Briefly, the standard deviation in pixel intensities over time can be computed from high frame-rate time-series and used to quantify the mobility of each filament type. Using this method, Reference [18] showed that the mobility of both actin and microtubules in co-entangled composites is greatest in equimolar composites (ϕ_T = 0.5). This surprising result, which aligns with the post-strain relaxation behavior (described in Section 3.3), arises from an interplay between varying mesh sizes and filament rigidity. Namely, as the fraction of microtubules in composites increases so does the mesh size, allowing for larger voids for filaments to move through (increasing mobility). However, increasing ϕ_T eventually comes at a cost as the majority of filaments are rigid rods rather than semiflexible filaments, which hinders bending modes and fluctuations and ultimately reduces mobility.

3D stacks of images can also be used to determine network structure and connectivity. Evaluating these types of images has shown that the actin and microtubule networks comprising composites are isotropic, entangled, and well-integrated with one another.

More recently developed in situ labeling methods (Section 4.1.2) can more accurately depict network architecture [23] and can be analyzed to determine network correlation lengthscales and fluctuation rates.

4.3 Molecular-tracking microrheology

To directly track filament motion during and following strain, one can incorporate labeling technique (3) into cytoskeleton networks. This method results in punctile segments along filaments that can be tracked over time to determine filament trajectories. Incorporating fluorescence imaging and particle-tracking algorithms into an optical tweezers setup allows for imaging of these segments during micorheology measurements [19, 28].

This method has been used to couple filament deformations and strain propagation to force response in entangled and crosslinked networks of actin [19, 28]. One key result of this work was to determine the origin of stress stiffening and softening in crosslinked actin networks (see Section 3.2). In particular, these studies showed that initial stiffening arises from acceleration of strained filaments due to molecular extension along the strain path, while softening and yielding is coupled to filament deceleration, halting, and recoil. Networks also display a surprising non-monotonic dependence of filament deformation on crosslinker concentration. Namely, networks with no crosslinks or substantial crosslinks both exhibit fast initial filament velocities and reduced molecular recoil while intermediate crosslinker concentrations display reduced velocities and increased recoil. These collective results arise from a balance of network elasticity and force-induced crosslinker unbinding and rebinding. In accord with recent simulations [28], this work also showed that post-strain stress can be long-lived in crosslinked networks by distributing stress to a small fraction of highly strained connected filaments that span the network and sustain the load, while the rest of the network is able to recoil and relax.

5. Conclusions

As described in the preceding sections, several recent advances in in vitro network design and microrheological measurement techniques have enabled key insights into the mechanics and mobility of cytoskeleton networks.

The engineered networks include actin and microtubule networks with well-defined, versatile crosslinking motifs; networks of actin bundles mediated by counterion crossbridges, and composite networks of sterically and chemically interacting actin filaments and microtubules. The protocols and design schemes for these networks are highly modular to facilitate introducing higher levels of complexity and expanding the phase space of molecular constituents and structures. The versatile fluorescence labeling and imaging methods described allow for robust characterization of network dynamics and structure, while the active microrheology studies described can characterize the linear and nonlinear mechanical properties of these networks at the molecular and cellular scales. Some of the key findings this body of work has revealed include: the existence of critical strain rates and concentrations for actin networks to exhibit nonlinear mechanics, the inhomogeneous nature of stress propagation throughout crosslinked actin networks, the important role that actin plays in suppressing the buckling of microtubules, and the elegant competition between mesh size and polymer stiffness that leads to emergent dynamics in actin-microtubule networks.

While many open questions remain, these presented advances open the door for a wide range of highly-controlled new experiments to explore the vast phase space of mechanical and structural properties of diverse cytoskeleton networks.

Acknowledgements

Authors would like to thank Prof. Jennifer Ross (University of Massachussetts, Amherst), Prof. Moumita Das (Rochester Institute of Technology), Robert Fitzpatrick, Dr. Tobias Falzone, and Dr. Manas Khan for their contributions to the described work. This work was funded by an NSF CAREER Award (no. 1255446), an NIH-NIGMS Award (no. R15GM123420), Research Corporation & Gordon & Betty Moore Foundation Collaborative Innovation Award, and a W.M. Keck Foundation Research Grant.

Conflict of interest

Authors declare no conflict of interest.

Author details

Shea N. Ricketts, Bekele Gurmessa and Rae M. Robertson-Anderson*
Department of Physics and Biophysics, University of San Diego, San Diego, California, United States

*Address all correspondence to: randerson@sandiego.edu

IntechOpen

© 2019 The Author(s). Licensee IntechOpen. This chapter is distributed under the terms of the Creative Commons Attribution License (http://creativecommons.org/licenses/by/3.0), which permits unrestricted use, distribution, and reproduction in any medium, provided the original work is properly cited. (cc) BY

References

[1] Pollard TD. The cytoskeleton, cellular motility and the reductionist agenda. Nature. 2003;**422**:741-745

[2] Gardel ML, Kasza KE, Brangwynne CP, Liu J, Weitz DA. Mechanical response of cytoskeletal networks. Methods in Cell Biology. 2008;**89**: 487-519

[3] Gardel ML, Shin JH, MacKintosh FC, Mahadevan L, Matsudaira P, Weitz DA. Elastic behavior of cross-linked and bundled actin networks. Science. 2004; **304**:1301

[4] Murrell MP, Gardel ML. F-actin buckling coordinates contractility and severing in a biomimetic actomyosin cortex. PNAS. 2012;**109**:20820-20825

[5] Dogterom M, Koenderink GH. Actin-microtubule crosstalk in cell biology. Nature Reviews Molecular Cell Biology. 2019;**20**:38-54

[6] Preciado López M, Huber F, Grigoriev I, Steinmetz MO, Akhmanova A, Dogterom M, et al. In vitro reconstitution of dynamic microtubules interacting with actin filament networks. Methods in Enzymology. 2014;**540**:301-320

[7] Fletcher DA, Mullins RD. Cell mechanics and the cytoskeleton. Nature. 2010;**463**:485-492

[8] Hoffman BD, Crocker JC. Cell mechanics: Dissecting the physical responses of cells to force. Annual Review of Biomedical Engineering. 2009;**11**:259-288

[9] Jensen MH, Morris EJ, Weitz DA. Mechanics and dynamics of reconstituted cytoskeletal systems. Biochimica et Biophysica Acta (BBA)—Molecular Cell Research. 2015;**1853**: 3038-3042

[10] Huber F, Boire A, López MP, Koenderink GH. Cytoskeletal crosstalk: When three different personalities team up. Current Opinion in Cell Biology. 2015;**32**:39-47

[11] Hawkins T, Mirigian M, Selcuk Yasar M, Ross JL. Mechanics of microtubules. Journal of Biomechanics. 2010;**43**:23-30

[12] Yang Y, Bai M, Klug WS, Levine AJ, Valentine MT. Microrheology of highly crosslinked microtubule networks is dominated by force-induced crosslinker unbinding. Soft Matter. 2012;**9**:383-393

[13] Gardel ML, Nakamura F, Hartwig J, Crocker JC, Stossel TP, Weitz DA. Stress-dependent elasticity of composite actin networks as a model for cell behavior. Physical Review Letters. 2006;**96**:088102

[14] Moeendarbary E, Valon L, Fritzsche M, Harris AR, Moulding DA, Thrasher AJ, et al. The cytoplasm of living cells behaves as a poroelastic material. Nature Materials. 2013;**12**:253-261

[15] Tsuda Y, Yasutake H, Ishijima A, Yanagida T. Torsional rigidity of single actin filaments and actin–actin bond breaking force under torsion measured directly by in vitro micromanipulation. PNAS. 1996;**93**:12937-12942

[16] Strehle D, Schnauß J, Heussinger C, Alvarado J, Bathe M, Käs J, et al. Transiently crosslinked F-actin bundles. European Biophysics Journal. 2011;**40**: 93-101

[17] Kim T, Gardel ML, Munro E. Determinants of fluidlike behavior and effective viscosity in cross-linked actin networks. Biophysical Journal. 2014; **106**:526-534

[18] Ricketts SN, Ross JL, Robertson-Anderson RM. Co-entangled

actin-microtubule composites exhibit tunable stiffness and power-law stress relaxation. Biophysical Journal. 2018; **115**:1055-1067

[19] Gurmessa B, Ricketts S, Robertson-Anderson RM. Nonlinear actin deformations lead to network stiffening, yielding, and nonuniform stress propagation. Biophysical Journal. 2017; **113**:1540-1550

[20] Gurmessa BJ, Bitten N, Nguyen DT, Saleh OA, Ross JL, Das M, et al. Triggered disassembly and reassembly of actin networks induces rigidity phase transitions. Soft Matter. 2018. 2019;**15**: 1335-1344. DOI: 10.1039/C8SM01912F.

[21] MS e S, Depken M, Stuhrmann B, Korsten M, MacKintosh FC, Koenderink GH. Active multistage coarsening of actin networks driven by myosin motors. PNAS. 2011;**108**:9408-9413

[22] Mizuno D, Tardin C, Schmidt CF, MacKintosh FC. Nonequilibrium mechanics of active cytoskeletal networks. Science. 2007;**315**:370-373

[23] Regan K, Wulstein D, Rasmussen H, McGorty R, Robertson-Anderson RM. Bridging the spatiotemporal scales of macromolecular transport in crowded biomimetic systems. Soft Matter. 2018. 2019;**15**:1200-1209. DOI: 10.1039/ C8SM02023J

[24] https://docs.google.com/document/ d/1QfCAac1OFhBnF-D9IZc 7NvSnrUJNXwsm-ZuVjZKJDfl/edit? usp=sharing

[25] Robertson-Anderson RM. Optical tweezers microrheology: From the basics to advanced techniques and applications. ACS Macro Letters. 2018;7: 968-975

[26] Falzone TT, Blair S, Robertson-Anderson RM. Entangled F-actin displays a unique crossover to microscale nonlinearity dominated by entanglement segment dynamics. Soft Matter. 2015;**11**:4418-4423

[27] Gurmessa B, Fitzpatrick R, Falzone TT, Robertson-Anderson RM. Entanglement density tunes microscale nonlinear response of entangled actin. Macromolecules. 2016;**49**:3948-3955

[28] Falzone TT, Robertson-Anderson RM. Active entanglement-tracking microrheology directly couples macromolecular deformations to nonlinear microscale force response of entangled actin. ACS Macro Letters. 2015;**4**:1194-1199

[29] de Gennes P-G, Gennes PP-G. Scaling Concepts in Polymer Physics. Ithaca, NY: Cornell University Press; 1979

[30] Doi M, Edwards SF. The Theory of Polymer Dynamics. Oxford, UK: Clarendon Press; 1988

[31] Sussman DM, Schweizer KS. Microscopic theory of the tube confinement potential for liquids of topologically entangled rigid macromolecules. Physical Review Letters. 2011;**107**:078102

[32] Wang S-Q, Ravindranath S, Wang Y, Boukany P. New theoretical considerations in polymer rheology: Elastic breakdown of chain entanglement network. The Journal of Chemical Physics. 2007;**127**:064903

[33] Sussman DM, Schweizer KS. Entangled polymer chain melts: Orientation and deformation dependent tube confinement and interchain entanglement elasticity. The Journal of Chemical Physics. 2013;**139**:234904

[34] Sussman DM, Schweizer KS. Entangled rigid macromolecules under continuous Startup shear deformation: Consequences of a microscopically anharmonic confining tube. Macromolecules. 2013;**46**:5684-5693

[35] Sussman DM, Schweizer KS. Microscopic theory of quiescent and deformed topologically entangled rod solutions: General formulation and relaxation after nonlinear step strain. Macromolecules. 2012;45:3270-3284

[36] Kalcioglu ZI, Mahmoodian R, Hu Y, Suo Z, Van Vliet KJ. From macro- to microscale poroelastic characterization of polymeric hydrogels via indentation. Soft Matter. 2012;8:3393

Chapter 12

The Mitosis of *Entamoeba histolytica* Trophozoites

Eduardo Gómez-Conde, Miguel Ángel Vargas Mejía,
María Alicia Díaz y Orea, Luis David Gómez-Cortes and
Tayde Guerrero-González

Abstract

The mechanisms of mitosis in higher eukaryotic organisms are very well studied; however, regarding protozoa, there are still many questions in need of an answer. Because of the complexity with which it carries out this process, many forms of mitosis exist, such as open orthomitosis, semi-open orthomitosis, semi-open pleuromitosis, closed intranuclear pleuromitosis, closed intranuclear orthomitosis, and closed extranuclear pleuromitosis. The fascinating aspect about the mitosis of *Entamoeba histolytica* trophozoites is that it falls out of the context of this classification, but not entirely. The *Entamoeba histolytica* trophozoites first carry out karyokinesis and then cytokinesis. The mitosis of this parasite is comprised of the following phases: prophase, metaphase, early and late anaphase, early and late telophase, and karyokinesis. The difference lies in the mechanism by which it carries out the distribution of the genetic material because it forms three mitotic spindles: two radial spindles that practically surround every group of chromosomes and one that we call inter microtubule-organizing centers (IMTOCs). The latter transports each group of chromosomes at each of the nucleus poles. Based on these observations, we propose that *Entamoeba histolytica* trophozoites carry out a type of mitosis we have called modified intranuclear pleuromitosis open.

Keywords: *Entamoeba histolytica*, mitosis, chromatin, mitotic spindle

1. Introduction

Mitosis in the cells of living beings guarantees the cells' multiplication during the processes of tissue replacement and repair. However, in some protozoa it carries out the purpose of maintaining the species, such as in the case of *Entamoeba histolytica* trophozoites. Differences in the intracellular structures of the mitotic apparatus of human somatic cells [1] (**Figure 1a**) and of *E. histolytica* trophozoites [2–6] (**Figure 1b**) generate the need to briefly review what the cell cycle of the former is like. This will serve as a basis for explaining the equivalence of the intracellular structures of mitosis between the cells of these two species of organisms so distant in evolution.

In order to understand how mitosis occurs in *E. histolytica* and the structures involved, in this chapter we first present a brief review of the cell cycle and mitosis in higher eukaryotes, schematized in **Figures 2** and **3**, which will serve as basis

IntechOpen

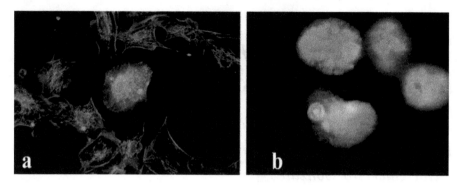

Figure 1.
Higher eukaryotic cells (a) and trophozoites of Entamoeba histolytica *(b).*

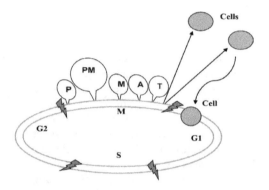

Figure 2.
Schematic diagram representing the cell cycle phases of higher eukaryotic cells. G1, growth 1; S, synthesis; G2, growth 2; and M, mitosis. Prophase (P), prometaphase (PM), metaphase (M), anaphase (a), and telophase (T) occur during mitosis.

used to compare with the mitosis of lower eukaryotes. Afterward, we explain the cell cycle in protozoa and the different mitotic models that occur in them based on different authors, observations masterfully compiled by Raikov IB. In addition, we relate information about the cell cycle of *E. histolytica* and explicitly the mitosis of this protozoan. Regarding the mitosis of *E. histolytica*, we considered scientific evidence published by other authors and our own observations obtained through phase-contrast techniques, video microscopy, acridine orange vital stain, and immunofluorescence, all of which allow us to propose a mechanism on how the mitotic process occurs in this protozoan parasite found in humans.

2. The cell cycle of higher eukaryotes

The cell cycle phases have been divided into interface and M phase (mitosis). During the interface, the cell performs functions of the tissue in which it differentiated into (phenotype) in order to stay alive (G1 phase), duplicate its genetic material (S phase), and prepare for mitosis (G2 phase). During the G1 phase, the cell maintains its biochemical integrity, expresses its phenotype, and synthesizes elements necessary for the duplication of genetic material. In the S phase, the cell carefully duplicates its genetic material so that each chromosome is doubled. During the G2 phase, the cell prepares for the M phase. Sometimes, some cells that are in the G1 phase enter a state of latency or rest, known as the G0 phase [1].

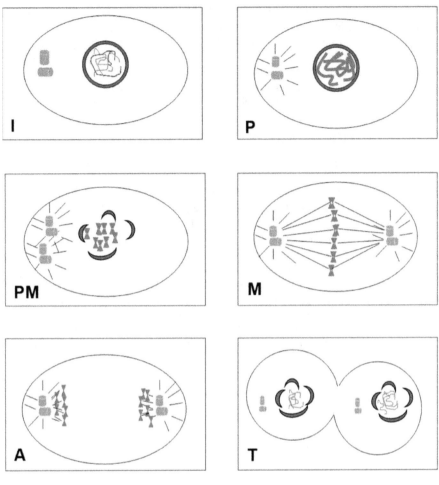

Figure 3.
Schematic diagram depicting the phases of mitosis in a higher eukaryotic cell. (I) Interface, (P) prophase, (PM) prometaphase, (M) metaphase, (A) anaphase, and (T) telophase.

The G1 phase covers the end of the M phase up until the beginning of the S phase. The S phase follows at the end of the G1 phase and ends at the beginning of the G2 phase. The G2 phase starts at the end of the S phase and finishes at the beginning of mitosis (**Figure 2**).

The duration of the interface is longer than the M phase, which lasts only 1 h. However, in the embryonic cells of higher eukaryotic organisms, the S phase is reduced; consequently these cells' cycle is short [1]. The cell cycle of embryonic cells explains the accelerated cell multiplication and the rapid growth of the embryo. The cell cycle of fruit fly embryos lasts only 8 h in contrast to the cell cycle of mammals which lasts 24 h [1].

The duration of the cell cycle varies but the process is similar in all cases. It involves the preparation of the cell in order to give rise to a new organism, as it occurs in unicellular organisms, or to form two identical cells during embryonic development or cell regeneration. Although the two newly formed cells of multicellular organisms are identical, during their cell cycle, each one can modify its phenotype to specialize in a specific function, as it occurs during the advanced stages of the embryonic development of higher eukaryotic organisms [1].

Before a cell initiates mitosis, it needs to duplicate its genetic material and prepare optimal cytoplasmic conditions that will allow it to form two identical cells. Mitosis of higher eukaryotic cells begins with prophase (P), during which the chromatin gradually condenses until the duplicated chromosomes are visible, each with its two sister chromatids joined by the centromere. The microtubules of the cytoskeleton are disassembled, and the formation of the mitotic spindle begins in between the centrosomes that move away from each other. In this phase, the nucleolus is disorganized and not visible during the entire mitosis. Prometaphase (PM) begins abruptly with the disorganization of the nuclear envelope that remains in the form of small vesicles around the mitotic spindle during mitosis. Several protein complexes called kinetochores mature and assemble in the centromere of each chromatid. The fibers of the mitotic spindle that are attached to these structures are called microtubules of the kinetochore; the fibers that do not bind to the kinetochore are known as polar microtubules, and the fibers that are outside the spindle are called astral microtubules. When changing to metaphase (M), the microtubules of the kinetochore align the condensed chromosomes into an equatorial plate. The other end of the kinetochore microtubules attaches to the centrosome of each pole opposite the spindle. Anaphase (A) begins exactly at the moment where the kinetochore pair separates, aided by the microtubules of the mitotic spindle, and is directed toward the opposite poles of the nucleus. The polarization of the chromosomes produces shortening of the kinetochore microtubules, whereas the polar microtubules become longer. During telophase (T) the daughter chromosomes reach the poles of the nucleus, and the kinetochore microtubules disappear. The polar microtubules have lengthened further, and the nuclear envelope begins to organize around the daughter chromosomes. In this phase the nucleolus reappears [1]. During cytokinesis, the cytoplasm divides, and the cell membrane is strangulated in the middle portion of the cell by myosin rings causing the cell to separate, forming two daughter cells (**Figure 3**).

3. The cell cycle in protozoa

For their survival, unicellular organisms also need to duplicate their DNA, divide, and, thus, give origin to a new organism [7]. Like in the cell cycle of higher eukaryotic organisms, in the protozoa interphase (I) and mitosis (M) also occur. The phases (G1), (S), and (G2) are also present in interphase. The phases of mitosis are the same as those in higher eukaryotic cells [7]. The duration of the M phase, as well as each of its phases, depends on the culture conditions. However, the beginning of the S phase and its duration and culmination are evidently regulated by the genetic material [7]. For example, the cell cycle of the *Entamoeba histolytica* clone L-6 lasts from 15 to 18 h: G1 lasts 1 h; the S phase lasts 6 h; and the G2 phase lasts 3 h [8]. The cell cycle of protozoa is very similar to that of prokaryotic organisms because both have states of inactivity in situations of environmental stress, for example, the cystic form in some protozoa and the formation of spores in bacteria, which suggests that they have alternating functional states during the G1 phase [9].

The presence of cyclin-dependent protein kinases related to human cdc2 in some parasites such as *Trypanosoma brucei* (tbcrk1–3) and *Paramecium tetraurelia* suggests their participation in cell cycle regulation of lower eukaryotic organisms [10, 11]. Variation in cytoplasmic calcium concentrations has also been found to be involved in cell cycle regulation in trypanosomes [10]. In particular, it regulates the expression of procyclin mRNA during the differentiation of elongated forms into short ovoid forms [12]. In *Plasmodium falciparum*, the Pfcrk-1 gene has been identified; it encodes a cdc2-related protein kinase that is regulated during the development of the parasite [13].

The cell cycle can be interrupted experimentally with drugs that inhibit the activity of proteasomes such as lactacystin which maintains the procyclic forms of *T. brucei* in the G2 + M phases [14] or with drugs that induce morphological changes and rapid and effective inhibition of DNA synthesis such as sinefungin, which blocks the beginning of the S phase of *Leishmania donovani* promastigotes, stopping them in the G1 phase [15], or with drugs that stabilize the microtubules of the mitotic spindle of *L. donovani* such as taxol that interferes with the progression of G2/M [15].

Mitosis is the main type of nuclear division of protozoa. The fundamental characteristic of mitosis is that the two copies of chromosomes or chromatids are equally distributed between the two daughter nuclei. Consequently, each daughter nucleus receives a complete series of chromosomes. The details of mitotic mechanisms vary widely, particularly in lower eukaryotes including protozoa. In protozoa the level of development of the spindle and centrioles (or structures that are functionally similar to them, such as the microtubule-organizing centers (MTOC)) and the behavior of the nucleolus during mitosis vary widely. In spite of the variants, the two chromatids of each replicated chromosome migrate toward the daughter nucleus while conserving the fundamental characteristic of mitosis [7].

The mitosis observed in protozoa has been classified according to the site in which the formation of the mitotic spindle occurs, the appearance of a complete spindle or formation of two half spindles, and the disintegration, or not, of the nuclear envelope. If the mitotic spindle forms inside the nucleus, it is an intranuclear mitosis, whereas if the spindle forms outside the nucleus, it is said to be an extranuclear mitosis. If a complete spindle is formed, it is an orthomitosis; on the other hand, if two half spindles are formed, it is called pleuromitosis [7]. Finally, if the nuclear envelope remains intact, it is a closed mitosis; if it partially disintegrates, it is said to be a semi-open mitosis, but if it disintegrates completely, it is called a eumitosis, which is equivalent to the mitosis of the higher eukaryotic cells [7]. The combination of these events, during the reproduction of the protozoa, allows the mitosis to be classified into six types: (1) open orthomitosis, (2) semi-open orthomitosis, (3) semi-open pleuromitosis, (4) intranuclear pleuromitosis, (5) intranuclear orthomitosis, and (6) extranuclear pleuromitosis [7] (**Table 1**).

Open orthomitosis has all the characteristics of prototypic mitosis of eukaryotic organisms: the nuclear envelope disorganizes, the nucleolus disappears, and a bipolar, axial, and symmetric spindle with chromosomal fibers joined to the kinetochore forms. Also, the MTOC is located in the cytoplasm where the formation of an equatorial chromosome plate occurs. This type of division occurs in *Phytomastigophora*, *Sarcodina*, *Labyrinthomorpha*, *Gregarines, and Dinoflagellates* [16].

Semi-open orthomitosis is peculiar in the way in which the filaments of the mitotic spindle pass through the nuclear membrane via fenestrations located at the poles of the nucleus. The spindle is symmetric and bipolar and contains continuous chromosomal fibers. Chromatin is poorly condensed and formation of the equatorial plate varies. This form of division is found in green flagellates [7].

In **semi-open pleuromitosis**, two identical half spindles are formed with radial and chromosomal fibers that pierce the nuclear membrane before the centrioles occupy the poles of the nucleus. The microtubules penetrate through fenestrations formed in the nuclear envelope. In this type of division, there is no formation of an equatorial plate. It is common in *Gregarines, Coccidia, Toxoplasmids, and Sarcosporidia* [7].

Closed intranuclear pleuromitosis displays two symmetrical half spindles inside the nucleus, each one originating in a MTOC. The chromosomes are less condensed, and there is no formation of the equatorial plate. It is observed in *Microsporidia, Kinetoplastid, Oximonadida, Foraminifera, Radiolarians*, and some green flagellates [7].

Types of mitosis	Spindle	Nuclear envelope	MTOC	Nucleolus	Chromatin
Open orthomitosis	Bipolar, axial, and symmetrical	Disorganized and not observable	Yes	Disorganized and not observable	Condensed
Semi-open orthomitosis	Bipolar and symmetric	Perforated at the core poles	Yes	¿?	Less condensed
Semi-open Pleuromitosis	Two identical hemi-spindles	Perforated near spindle formation	Yes	¿?	Less condensed
Closed intranuclear pleuromitosis	Two intranuclear symmetrical hemi-spindles	Whole	Yes	Yes	Less condensed
Closed intranuclear orthomitosis	Axial, bipolar, symmetrical, and intranuclear	Whole	Yes	¿?	Condensed
Closed extranuclear pleuromitosis	Two extranuclear mitotic hemi-spindles	Whole	Yes	Remains	Condensed

¿?: Absent.

Table 1.
Types of mitosis in protozoa. Microtubule-organizing center.

Closed intranuclear orthomytosis is characterized by the formation of a symmetric, axial, bipolar, and intranuclear spindle. The chromosomes form an equatorial plate which occurs in *Rhizopoda, Gregarines, Euglenids, and the micronucleus of the ciliates* [7].

Closed extranuclear pleuromitosis presents an intact nuclear envelope with the formation of two extranuclear mitotic half spindles, adjacent to the nucleus. The kinetochores are found in the nuclear envelope, which allow interaction with spindle fibers and the distribution of chromosomes during nuclear strangulation. It has been observed to occur in *Trichomonadida and Hypermastigida* [7].

The structures similar to the centrioles of kingdom Protista, currently known as MTOC, have received different names such as centrosphere, rhizoplast, spindle polar body, kinetosome, atractophores, or organelle associated with the nucleus [17]. Even though they present great diversity in their arrangement, they adequately participate in the spatial organization and behavior of microtubules during the cell cycle. In *E. histolytica*, the presence of a MTOC has been observed in the center of the nucleus and in one of the poles during mitosis [3, 4, 6].

Apparently there is just one MTOC in this protozoan. However, the binding of recombinant anti-tubulin γ antibodies, from the amoeba, at the MTOC site, suggests that this structure is doubled and polarized, respectively, during anaphase and telophase [18].

The chromatin of the protozoa during interphase is in a decondensed and condensed form. In some protozoa, chromatin is dispersed, while in others it is condensed forming peripheral groups, reticular fibers, individual chromosomes, chromocenters, karyosome, or a dense mass that occupies the whole nucleus [7].

The level of compaction of chromatin mainly varies from one species to another. (i) Finely dispersed chromatin has been found in protozoa that have very large nuclei as seen in *Gregarines and Coccidia* (ii) Granular chromatin is very rare and has only been observed in organisms such as *Trichomonadida*.

(iii) Dispersed chromatin is characteristic of protozoa such as *Amoeba proteus* and *Chaos illinoisensis*. (iv) The compacted chromatin is located at the periphery of the nucleus in the form of a continuous plate or as individual chromocenters. Its structure can be finely granular as it occurs in the kinetoplastids, Foraminifera gametes, and life cycle dispersive states of *Sporozoa* (sporozoites, merozoites, and endozoites). Chromatin that is located in the periphery can be decondensed during the transformation from sporozoites or merozoites to active growth states such as trophozoites or gametocytes [7]. The structure of the chromatin in the form of filaments is located in the central portion of the nucleus of Foraminifera, Mixoteca, and Alogramia gametes. At the ultrastructural level, they form blocks and chains that give the appearance of a reticle. The filamentous structure becomes decondensed during the encystment of *A. schizopyrenidae and Naegleria fowleri*. (vi) Highly condensed chromatin is observed in *euglenids*. The level of compaction varies according to the conditions of the medium and exposure to light. The Euglena chromosomes maintained in darkness are very compact, while exposed to light are very dispersed. (vii) Permanently condensed chromatin is found in chromosomes that are linked by the kinetochore to the internal face of the nuclear envelope of organisms such as *Trichonympha, Barbulanympha, and Spirotrichonympha*. (viii) Especially compacted chromatin is found in holomastigotes where they acquire a clearly defined spiral structure [7].

Due to the fact that some protozoa have chromatin organized in a similar way to that of prokaryotes, it has led to classify this phylum in (a) mesocarion and (b) eukaryotes. Both types have a well-defined nuclear envelope, but the former possess chromatin arranged in fibers aggregated in a similar way to bacteria [7].

(a) Mesocarion protozoa include organisms of the *dinoflagellates'* order, and (b) eukaryotes include organisms of the Plasmodroma and Ciliophora subphylum. Dinoflagellates are protozoa with well-formed nucleus, of which its chromatin remains compacted during all the phases of the cell cycle. The chromosomes of the dinoflagellates have a shape similar to coarse threads or fibrillar rods. In some species, chromosomes are decondensed with a structure similar to the nuclei of prokaryotic organisms (noctiluca and parasitic dinoflagellate forms) and appear like strands of DNA lacking histones [19].

The number of chromosomes of protozoa has been determined by applying electrophoresis in a pulse field gradient (PFG) and obtaining karyotypes through cellular explosion. By means of the PFG, the DNA size of the chromosome in two species of fish microsporidia has been established. The molecular karyotype of *Glugea atherinae* shows 16 bands of DNA from 240 to 27,000 kb, and *Spraguea lophii* (the smallest nuclear genome of eukaryotic organisms) has 12 bands of 230 to 980 kb [20]. It has also been found that *G. duodenalis* presents 4 to 6 chromosomal bands between 1 and 4 Mb [21] and *Leishmania* has 20 to 28 chromosomal bands from 250 to 2600 [22]. In *Entamoeba histolytica*, 6 to 9 chromosomal bands have been identified of approximately 2000, 1140, 800, 575, 490, 400, 340, and a doublet of 280 Kb [23] and *Plasmodium falciparum* has 7 chromosomal bands ranging from 750 to 2000 kb [24]. In *T. vaginalis* six chromosomal bands of 5700, 4700, 3500, 1200, 1100, and 75 kbp have been identified [25].

In general, the chromatin of the flagellates is compacted, although there are variations of condensation sometimes forming dense rods that touch the nuclear envelope [26]. In functional terms, decondensed chromatin is considered transcriptionally active [27]. Its arrangement is fibrillar with the formation of aggregates of granular appearance as it occurs in organisms of the *Cryptomonadida* order. In some cases, it forms a fibrous sheet as in *E. invadens* [28]. In *A. proteus* it is identified as dispersed chains of 80–90 nm [29]. In *Leishmania*, it has been proposed that chromatin comprises long diploid holochromosomes that contain all functional structures, such as telomeres, centromeres, and replication origins [30].

In the ciliated protozoa, the genetic material is stored in the macro- and micronucleus. The DNA contained in the macronucleus is transcriptionally active unlike the content in the micronucleus which is inactive [31]. Both nuclei contain DNA and RNA [32]. The chromatin of the macronucleus of the ciliated protozoa is commonly organized into numerous discrete masses called "small bodies" [33] although it has also been observed in the form of spongy masses [34], reticular formations, long chains of chromatin thin plexuses [7], discretely elongated bodies [35], compact spheres, spherical masses, and clear halo granules [28]. The macronucleus of these protozoa contains a structure made visible by light microscope called the replication band, which is a specific site of DNA replication that migrates from the macronucleus and advances along the edge of this band generating the rearrangement of the chromatin in two zones: the proximal and the distal. The proximal reorganizes the chromatin for the synthesis of DNA, and the distal carries it out [36]. Apparently in these organisms, chromosomal fragmentation and the elimination of internal sequences as a route of DNA processing occur [37].

4. Cell cycle of the trophozoites of *Entamoeba histolytica*

One of the main problems in studying the cell cycle and the mitosis of the trophozoites of *Entamoeba histolytica* has been how difficult it is obtaining synchronized cultures. Even when good synchronization with hydroxyurea and nucleotide starvation is obtained, the viability of the trophozoites is low. The synchronization of the cultures of trophozoites of *Entamoeba histolytica* of clone L6 with high doses of colchicine and tritiated thymidine labeling allowed to identify that the phases G1, S, and G2 last 5, 6, and 3 h, respectively [38].

4.1 Mitosis in the trophozoites of *Entamoeba histolytica*

Studies on the organization of the nucleic acids of live trophozoites *of Entamoeba histolytica* with acridine orange stain [5] and those fixed with paraformaldehyde and observed by phase-contrast microscopy (**Figure 4**) show six mitotic phases: prophase, metaphase, early anaphase, late anaphase, early telophase, and late telophase (**Figure 4**).

Unlike the mitosis of the higher eukaryotic cells, the nuclear envelope of the *Entamoeba histolytica* trophozoites remains present during all phases. Another important observation is that the intranuclear RNA located near the nuclear envelope (**Figure 5a** and **b**) remains present during all the phases of mitosis and is fragmented and distributed between the two daughter nuclei [5].

The permanence of the nuclear envelope of *Entamoeba histolytica* trophozoites throughout the whole process of mitosis suggested that the nucleus is first divided (karyokinesis) and then the cell (cytokinesis), resulting in two daughter cells. The chromatin (DNA and RNA) of *Entamoeba histolytica* trophozoites apparently does not show changes of condensation during the phases of mitosis. It is observed as large and small spherical structures (**Figure 5a**). Nuclei during interphase show large chromosomes in the center of the nucleus and the RNA near to the inner face of the nuclear envelope.

During prophase, the oval nucleus shows 5 to 6 chromosomes and 16 to 18 small chromosomes. The chromosomes are observed to be arranged around the microtubule-organizing center (**Figures 4b, 5c** and **d**) in the center of the nucleus, and the RNA is located around the periphery in a ring shape [5].

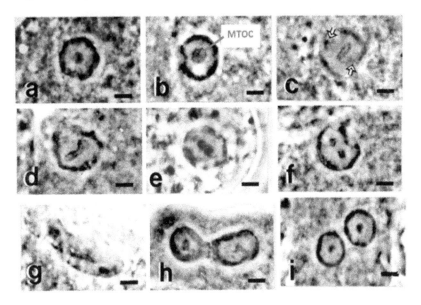

Figure 4.
Phases of mitosis in the nuclei of Entamoeba histolytica. *Trophozoite (a) interface, (b) prophase, (c) metaphase, (d) early anaphase, (e) delayed anaphase, (f) early telophase, (g) late telophase, (h) early karyokinesis, and (i) late cytokinesis. MTOC, microtubule-organizing center.*

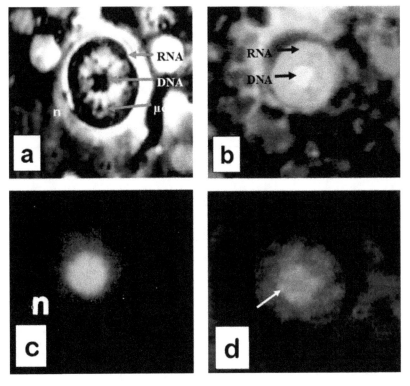

Figure 5.
Interphase and prophase nuclei of Entamoeba histolytica *trophozoites. (a) Phase-contrast microscopy, (b) stained with orange acridine and observed in the fluorescence microscope. (c) Tubulin β in the microtubule-organizing center (green color). (d) Vital stain with orange acridine which are seen in spherical chromosomes (arrow) of green color arranged in a hexagon. μc, microchromosomes.*

Mitotic apparatus	Human cells [1]	*E. histolytica* trophozoites
Spindle:		
Number.	One	Three
Types	Bipolar, axial, and Symmetric	Two radial and one inter MTOCs
Location	Centrosome-kinetochore) Cytoplasmic	Two radial are intranuclear, The inter MTOCs is intranuclear and cytoplasmic [2] Bipolar spindles [39]
Origin of spindle microtubules	Centrosome	Duplicated MTOC
Tubulins:		
γ	Centrosome	MTOC
α and β	Cytoplasmic	Intranuclear and Cytoplasmic
Nuclear envelope	Disorganized during Mitosis	Remains during mitosis
Nucleolus	Disorganized during mitosis and not observable	No nucleolar structure has been demonstrated
RNA	Disorganized and not Observable	It remains condensed [5]
Chromatin	Condensed in the metaphasic chromosomes	It remains condensed throughout mitosis
DNA	Condensed and Decondensed	It remain condensed
Chromosomes:		
Number	46	Indeterminate:
	44 autosomes	24–32 [23]
	2 sex chromosomes	6 [4]
		5 [40]
		6 [5]
		30–50 [41]
		24–32 [42]

Table 2.
Differences in the structures of the mitotic apparatus between human somatic cells and Entamoeba histolytica trophozoites.

In metaphase, the round nucleus increases in size, and the chromosomes move further away from the center of the nucleus. The side view of the duplicated chromosomes shows two parallel rows of round bodies. The RNA ring breaks and forms two to three oval portions located in opposite poles (**Figure 4c**).

Early and late anaphase is characterized by the separation of the chromosomes into two apparent equal parts, each with six chromosomes. In this phase, the nucleus is observed to be elongated with an unchanged RNA (**Figure 4d** and **e**).

In early and late telophase, the nucleus size is 21 μm. Each group of six chromosomes, with the respective small chromosomes, is located in the opposite poles of the nucleus arranged in a ring shape, while the RNA forms small condensations evenly distributed between the two daughter nuclei (**Figure 4f, g**, and **h**).

During karyokinesis, the daughter nuclei separate, each with their own DNA and RNA, and in the end they are observed to be joined by a cytoplasmic filament [5] (**Figure 4h** and **i**).

As mentioned at the beginning of this chapter, there are variations in the types and in the location of the mitotic spindles in different protozoa. By transmission electron microscopy [3] and immunofluorescence studies [39, 2], the mitotic spindle of *Entamoeba histolytica* trophozoites is shown to be intranuclear. In this chapter we not only show the presence of three intranuclear mitotic spindles in this parasite, but we propose a model that explains how the spindle microtubule fibers distribute the chromosomes into the two daughter nuclei.

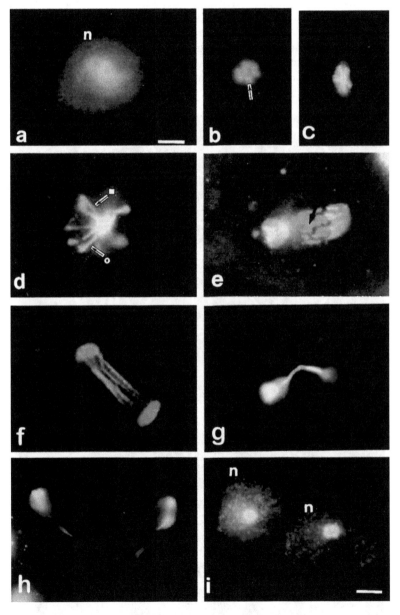

Figure 6.
Structural organization of the mitotic spindles of the nucleus of Entamoeba histolytica *trophozoites during the mitosis phases. (a) Interphase, (b and c) prophase, (d) metaphase, (e) anaphase, (f–g) telophase, and (h–i) karyokinesis. Nucleus treated with RNAse, incubated with anti-β-tubulin antibodies, and contrasted with propidium iodide.*

The MTOC of the protozoa is equivalent to the centrosome of the higher eukaryotic organisms (**Table 2**).

During prophase, the formation of many radially arranged microtubule fibers is observed in the MTOC located in the center of the nucleus [3] (**Figures 6b** and **c**, **7b** and **c**). In metaphase, the MTOC is duplicated, and radial microtubule fibers directed toward the nuclear envelope (radial spindles) emerge from each one. MTOC fibers also arise from transverse microtubules that go from one MTOC to the other (spindle inter MTOC). It is possible to appreciate in the nuclei of the *Entamoeba histolytica* trophozoites during mitosis three mitotic spindles: two radial and one inter MTOC from their MTOC (**Figure 8a**). Apparently, each radial spindle guides the free end of its microtubule fibers toward the nucleus poles, surrounding each group of chromosomes in a mesh (**Figure 8b**). The spindle that forms between the two MTOCs serves to transfer the groups of chromosomes trapped by the radial spindles toward the opposite poles of the nucleus. During anaphase, each group of

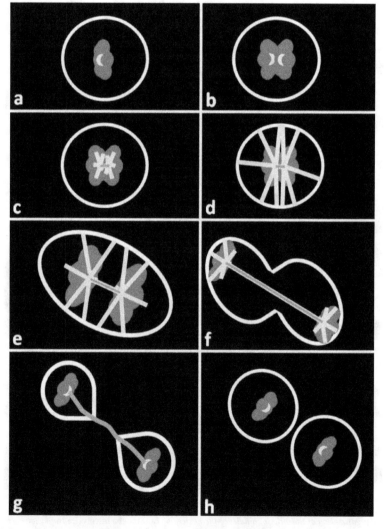

Figure 7.
Diagram of the organization of the mitotic spindles in the nucleus of Entamoeba histolytica *trophozoites. (a) Interphase, (b and c) prophase, (d) metaphase, (e) anaphase, (f) telophase, and (g–h) karyokinesis.*

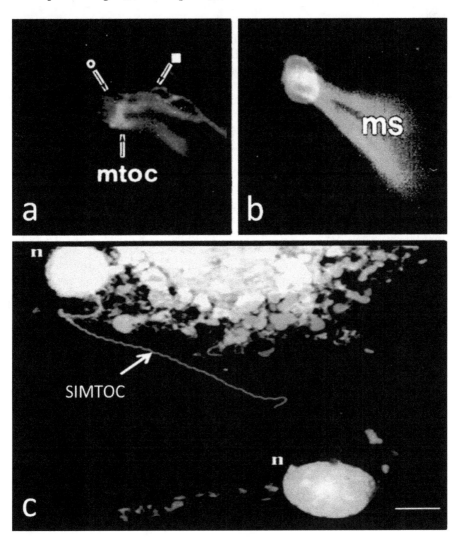

Figure 8.
Nuclear pole of Entamoeba histolytica *trophozoites during telophase and spindle inter microtubule-organizing center (SIMTOC). (a) Nucleus treated with RNAse and incubated with anti-β-tubulin antibodies. (b) Nucleus treated with RNAse, incubated with anti-β-tubulin antibodies, and contrasted with propidium iodide. O, radial spindle at one of the poles. o, part of the spindle inter microtubule-organizing center. (c)* Entamoeba histolytica *trophozoites stained with orange acridine, hypotonized with KCL 0.075 M, and observed with fluorescence microscope during karyokinesis. Spindle inter microtubule-organizing center in cord form.*

chromosomes is surrounded by fibers of the radial spindles, and the MTOC spindle increases in length, leading the chromosomes toward the opposite poles of the nucleus (**Figures 6e** and **7e**). In telophase each group of chromosomes is located at opposite poles of the nucleus. Each group of chromosomes surrounded by radial spindles has the appearance of a round pumpkin with linear marks. Karyokinesis begins with the separation of the nuclei that are still joined by microtubule fibers of the spindle inter MTOCs (**Figures 6h–i, 7g–h, 8c**). Apparently the spindle remains even when the nuclei have been divided; it is still unknown if it perforates the nuclear envelope or if this cord remains surrounded by it. An interesting observation occurs when the *Entamoeba histolytica* trophozoites are vitally stained with acridine orange and hypotonized with 0.075 M KCL. Under these conditions it is possible to observe microtubular structures during mitosis (**Figure 8c**).

After karyokinesis, cytokinesis begins; the trophozoite with two nuclei begins to divide by narrowing the cytoplasm in its middle part [5]. This process is relatively slow and occurs gradually through stretching with intervals of rest. The cytoplasm of the middle part of the trophozoite thins until it forms a very thin filament which then breaks and results in two trophozoites of *Entamoeba histolytica* with a nucleus in each of them. It is still unknown whether cytoplasmic DNA [38] duplicates during mitosis of trophozoites or if it is only genetic material with other functions. The description and observations realized in the different phases of mitosis in *E. histolytica* trophozoites using the phase-contrast microscopy technique are consistent with those described by acridine orange vital staining and transmission electron microscopy [3–6]. Peripheral RNA chromatin and central DNA chromatin behaved in a similar manner to the acridine orange staining described [5]. The data described and observed with the anti-β-tubulin antibodies of *E. histolytica* regarding the radial microtubule bundles correlate with the observations described with transmission electron microscopy of nuclei in prophase and prometaphase [3, 4, 6]. However, there is a discrepancy about the number of spindles that are present and observed between the two nuclei in formation [2, 3, 6]. The description of an inter-MTOC spindle independent of radial spindles was based on its observation with immunofluorescence (**Figure 8a**). An observation that brings forth new ways of studying the nuclear division in *E. histolytica* trophozoites is the presence of a green fluorescent internuclear cord obtained with the acridine orange staining and KCL-hypotonization.

5. Conclusions

The identification of β-tubulin bundles that surround the DNA nuclei in telophase suggests a mechanism of entrapment similar to a "hand-closure movement" that allows, along with the inter-MTOC spindle, the distribution of genetic material between the two newly formed nuclei.

The mitosis of *Entamoeba histolytica* trophozoites is a type of intranuclear pleuromitosis, closed or open? modified, since three spindles are formed: two radial and one inter MTOCs. In addition, these are found within the nucleus. It remains to be discovered if the spindle that apparently is outside the nucleus has a nuclear envelope or not.

Author details

Eduardo Gómez-Conde[1]*, Miguel Ángel Vargas Mejía[2], María Alicia Díaz y Orea[3], Luis David Gómez-Cortes[4] and Tayde Guerrero-González[5]

1 Laboratory of Research at Immunobiology, School of Medicine, Merciful Autonomous University of Puebla, Mexico

2 Molecular Biomedicine Department, Center for Research and Advanced Studies of the National Polytechnic Institute, Mexico City, Mexico

3 Laboratory of Research at Experimental Immunology, School of Medicine, Merciful Autonomous University of Puebla, Mexico

4 School of Biology, Merciful Autonomous University of Puebla, Mexico

5 Hospital "1ro of October", Institute of Security and Social Services for State Workers, Mexico City, Mexico

*Address all correspondence to: gom_cond@yahoo.com

IntechOpen

© 2019 The Author(s). Licensee IntechOpen. This chapter is distributed under the terms of the Creative Commons Attribution License (http://creativecommons.org/licenses/by/3.0), which permits unrestricted use, distribution, and reproduction in any medium, provided the original work is properly cited. (cc) BY

References

[1] Bruce A, Johnson A, Lewis J, Raff M, Walter P. The Mechanics of Cell Division. Molecular Biology of the Cell. Fifth ed. New York London, U.S.A: Garland Publishing Inc; 2008. pp. 1060-1092

[2] Dastidar PG, Majumder S, Lohia A. Eh Klp5 is a divergent member of the kinesin 5 family that regulates genome content and microtubular assembly in *Entamoeba histolytica*. Cellular Microbiology. 2007;**9**:316-328. DOI: 10.1111/j.1462-5822.2006.00788.x

[3] Solis JF, Barrios R. *Entamoeba histolytica*: Microtubule movement during mitosis. Experimental Parasitology. 1991;**73**:276-284. PMID: 1915743

[4] Argüello C, Valenzuela V, Rangel E. Structural organization of chromatin during the cell cycle of *Entamoeba histolytica* trophozoites. Archives of Medical Research. 1992;**23**:77-80. PMID: 1285087

[5] Gómez-CondeE,Hernández-JaureguiP, González-Camacho M, Orozco E, López CA. Chromatin organization during the nuclear division stages of live *Entamoeba histolytica* trophozoites. Experimental Parasitology. 1998;**89**:122-124. PMID: 9603497

[6] Gicquaud RC. Étude de la ultrastructure du noyau et de la mitose de *Entamoeba histolytica*. Biology Cellulaire. 1979;**35**:305-312

[7] Raikov IB. The Protozoan Nucleus, Morphology and Evolution. Vol. 9. New York: Springer–Verlag; 1982. p. 73

[8] Orozco E, Solís FJ, Domínguez J, Chávez B, Hernández F. *Entamoeba histolytica*: Cell cycle and nuclear division. Experimental Parasitology. 1988;**67**:85-95. PMID: 2901981

[9] Kaul SC. Effect of heat shock on growth and division of *Stylonichia mytilus*. Biochemistry and Cell Biology. 1991;**69**:23-28. PMID: 2043340

[10] Mottram JC, Smith G. A family of trypanosome cdc2-related protein kinases. Gene. 1995;**162**:147-152. DOI: 10.1016/0378-1119(95)00350-f

[11] Tang L, Pelech SL, Berger JD. Isolation of the cell cycle control gene cdc2 from *Paramecium tetraurelia*. Biochimica et Biophysica Acta. 1995;**1265**:161-167. DOI: 10.1016/0167-4889(94)00206-t

[12] Stojdl DF, Clarke MW. *Trypanosoma brucei*: Analysis of cytoplasmic Ca^{2+} during differentiation of bloodstream stages in vitro. Experimental Parasitology. 1996;**83**:134-146. DOI: 10.1006/expr.1996.0057

[13] Doerig C, Doerig C, Horrocks P, Coyle J, Carlton J, Sultan A, et al. Pfcrk-1, a developmentally regulated cdc2-related protein kinase of *Plasmodium falciparum*. Molecular and Biochemical Parasitology. 1995;**70**:167-174. PMID: 7637697

[14] Mutomba MC, To WY, Hyun WC, Wang CC. Inhibition of proteasome activity blocks cell cycle progression at specific phase boundaries in African trypanosomes. Molecular and Biochemical Parasitology. 1997;**90**:491-504. PMID: 9476796

[15] Mounlay L, Robert-Gero M, Brown S, Gendron MC, Tournier F. Sinefungin and taxol effects on cell cycle and cytoskeleton of *Leishmania donovani* promastigotes. Experimental Cell Research. 1996;**226**:283-291. DOI: 10.1006/excr.1996.0229

[16] Perret E. Microtubular spindle and centrosome structures during the cell

cycle in a dinoflagellate *Crypthecodinium cohnii*: An immunocytochemical study. Bio Systems. 1991;**25**:53-65. PMID: 1854914

[17] Brinkley BR. Microtubule organizing centers. Annual Review of Cell Biology. 1985;**9**:145-172. DOI: 10.1146/annurev.cb.01.110185.001045

[18] Gómez-Conde E, López–Robles MC, Hernández-Rivas R, Guillen N, Hernández-Jauregui P, Vargas-Mejía M. Structural organization of gamma-tubulin in microtubule organizing center (MTOC) during the nuclear division of *Entamoeba histolytica* trophozoites. Archives of Medical Research. 2000;**31**:S205-S206 PMID: 11070285

[19] Ris H, Kubai DF. Cromosome structure. Annual Review of Genetics. 1970;**4**:263-294. DOI: 10.1146/annurev.ge.04.120170.001403

[20] Biderre C. On small genomes in eukaryotic organims: Molecular karyotypes of two microsporidions species (Protozoa) parasites of vertebrates. California Academy of Sciences. 1994;**317**:399-404. PMID: 7994619

[21] Sarafis K, Isaac-Renton J. Pulsed-field gel electrophoresis as a method of biotyping of *Giardia duodenalis*. The American Journal of Tropical Medicine and Hygiene. 1993;**48**:134-144. DOI: 10.4269/ajtmh.1993.48.134

[22] Bastien P, Blaineau C, Pages M. Molecular karyotype in Leishmania. Sub-Cellular Biochemistry. 1992;**18**:131-187. PMID: 1485351

[23] Valdés J, Ocádiz R, Orozco E. Identification of *Entamoeba histolytica* chromosomes by pulsed field gradient electrophoresis. Archivos de Investigación Médica. 1990;**21**:229-231. PMID: 2136489

[24] Van Der Ploeg LHT, Smits M, Ponnudurai T, Vermeulen A, Meuwissen JHET, Langsley G. Chromosome-size DNA molecules of *Plasmodium falciparum*. Science. 1985;**229**:658-661

[25] Lehker MW, Alderete JF. Resolution of six chromosomes of *Trichomonas vaginalis* and conservation of size and number among isolates. The Journal of Parasitology. 1999;**85**:976-979. PMID: 10577741

[26] Roger TD, Scholes VE, Schlichting HE. An ultrastructural comparison of *Euglena gracilis* klebs, Bleanched euglena and Astasia Langa Pringsheim. The Journal of Protozoology. 1972;**19**:133-139. PMID: 4621518

[27] Lynch MJ, Leake RE, O'Conell KM, Buetow DE. Isolation, fractionation and template activity of the continuosly condensed chromatin of *Euglena gracilis*. Experimental Cell Research. 1975;**91**:349-357. DOI: 10.1016/0014-4827(75)90114-7

[28] Jiménez-García LF, Elizundia JM, Lólez-Zamerano B, Maciel A, Zavala G, Echeverría OM, et al. Implications for evolution of nuclear structures of animal, plants, fungi and protoctists. BioSystem. 1989;**22**:103-116. PMID: 2720137

[29] Wisw GE, Goldstein L. Localization and characterization of chromatin within the interphase nucleus of Amoeba proteus by means of in situ centrifugation and radioautography. Chromosoma. 1972;**36**:176-192

[30] Galindo I, Argüello C, Ramírez JL. What is a chromosome like in Leishmania? Biological Research. 1993;**26**:115-120. PMID: 7670523

[31] Prescott DM. The c-value paradox and genes in ciliated protozoa. Modern

Cell Biology. Mc Intosh JR ed. New York: Alan R Liss Inc; 1983. P.329-362.

[32] Moses MJ. Nucleic acids and proteins of the nuclei of paramecium. Journal of Morphology. 1950;**87**:493-595. PMID: 24539338

[33] Lipps HJ, Morris NR. Chromatin structure in the nuclei of the ciliate *Stylonichia Mytilus*. Biochemical and Biophysical Research Communications. 1977;**74**:230-234

[34] Kennedy JR. The morphology of *Blepharisma undulans* stein. The Journal of Eukaryotic Microbiology. 1965;**12**:542-561. DOI: 10.1111/j.1550-7408.1965.tb03254.x

[35] Seshachar BR. Observations on the fine structure of the nuclear apparatus of *Blepharisma intermedium* bhandary (Ciliata: Spirotricha). The Journal of Protozoology. 1964;**11**:402-409

[36] Olins AL, Olins DE, Franke WW, Lipps HJ, Prescott DM. Stereo-electron microscopy of nuclear structure and replication in ciliated protozoa (hypotricha). European Journal of Cell Biology. 1981;**25**:120-130. PMID: 6793369

[37] Amar L. Chromosome end formation and internal sequence elimination as alternative genomic rearrangements in the ciliate paramecium. Journal of Molecular Biology. 1994;**236**:421-426. DOI: 10.1006/jmbi.1994.1154

[38] Orozco E, Gharaibeh R, Riverón AM, Delgadillo DM, Mercado M, Sánchez T, et al. A novel cytoplasmic structure containing DNA networks in *Entamoeba histolytica* trophozoites. Molecular & General Genetics. 1997;**254**:250-257. PMID: 9150258

[39] Mukherjee C, Majumder S, Lohia A. Inter-cellular variation in DNA content of *Entamoeba histolytica* originates from temporal and spatial uncoupling of cytokinesis from the nuclear cycle. PLoS Neglected Tropical Diseases. 2009;**3**:409;1-409;40911. DOI: 10.1371/journal.pntd.0000409

[40] Solís FJ, Córdova LG. The chromosomes of *Entamoeba histolytica*. Archives Medical Research. 2000;**31** (4 Suppl):S202-S204. PMID: 11070284

[41] Willhoeft U, Tannich E. Fluorescence microscopy and fluorescence in situ hybridization of *Entamoeba histolytica* nuclei to analyse mitosis and the localization of repetitive DNA. Molecular Biochemical Parasitology. 2000;**105**:291-296. PMID: 10693751

[42] Chávez-Munguía B, Tsutsumi V, Martínez-Palomo A. Entamoeba histolytica: Ultrastructure of the chromosomes and the mitotic spindle. Experimental Parasitology. 2006;**114**:235-239. PMID: 16631745

State of the Art in Parasitic Infections

Chapter 13

Challenges for the Control of Poultry Red Mite (*Dermanyssus gallinae*)

José Francisco Lima-Barbero, Margarita Villar, Ursula Höfle and José de la Fuente

Abstract

The Poultry Red Mite, *Dermanyssus gallinae*, is an ectoparasite which is considered the major pest for the egg-laying industry. The mite hides in crevices and cracks during daylight and feed on the blood of the hens in the darkness. It can also parasitize other bird and mammal species, including man that can develop gamasoidosis when bitten at work or private residences. The control of the mite infestations has relied in synthetic acaricides, but the development of resistances and the restricted list of authorized products make fundamental the development of novel control measure. The combination of alternative control measures, such as monitoring of the mite infestation, plant-derived products, inner dusts, biological control and vaccines, poses as the best way for achieving satisfactory results.

Keywords: *Dermanyssus*, poultry, mite, zoonosis, control, vaccines

1. Introduction

The poultry red mite (PRM), *Dermanyssus gallinae* (De Geer, 1778), is a hematophagous mite that affects mainly poultry [1] but also parasitizes other avian [2] and mammalian hosts [3–5], including humans [6]. PRM has a worldwide distribution and it constitutes a serious problem for the European egg-laying industry where the average prevalence is 80% with some countries reaching a prevalence higher than 90% of the farms affected [1]. PRM infestation is associated with severe economic losses in the egg production industry [7], also causing health and welfare issues in the hens [7–9]. Additionally, the PRM has shown to be a mechanical vector for multiple pathogenic viruses and bacteria [1].

The control of PRM is mainly based on the use of synthetic acaricides. However, synthetic acaricides have important limitations such as the development of resistant mite populations, environmental contamination and limited efficacy for controlling already settled infestations [1, 10]. Thus while research focused on *D. gallinae* was previously scarce, it increased significantly in recent years probably due to the support received due to the growing impact of mite infestations on the egg-laying industry [10]. The limitations of the conventional control measures make research on alternative control measures as one of the leading research topics in recent years. Amongst those control measures, vaccination poses a promising effective and environmentally sound intervention.

IntechOpen

The aim of the present review is to show the current knowledge about the PRM, the challenges it poses from the One Health perspective for both human and animal health and the future possibilities for the control and prevention of PRM infestations.

2. Biology

Dermanyssus gallinae is taxonomically assigned to the Dermanyssidae family englobed in the order Mesostigmata of the Arachnida Class. There are 14 other mite species that affect birds and are morphologically very similar to *D. gallinae* which may be misidentified when identification is solely based on morphological characteristics [11]. Recent advances in molecular tools as gene sequencing or DNA barcoding, combined with morphological features is allowing a proper mite identification, including *D. gallinae* identification [12–14] (**Figure 1**).

Dermanyssus gallinae is an obligatory ectoparasite that feeds on the blood of the host. It has a global distribution [15]. In contrast with other *Dermanyssus* spp., *D. gallinae* is a generalist species with a low host specificity [16]. The PRM is a pest in the egg-laying farms [1], but can also be found parasitizing more than 30 wild and domestic bird species [11] and mammals [3–5], including humans [6]. The life cycle for *D. gallinae* includes five developmental stages: egg, larvae, protonymph, deutonymph and adult (**Figure 2**). Larvae have three pairs of legs while the rest of the stages have four pairs of legs. The PRM requires a blood meal for molting from protonymph to deutonymph, to adult and for egg-laying [17] (**Figure 2**). The color of the fed stages varies from bright red to brown, depending on the digestion of the blood inside de mite, while unfed stages are white. Adults and fed deutonymphs are

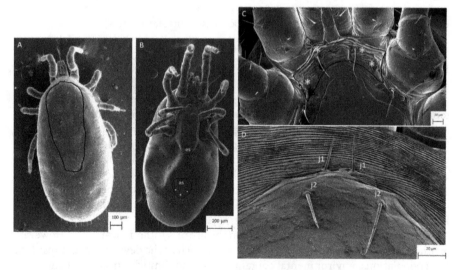

Figure 1.
SEM images from several morphological characteristics useful for the identification of D. gallinae *and differentiation from other similar species. Morphological characteristics shown are present in adult females according to Di Palma et al. [14]. (A) Dorsal overview. Dorsal shield (outline traced) with prominent shoulder. (B) Ventral overview. Epigynal (es) and anal (as) shields are rounded posteriorly. Anal shield with three anal setae (*). (C) Detail of the sternal shield. The sternal shield is wider than long and containing two pairs of setae (*). (D) Detail of dorsal shield. The two pairs of setae (j1 and j2) are on the dorsal shield. See methodology for additional information.*

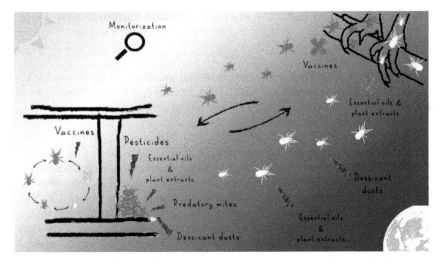

Figure 2.
Graphical representation of the PRM biological cycle and points of action for different control measures. Iconography explanation: large red mites = fed adult mites; small red mites = fed nymphal stages; large white mites = starved adults; small white mites = starved nymphal stages; cross = points where the treatment can interrupt the mite cycle; thunderbolt = points of action for the different treatment options. New control interventions such as vaccination, predatory mites or plant extracts are shown. See methodology for information source.

visible with the naked eye. Life cycle usually takes 2 weeks to complete, but it can be shorter when ideal conditions are provided (25–27°C and high relative humidity) [17–19]. Long-time emptied hen houses have been reported to remain infested. This finding is justified by the ability of the mite to survive without any blood meal for up to 9 months if the environment is suitable. However, desiccation and high temperatures (>45°C) are lethal [19]. Oviposition is carried out only by adult female mites. A maximum of approximately 30 eggs can be laid by a single female in her lifetime, usually in clutches of 4–8 eggs after a blood meal [20].

The PRM lacks real eyes and it can senses changes in the luminosity of the environment with photocells [21]. During daylight hours, mite is usually hidden in cracks and crevices where it is out of the reach of the hen. In these shelters, it gathers with more mites until they can form a cluster of hundreds of mites of different stages. This behavior is driven by aggregation pheromones [22]. It is in the darkness when the PRM comes out of their refuges to feed on the host. The host-seeking process is multifactorial, but temperature has been proven to play an important role as the PRM is highly sensitive to even minor changes in temperature and starved mites have an increased sensibility [23, 24]. *D. gallinae* increases its activity when exposed to substrate vibrations which are supposed to be used for host localization [23]. Surface skin lipids are also involved in the host identification and stimulation [22, 25]. These lipids are used to improve feeding rates in artificial feeding devices when synthetic membranes are used [26] and have provided possibilities for the use of essential oils in the control of PRM infestations in layer houses. In contrast with other hematophagous ectoparasites that utilize CO_2 to identify their hosts, CO_2 did not induce any host seeking response in *D. gallinae* under laboratory conditions but induced immobility under light conditions, which is interpreted as a survival strategy to avoid being eaten by the host [23]. Nymphal and adult stages stay on the host for feeding for 30–60 min [27]. According to this behavior, PRM can be considered as a micro predator [16].

3. One health: poultry industry, environment and human health

3.1 Poultry industry

The PRM is not a significant issue in the broiler industry, mainly due to its short production cycle, but it poses a substantial threat to the egg-laying industry world-wide, except for layer farms in the USA where *Ornythonyssus sylviarum* is the main mite species affecting layer hens [28]. However, recent reports suggest significant increase of *D. gallinae* infestations in the USA [15]. Although *O. sylviarum* is also present in wild birds of European countries, *D. gallinae* is the specie responsible for farm infestations. However, mixed infestations have been reported in countries out of Europe [29]. Infestations can reach high prevalence in Europe, where the aver-age prevalence is more than 80% with several countries reaching higher than 90% [30]. However, PRM prevalence can be more related to certain areas rather than a country as different prevalence has been observed in different regions of the same country [31]. PRM infestations have been described in every production system. Less-intensive farming systems present higher risks of infestation which usually is inversely proportional to the level of intensification [32]. Therefore, PRM preva-lence is generally higher in backyard and free-range units, followed by barns and, ultimately, by enriched systems [33]. Enriched cages usually show higher levels of infestation when compared to traditional pens in those countries where they are still allowed [32]. These systems improve mite survival by providing more safe areas to the mite far from the reach of the hens and the treatments at the same time as they promote hen welfare.

Temporal dynamics of PRM infestations vary greatly between laying hen houses. Specific environmental conditions and differences in laying hen house management are responsible for these variations. The age of the flock is another modulating factor according to a model developed for forecasting the population dynamics in a hen house [34]. The age of the flock has a negative effect on the growth of the mite population as mite populations decline as the age of the hens increases despite the fact that the immune response of the hen against a PRM infestation has not been well characterized. An experimental infestation developed an increase of the serum amyloid-A [35], but hens do not generate natural potent immunoprotective responses [36]. The development of an immune response by the bird after a chronic exposure is a plausible explanation which has been proposed that requires further research [34, 37]. The type of hen hybrid and how they were raised as pullets seem to have some effects on the vertical distribution of the mite infestation in aviaries, which is explained by differences in the space use by differ-ent hybrids [38].

Infestation levels vary seasonally [38]. Seasons prone to more severe infestations also differ depending on the climate of each region [38]. Usually, seasons with mild temperatures and high relative humidity can be correlated with lower fluctuations of these parameters inside the layer house, providing more ideal conditions for the mite to grow and therefore show more severe infestations. In this way, in northern countries the infestation peak usually happens in summer months while in more temperate climates the most prevalent seasons are spring and autumn.

Moderate and low infestations do not seem to have an effect on the produc-tion parameters independently of the layer hen productive system [39]. Instead, severe infestations are associated with important production losses albeit varia-tions between housing systems [21]. Therefore, PRM has been demonstrated to negatively affect the proportion of laying hens, egg weight and the amount of first-choice eggs in enriched cages facilities while detrimental effects have been observed on egg mass, first-choice eggs and bodyweight of hens housed in aviary systems [39]. The impact on egg production can cause reductions of up to 20% [8]. PRM infestations are also responsible for devaluation of eggs when these are blood spotted. The spots are the result of fed mites getting crushed beneath the eggs while walking or hiding on the conveyor belt [40].

PRM is also responsible for health and welfare issues for egg-laying hens. When asked, most egg-producers commonly state that PRM is the major issue concerning hen welfare [41]. The main sign of a severe infestation is the anemia observed in the birds. An adult mite can ingest 0.2 μl of blood in a blood meal [42]. It is described that a laying hen can lose more than 3% of its blood volume every night [8]. In cases of severe infestations, increased bird mortality is observed due to exsanguination. The mortality due to a PRM infestation has been estimated to increase between 4 and 50% [43], and correlates with an increased mite burden. Several studies find significant relationships between PRM infestation and hen mortality [7, 44]. PRM infestation increases food and water intake. Hens under infestation suffer restlessness, agitation, sleep deprivation and increased preening and feather pecking [9, 45]. Thus, the infestation puts the hens into chronic distress making them more susceptible to diseases and reducing vaccine efficacy.

Many dermanyssoid mites are confirmed vectors of bacterial and viral pathogens. Several pathogens have been isolated from *D. gallinae*, thus confirming its role as mechanical vector. Several reports have detected pathogenic bacteria in PRM such as *Coxiella burnetii, Erysipelothrix rhusiopathiae, Listeria monocytogenes, Pasterella multocida Mycoplasma gallisepticum, Chlamydophila psittaci* and Spirochetes [46–48]. However, its role as a biological vector for these pathogens is not yet fully elucidated and requires further research. The PRM has been demonstrated under laboratory conditions to act as a vector for *Salmonella enteritidis* where they showed the oral transmission after ingestion of washed mites contaminated by cuticular contact or during blood meal [49]. Additionally, *S. enterica* subsp. *enterica* serovar gallinarum biovar gallinarum (*S. gallinarum*), the etiological agent of the fowl typhoid, was found to survive for up to 4 months in infected mites [50]. Recently, Pugliese et al. [51] showed the maintenance of *S. gallinarum* in two different productive cycles where after an outbreak of fowl typhoid, the mites remained infected even after a sanitary break and vaccination of the second flock. An interesting finding of this work was that the number of bacteria found in the mites varied according to the antibody titers of the vaccinated hens. This finding illustrates the complex relationship between host, parasite and bacterial pathogen. PRM has an experimentally confirmed potential capacity for acting as a mechanical vector of avian influenza virus after a bloodmeal on infected hens [52]. Other viral agents such as avipox virus, fowl adenovirus, Marek's disease virus, avian paramyxovirus type I and the Eastern, Western and Venezuelan equine encephalomyelitis viruses have been isolated from PRM [7].

In summary, PRM is responsible for economic losses of around 231 million Euros annually in Europe considering the combination of the production losses, health issues and cost of mite infestation control [53]. Other reports estimate the economic impact of PRM infestations in Europe between 0.5 and 0.6 Euros per laying hen [54].

3.2 Environment and wildlife

Historically, wild birds were considered as the main source of the mite infestation in the poultry houses. However, mitochondrial cytochrome oxidase I (*mt-COI*) gene sequencing, which allowed secured *Dermanyssus* species identification, demonstrated that none of the *Dermanyssus* species that specifically parasitize wild birds were found in poultry farms and concluded that only *D. gallinae* harbored synanthropic populations [11]. Additionally, the same research described that the *D. gallinae* populations associated with poultry farms belong to different genetic lineages [11]. In addition, recent research on genetic differences between *Ornithonyssus sylviarum* present in wild sparrow nests and layer houses in the USA indicated the absence of mite exchange [55]. However, wild bird nests located in the proximities of the hen house can act as a reservoir of mites and thus allow re-infestation. Mul et al. [56] performed a risk analysis in which poultry farmers and employees, followed by hen cadavers and manure aeration, represented the highest risks of introduction and spread of PRM in the farm. If the manure belts are shared amongst barns, they constitute a severe risk of spreading the PRM [56]. Rodents and insects are potential carriers of mites, and although the role of pests in the introduction and spread of PRM in layer farms has not been fully elucidated, a case of phoresy of *D. gallinae* has been described in a beetle [57].

In a recent questionnaire by free-range farmers in the UK, antiparasitics were reported as one of the three most commonly used medicines against PRM [41]. A recent scandal on the discovery of an unauthorized product in food-producing animals (Fipronil, $C_{12}H_4Cl_2F_6N_4OS$) in contaminated eggs from farms in 45 coun-tries worldwide. The concentration in the contaminated product did not reach toxic doses for humans, but a mediatic Public Health alert was raised, and a food fraud investigation was started by European authorities [58]. Only two compounds are specifically labeled to control PRM infestations while birds are present (Phoxim, $C_{12}H_{15}N_2O_3PS$ and Spinosad, $C_{41}H_{65}NO_{10}$ (A); $C_{42}H_{67}NO_{10}$ (D)) by the European Union (EU), and recently a new compound (Fluralaner, $C_{22}H_{17}Cl_2F_6N_3O_3$) has been approved [59, 60]. Authorized products do not penetrate the whole egg but improper handling when breaking the shell can lead to food contamination [61]. Risks of residues of traditional and unlabeled pesticides entering the food chain are due to its presence in body tissues of hens that are slaughtered for human consump-tion [60]. A withdrawal period has been suggested for the skin tissue after applica-tion of Spinosad and Abamectin ($C_{48}H_{72}O_{14}$ (B_{1a}); $C_{47}H_{70}O_{14}$ (B_{1b})), an acaricide with available formulations for spray application in some European countries, due to the detection of residues in this tissue [62]. The chemicals used to control PRM may also have adverse effects for workers directly exposed while applying the treat-ment. The limited availability of tools and the increase of resistance are forcing the farmers to turn to non-authorized products to face PRM infestations and underline the necessity for alternative control methods.

3.3 Zoonotic risks

D. gallinae is known as a bird ectoparasite but it has low host specificity [16]. This lack of specificity allows the mite to feed on mammals, including humans, when the natural host is not available [6]. Human parasitosis due to PRM is called gamasoidosis or dermanyssosis. Skin erythematous papules are the usual clinical signs for gamasoidosis and urticarial lesions have been also described [6]. Skin lesions are usually pruriginous and can be distributed throughout the entire body, but are more frequently located in the arms, legs and the upper trunk [6]. Regarding human gamasoidosis associated with *D. gallinae*, two epidemiological scenarios are described: urban cases and occupational cases [6]. *D. gallinae* is the most commonly ectoparasite identified as the causal agent of gamasoidosis, but the cases assigned to *D. gallinae* can be misdiagnosed due to the difficulty of species determination for non-trained practitioners. The geographical expansion of other similar mite species such as *Ornythonyssus* spp. [63] due to climate change, host expansion and globaliza-tion will require more precise analysis.

Occupational cases are those related to poultry workers. The infestation can occur both in professional workers and hobbyists. These mite attacks usually happen during the daytime, while the workers are handling birds, cages or collecting eggs or when cleaning the premises. High levels of mite infestation and lack of proper protective clothing increases the risk of mite bites. Despite the high prevalence of infestation in egg-laying farms and continued exposure of the workers to the PRM, the number of reports of occupational cases is limited [6, 64]. The low number of reported cases can be explained by the fact that the attacks occur under specific conditions (severe infestation and lack of protection) or because workers do not report the attacks.

Urban cases are not associated with poultry workers. These cases are usually linked to familiar homes or public buildings such as hospitals and halls. In these cases, synanthropic birds, generally pigeons, are the source of the infestation [6]. Most of them occur when the host has left the nest after the breeding season. At that moment, the mites search for a new host to obtain a bloodmeal. Recent investigations suggest the existence of a pigeon specific lineage (*D. gallinae* L1) that is more frequently involved in human gamasoidosis [65]. Skin lesions in urban cases tend to be more severe than those in occupational cases, basically due to extended exposure.

Reports of gamasoidosis are scarce but their frequency has increased in the recent years [6]. PRM gamasoidosis is still an underdiagnosed parasitosis mainly due to un-specific signs which do not lead the practitioners to a certain diagnosis and, generally, the fact that PRM bites cause only light to mild clinical symptoms, indistinguishable from other bug bites and do not put the patient in need of seeking medical assistance. Recently, the bacterial genera *Tsukamurella* has been identified as part of the microbiome of the PRM with an endosymbiotic relationship suggested [66]. *Tsukamurella* species are foremost saprophyte bacteria that have occasionally been identified as opportunistic organisms associated with postoperative infections [67]. This, and the avian pathogens listed earlier, together with reports of *D. gallinae* infestations in hospitals [68] highlight potential zoonotic risks associated with PRM. Thus, because of the potential vector role of PRM for zoonotic pathogens it should be included in routine medical differential diagnosis for skin lesions.

4. Control measures

Treatment and control of PRM infestations have until recently relied on the spraying of chemical acaricides in infested premises, and mostly still occurs despite the limited list of products licensed to be used against the PRM in the EU. In general, traditional control actions achieve only temporary effects and mite populations return to levels prior to treatment soon after treatment application. One of the main limitations in the use of pesticides is the incapacity to apply the product to a degree that does not allow the target to escape from exposure by hiding in cracks and crevices [38]. Another significant problem in the use of pesticides is the emergence of resistances [69]. The number of PRM populations with reduced sensibility to traditional pesticides as λ-Cyhalothrin or Amitraz has grown especially after 2012. In the case of Phoxim, which has been considered a highly effective compound, highly resistant populations have been detected since 2015 [70]. This is probably related to withdrawal of most of the labeled compounds from the marked and subsequent overuse and misuse of the only remaining products available. The single chemical pesticide that shows satisfactory results is a recent labeled to be used as poultry isoxazoline, Fluralaner. Fluralaner has demonstrated a nearly

100% efficacy after two applications in poultry farms [71]. The key for this product is that with the oral administration the treatment reaches the whole mite population when the mites feed on the hens. This delivery method avoids the necessity to spray the product, a way of administration that has been proven of low efficacy for the control of PRM as there are mites that escape from the treatment.

An often-neglected tool for the control of PRM infestations in a layer hen house is the monitorization of the population. Many treatments do not show the expected results because they have not been applied at the right moment. The decision for applying treatment is traditionally taken when the farm employees announce a severe infestation, which is usually too late to allow successful control [72]. A proper monitorization routine can promote early detection and quantification of the infestation level and thus allowing proper programming of control measures. There are multiple methodologies that can be used for monitorization, including both quantitative and qualitative techniques. A description of the most commonly used monitoring methods has been recently reviewed [73]. Many monitoring systems are based on the placement of traps that emulate the hiding places of the mites and that are checked periodically. In this way, depending on the technique the farmer can obtain an estimate of the mite population in the hen house and/or a trend for the mite population evolution. There appears not be a single best choice for a monitoring method as it depends on the time and resources available in the farm. However, farms with monitoring programs in place can improve their capacity of PRM control [74].

Development of new control interventions is currently a priority in PRM research as a consequence of the severe impact of the mite in the egg-laying industry and the scarce resources for its control (**Figure 2**). Amongst those novel methods, treatments with essential oils and plant extracts have received significant attention. There are many studies on the effects of essential oils against PRM, but variable efficacy is observed [75]. Benefits of plant extracts and essential oils include their low mammalian and bird toxicity and short environmental persistence [75]. Several plant-based products are already commercialized against veterinary pests, and many others are in research phase. Essential oils are traditionally used for their repellence of pest arthropods [75]. The effect of essential oils can be due the influence of a number of volatile organic compounds (VOCs) in the host-recognition process [20]. Recent research found that the odor emitted by the hens can be modified through addition of plant-originated VOCs to the food and that some of those VOCs showed repellent activity against the PRM, making the hens less attractive to the mites [76]. The other approach for the use of plant derived compounds is using its insecticide properties for treating the hen house environment. Amongst those substances, neem oil is receiving special attention from researchers [75, 77]. Neem oil preparations are made of essential oil obtained from an Indian tree (*Azadirachta indica*) and have shown promising effects in PRM population reductions [77]. A disadvantage of neem oil application is the possible effects of the oily film on the farm installations and eggs, but technological improvements such as reducing the volume of solution or the droplet size can be applied to reduce these adverse effects [77].

Mite communities constituted by different mite species are able to establish themselves in layer farm buildings, mainly associated with manure [78]. These communities include mite species that are predators of free-living nematodes and arthropods, including mites [78]. Some *Hypoaspis* species identified in starling nests are considered putative predators of *D. gallinae* [79] and two mite species are already commercialized to be used in layer farms: *Androlaelaps casalis* (Androlis, APPI-group Koppert. France) and *Cheyletus eruditus* (Taurrus,

APPI-group Koppert. France). *A. casalis* have shown to control, but no to eradicate, PRM populations under laboratory conditions but was more efficient at temperatures under 30°C [80]. The authors suggested that predation can occur over other mite species when *D. gallinae* is hiding in safe places, basically at different heights (*D. gallinae* was on high areas of the cages while predators remained on the floor) [80]. Predatory mites are already effectively used in the control of phytophagous mites in greenhouses and in pig farms for the control of non-hematophagous arthropods. Biocontrol of PRM in layer farmhouses is based upon the massive release of predatory mites. The effectivity of predatory mites to control PRM infestations is variable, probably due to variations in environmental conditions [79]. The main disadvantage of using predatory mites as a control tool of *D. gallinae* is their high sensitivity to acaricides used to treat PRM infestations [78]. Thus, biocontrol using predatory mites is not compatible with the use of acaricides.

Another control method is based upon a perch design (Q-perch), which prevents the mite from reaching the hens by an electrified wire placed just beneath the perch where the bird is roosting [81]. Various desiccant dusts, diatomaceous earth and synthetic silica products are commonly used in commercial layer farms [74]. Generally, it is a measure used as a temporal constraint of PRM infestation and to reduce the number of treatments with synthetic acaricides. Inert dust kills the mite by dehydration and probably, by cuticle damage by destroying its protective wax layer [82]. The main limitation of the use of inert dusts is the limited efficacy in environments with high levels of relative humidity [82]. A synergistic effect between inert dusts and entomopathogenic fungi have been described [83]. The use of entomopathogenic fungus for the control of PRM is recent and there is limited research. Laboratory tests show promising results, and some have been tested with some success in field trials [84].

Vaccination against ectoparasites is not solely focused on the prevention of the infestation but also on the reduction of the parasite population [85]. Vaccination have demonstrated to provide high levels of protection against blood-feeding ecto-parasites by reducing cattle tick populations and prevalence of certain tick-borne pathogens [86]. The only commercial vaccines against ectoparasites (TickGard and Gavac) were developed with recombinant tick midgut antigens Bm86 and Bm95 and registered for the control of cattle tick infestations [87]. This vaccines demonstrated their efficacy for the control of tick infestations while reducing the use of acaracides and encourage further research for the identification of new effective protective antigens using different approaches [88].

Vaccine development relies on the identification of proteins that can act as protective antigens to which the host develops an immune response. The iden-tification of protective antigens in *D. gallinae* has been limited by the lack of molecular research about the mite. The description on the mite transcriptome [89] and, more recently, its genome [90] can enhance the understanding of the host–parasite relationship and the identification of protective antigens. Two approaches have been followed for PRM vaccines development, testing of mite extracts and the production of vaccines based on recombinant proteins (**Table 1**). Vaccination against PRM recombinant proteins has induced antigen specific IgY responses but variable results have been obtained when mites fed in *in vitro* tests on blood from immunized hens or blood enriched with antibodies extracted from egg yolk. Another limitation for the assessment of efficacy of a candidate antigen has been the high background effects observed in the *in vitro* tests due to the feed-ing physiology of the PRM. A recent optimization of an on-hen feeding device allows a more physiological evaluation of the vaccine effects allowing a better

Antigen	Type	Species	Adjuvant	Test	Effects (%)	Reference
Soluble protein mite extract	Native	*D. gallinae*	Incomplete Freund's	In vivo [92]	↑ 0.1 M	[92]
Soluble protein mite extract			QuilA	In vitro [93]	↑ 24 M	[94]
IEX Group 4					↑ 23.5 M*	[94]
IEX Group 5					↑ 11.4 M*	[94]
IEX Group 2					↓ 4.2 M	[94]
IEX Group 1					↑ 19.5 M*	[94]
IEX Group 3					↑ 13 M*	[94]
PBS soluble mite extract					↑ 10.1 M*	[93]
Membrane associated					↑ 2.2 M	[93]
Urea soluble					↑ 0.2 M	[93]
Integral membrane					↓ 1.5 M	[93]
Mite extract			ISA 50 V	In vitro [95]	↑ 50.7 M*	[95]
Soluble protein mite extract			ISA 207 VG	Field	↓ 78 Pop*	[96]
Akirin	Recombinant	*Aedes albopictus*	ISA 50 V	In vitro [95]	↑ 35.1 M*	[97]
Bm86		*Rhipicephalus microplus*			↑ 23 M*	[97]
Histamine release factor		*D. gallinae*	QuilA	In vitro [98]	↑ 4.1 M*	[99]
Cathepsin D-1				In vitro [93]	↑ 6.9 M*	[100]
Cathepsin L-1					↑ 2.6 M*	[100]
Unknown function protein 1					↑ 18.4 M*	[94]
Unknown function protein 2					↑ 0.6 M	[94]
Aspartyl proteinase					↑ 5.6 M	[94]

Antigen	Type	Species	Adjuvant	Test	Effects (%)	Reference
Phosphoglycerate dehydrogenase	Recombinant	D. gallinae	QuilA	In vitro [93]	↑4.1 M	[94]
Serpin-1					↑12 M*	[94]
Hemelipoglycoprotein-1					↑18.9 M*	[94]
Vitellogenin-1					↑21.9 M*	[94]
Peptidase C1A-like cysteine proteinase					↑14.5 M	[94]
Serpin-2					↓8.2 M	[94]
Unknown function protein 3					↑3.5 M	[94]
Paramyosin					↑20.1 M*	[101]
Tropomyosin					↑16.5 M*	[101]
Deg-SRP-1 + Deg-VIT-1 + Deg-PUF-1			ISA 70 VG	Field	—	[96]
Calumenin			ISA 71 VG	On hen [79]	↓35 O*	[102]
Akirin					↓42 O*	[103]
Cathepsin D-1					↓50 O*	[104]
Subolesin		Rhipicephalus microplus			↓44 O*	[102]
Cathepsin D-1	DNA	D. gallinae	chicken IL-21		—	[104]
Cathepsin D-1			Eimeria tenella		—	[104]

Abbreviations: M, mortality; O, Oviposition; ↑, increase; ↓, reduction.
*The effects are statistically significant.

Table 1.
Antigens tested as vaccine candidates against infestations by D. gallinae.

assessment of novel antigens [91]. Vaccines can be considered as an alternative and complementary intervention for PRM control, which can reduce the use of acaricides.

5. Conclusions and future directions

The negative impact of the PRM infestations have become more relevant with recent changes in the production systems, and it is expected to become worse as the market demands more welfare focused systems that reduce the options for controlling poultry infestations. These changes in the production procedures should include increased concerns in biosecurity and monitorization in order to achieve a better understanding of the mite ecology on each farm. PRM infestations constitute a challenge for the modern industry to guarantee hen welfare and prevention of risks for the workers.

Omics are a promising tool for enhancing the understanding of the mite-host interactions. These techniques are needed to resolve questions that are yet to be answered such as the determination of the role of the PRM as biological vectors for both poultry and human pathogens and the different mechanisms involved in the immune response in hens or if there are any on the mite side to modulate its host response. Alternative control methods and particularly vaccine are urgently needed for the effective and sustainable control of PRM infestations with the optimization and combination of different interventions.

See methodology for bibliometric analysis.

6. Methodology

6.1 Bibliometric analysis

A bibliometric analysis was performed in the web database Scopus (https://www.scopus.com) with the search code "dermanyssus AND gallinae" (date accessed: Sep 16, 2019). The search generated a total of 418 entries, from which 56 entries (14.4%) were published in the last 2 years (2018 and 2019). After the search was completed, we selected those references that addressed the main topics reviewed in this work.

6.2 Scanning electron microscope (SEM) imaging

Images obtained by scanning electron microscope (SEM) were used in **Figure 1** to show morphological characters that are useful for species identification [14]. The adult female mite used for SEM photography was dehydrated in absolute ethanol for 24 h. Specimens were mounted onto standard aluminum SEM stubs using conductive carbon adhesive tabs. Mites were observed and photographed with a field emission scanning electron microscope (Zeiss GeminiSEM 500, Oberkochen, Germany) operating in high vacuum mode at an accelerating voltage of 2 kV in the absence of metallic coating.

6.3 Points of action for control measures

The determination of the points of action for the different control measures was obtained based on the data available in previous works [1, 20, 22, 74–77, 79, 82, 103, 104].

Acknowledgements

JFLB was supported by Ministerio de Ciencia, Innovación y Universidades (Spain), Doctorado Industrial contract (DI-14-06917) and Sabiotec SA. MV was supported by the University of Castilla- La Mancha (Spain).

Author details

José Francisco Lima-Barbero[1,2], Margarita Villar[1,3], Ursula Höfle[1]
and José de la Fuente[1,4*]

1 SABIO, Institute for Game and Wildlife Research, Ciudad Real, Spain

2 SABIOTEC, Ciudad Real, Spain

3 Biochemistry Section, Faculty of Science and Chemical Technologies, and Regional Centre for Biomedical Research (CRIB), University of Castilla-La Mancha, Ciudad Real, Spain

4 Department of Veterinary Pathobiology, Center for Veterinary Health Sciences, Oklahoma State University, Stillwater, OK, USA

*Address all correspondence to: jose_delafuente@yahoo.com

IntechOpen

© 2020 The Author(s). Licensee IntechOpen. This chapter is distributed under the terms of the Creative Commons Attribution License (http://creativecommons.org/licenses/by/3.0), which permits unrestricted use, distribution, and reproduction in any medium, provided the original work is properly cited. (cc) BY

References

[1] Sparagano OAE, George DR, Harrington DWJ, Giangaspero A. Significance and control of the poultry red mite, *Dermanyssus gallinae*. Annual Review of Entomology. 2014;**59**:447-466. DOI: 10.1146/annurev-ento-011613-162101

[2] Roy L, Chauve CM. Historical review of the genus *Dermanyssus* Dugès, 1834 (Acari: Mesostigmata: Dermanyssidae). Parasite. 2007;**14**:87-100. DOI: 10.1051/parasite/2007142087

[3] Di Palma A, Leone F, Albanese F, Beccati M. A case report of *Dermanyssus gallinae* infestation in three cats. Veterinary Dermatology. 2018;**29**:348-e124. DOI: 10.1111/vde.12547

[4] Mignon B, Losson B. Dermatitis in a horse associated with the poultry mite (*Dermanyssus gallinae*). Veterinary Dermatology. 2008;**19**:38-43. DOI: 10.1111/j.1365-3164.2007.00646.x

[5] Declercq J, Nachtegaele L. *Dermanyssus gallinae* infestation in a dog. Canine Practice. 1993;**18**:34-35

[6] Cafiero MA, Barlaam A, Camarda A, Radeski M, Mul M, Sparagano O, et al. *Dermanysuss gallinae* attacks humans. Mind the gap! Avian Pathology. 2019;**48**:S22-S34. DOI: 10.1080/03079457.2019.1633010

[7] Sigognault Flochlay A, Thomas E, Sparagano OAE. Poultry red mite (*Dermanyssus gallinae*) infestation: A broad impact parasitological disease that still remains a significant challenge for the egg-laying industry in Europe. Parasites & Vectors. 2017;**10**:357. DOI: 10.1186/s13071-017-2292-4

[8] Cosoroaba I. Massive *Dermanyssus gallinae* invasion in battery-husbandry raised fowls. Revista de Medicina Veterinaria. 2001;**152**:89-96

[9] Kilpinen O, Roepstorff A, Permin A, Nørgaard-Nielsen G, Lawson LG, Simonsen HB. Influence of *Dermanyssus gallinae* and *Ascaridia galli* infections on behaviour and health of laying hens (*Gallus gallus domesticus*). British Poultry Science. 2005;**46**:26-34. DOI: 10.1080/00071660400023839

[10] Sparagano OAE, Tomley FM. The impact of the COREMI cost action network on the progress towards the control of the poultry red mite, *Dermanyssus gallinae*. Avian Pathology. 2019;**48**:S1. DOI: 10.1080/03079457.2019.1662175

[11] Roy L, Dowling APG, Chauve CM, Lesna I, Sabelis MW, Buronfosse T. Molecular phylogenetic assessment of host range in five *Dermanyssus species*. In: Control of Poultry Mites (*Dermanyssus*). Dordrecht: Springer Netherlands; 2009. pp. 115-142

[12] Young MR, Moraza ML, Ueckermann E, Heylen D, Baardsen LF, Lima-Barbero JF, et al. Linking morphological and molecular taxonomy for the identification of poultry house, soil, and nest dwelling mites in the Western Palearctic. Scientific Reports. 2019;**9**:5784

[13] Roy L, Chauve C. The genus *Dermanyssus* (Mesostigmata: Dermanyssidae): History and species characterization. In: Trends in Acarology. Dordrecht: Springer Netherlands; 2010. pp. 49-55

[14] Di Palma A, Giangaspero A, Cafiero MA, Germinara GS. A gallery of the key characters to ease identification of *Dermanyssus gallinae* (Acari: Gamasida: Dermanyssidae) and allow differentiation from *Ornithonyssus sylviarum* (Acari: Gamasida: Macronyssidae). Parasites

& Vectors. 2012;**5**:104. DOI:
10.1186/1756-3305-5-104

[15] Tomley FM, Sparagano O. Spotlight
on avian pathology: Red mite, a serious
emergent problem in layer hens. Avian
Pathology. 2018;**47**:533-535. DOI:
10.1080/03079457.2018.1490493

[16] Roy L, Chauve C, Buronfosse T.
Contrasted ecological repartition of
the northern fowl mite *Ornithonyssus
sylviarum* (Mesostigmata:
Macronyssidae) and the chicken
red mite *Dermanyssus gallinae*
(Mesostigmata: Dermanyssidae).
Acarologia. 2010;**50**:207-219. DOI:
10.1051/acarologia/20101958

[17] Kilpinen O. Activation of the
poultry red mite, *Dermanyssus gallinae*
(Acari: Dermanyssidae), by increasing
temperatures. Experimental and
Applied Acarology. 2001;**25**:859-867.
DOI: 10.1023/A:1020409221348

[18] Maurer V, Baumgärtner J.
Temperature influence on life
table statistics of the chicken
mite *Dermanyssus gallinae* (Acari:
Dermanyssidae). Experimental &
Applied Acarology. 1992;**15**:27-40. DOI:
10.1007/BF01193965

[19] Nordenfors H, Höglund J,
Uggla A. Effects of temperature and
humidity on Oviposition, molting, and
longevity of *Dermanyssus gallinae* (Acari:
Dermanyssidae). Journal of Medical
Entomology. 1999;**36**:68-72. DOI:
10.1093/jmedent/36.1.68

[20] Pritchard J, Kuster T, Sparagano O,
Tomley F. Understanding the biology
and control of the poultry red mite
Dermanyssus gallinae: A review. Avian
Pathology. 2015;**44**:143-153. DOI:
10.1080/03079457.2015.1030589

[21] Van Emous RA, Van TGCMF,
Mul MF. Red mites in theory and practice.
Praktijkrapport Pluimvee. 2005:17

[22] Koenraadt CJM, Dicke M. The
role of volatiles in aggregation and
host-seeking of the haematophagous
poultry red mite *Dermanyssus gallinae*
(Acari: Dermanyssidae). Experimental
& Applied Acarology. 2010;**50**:191-199.
DOI: 10.1007/s10493-009-9305-8

[23] Kilpinen O. How to obtain a
bloodmeal without being eaten by a
host: The case of poultry red mite,
Dermanyssus gallinae. Physiological
Entomology. 2005;**30**:232-240. DOI:
10.1111/j.1365-3032.2005.00452.x

[24] Kilpinen O, Mullens BA. Effect
of food deprivation on response
of the mite, *Dermanyssus gallinae,*
to heat. Medical and Veterinary
Entomology. 2004;**18**:368-371. DOI:
10.1111/j.1365-3032.2005.00452.x

[25] Zeman P. Surface skin lipids of
birds - a proper host kairomone and
feeding inducer in the poultry red mite,
Dermanyssus gallinae. Experimental &
Applied Acarology. 1988;**5**:163-173. DOI:
10.1007/BF02053825

[26] Harrington DWJ, Guy JH,
Robinson K, Sparagano OAE. Comparison
of synthetic membranes in the
development of an in vitro feeding
system for *Dermanyssus gallinae*.
Bulletin of Entomological Research.
2010;**100**:127-132. DOI: 10.1017/
S0007485309006865

[27] Maurer V, Bieri M, Foelsch DW.
Das Suchverhalten von *Dermanyssus
gallinae* in Huhnerstallen. Host-
finding of *Dermanyssus gallinae* in
poultry-houses. Eur. Poultry Science.
1988;**52**:209-215

[28] Mullens BA, Hinkle NC,
Robinson LJ, Szijj CE. Dispersal of
northern fowl mites, *Ornithonyssus
sylviarum*, among hens in an
experimental poultry house. Journal of
Applied Poultry Research. 2001;**10**:
60-64. DOI: 10.1093/japr/10.1.60

[29] Sreenivasa Murthy GS, Panda R. Prevalence of *Dermanyssus* and *Ornithonyssus* species of mites in poultry farms of Vikarabad area of Hyderabad. Journal of Parasitic Diseases. 2016;**40**:1372-1375. DOI: 10.1007/s12639-015-0693-x

[30] George DR, Finn RD, Graham KM, Mul MF, Maurer V, Moro CV, et al. Should the poultry red mite *Dermanyssus gallinae* be of wider concern for veterinary and medical science? Parasites & Vectors. 2015;**8**:178. DOI: 10.1186/s13071-015-0768-7

[31] Othman RA, Abdallah JM, Abo-Omar J. Prevalence of the red mite (*Dermanyssus gallinae*) in layer flocks in four districts in northern West Bank, Palestine. Open Journal of Animal Sciences. 2012;**2**:106. DOI: 10.4236/ojas.2012.22014

[32] Sparagano O, Pavlićević A, Murano T, Camarda A, Sahibi H, Kilpinen O, et al. Prevalence and key figures for the poultry red mite *Dermanyssus gallinae* infections in poultry farm systems. In: Control of Poultry Mites (*Dermanyssus*). Dordrecht, The Netherlands: Springer; 2009. pp. 3-10

[33] Sparagano OAE, Pavlićević A, Murano T, Camarda A, Sahibi H, Kilpinen O, et al. Prevalence and key figures for the poultry red mite *Dermanyssus gallinae* infections in poultry farm systems. Experimental & Applied Acarology. 2009;**48**:3-10. DOI: 10.1007/978-90-481-2731-3_2

[34] Mul MF, van Riel JW, Roy L, Zoons J, André G, George DR, et al. Development of a model forecasting *Dermanyssus gallinae*'s population dynamics for advancing integrated Pest management in laying hen facilities. Veterinary Parasitology. 2017;**245**:128-140. DOI: 10.1016/J.VETPAR.2017.07.027

[35] Kaab H, Bain MM, Bartley K, Turnbull F, Wright HW, Nisbet AJ, et al. Serum and acute phase protein changes in laying hens, infested with poultry red mite. Poultry Science. 2019;**98**:679-687. DOI: 10.3382/ps/pey431

[36] Harrington D, Robinson K, Guy J, Sparagano O. Characterization of the immunological response to *Dermanyssus gallinae* infestation in domestic fowl. Transboundary and Emerging Diseases. 2010;**57**:107-110. DOI: 10.1111/j.1865-1682.2010.01109.x

[37] Harrington DWJ, Robinson K, Sparagano OAE. Immune responses of the domestic fowl to *Dermanyssus gallinae* under laboratory conditions. Parasitology Research. 2010;**106**:1425-1434. DOI: 10.1007/s00436-010-1821-2

[38] Nordenfors H, Hoglund J. Long term dynamics of *Dermanyssus gallinae* in relation to mite control measures in aviary systems for layers. British Poultry Science. 2000;**41**:533-540. DOI: 10.1080/713654991

[39] Sleeckx N, Van Gorp S, Koopman R, Kempen I, Van Hoye K, De Baere K, et al. Production losses in laying hens during infestation with the poultry red mite *Dermanyssus gallinae*. Avian Pathology. 2019;**48**:S17-S21. DOI: 10.1080/03079457.2019.1641179

[40] Odaka M, Ogino K, Shikada M, Asada K, Kasa S, Inoue T, et al. Correlation between the proportion of stained eggs and the number of mites (*Dermanyssus gallinae*) monitored using a 'non-parallel board trap. Animal Science Journal. 2017;**88**:2077-2083. DOI: 10.1111/asj.12860

[41] Rayner AC, Higham LE, Gill R, Michalski J-P, Deakin A. A survey of free-range egg farmers in the United Kingdom: Knowledge, attitudes and practices surrounding antimicrobial use and resistance. Veterinary and Animal Science. 2019;**100072**. DOI: 10.1016/J.VAS.2019.100072

[42] Sikes RK, Chamberlain RW. Laboratory observations on three species of bird mites. The Journal of Parasitology. 1954;**40**:691-697

[43] Wójcik AR, Grygon-Franckiewicz B, Zbikowska E, Wasielewski L. Invasion of *Dermanyssus gallinae* (De Geer, 1778) in poultry farms in the Toruń region. Wiadomości Parazytologiczne. 2000;**46**:511-515

[44] Arkle S, Guy JH, Sparagano O. Immunological effects and productivity variation of red mite (*Dermanyssus gallinae*) on laying hens- implications for egg production and quality. World's Poultry Science Journal. 2006;**62**:249-257. DOI: 10.1079/WPS200594

[45] Kowalski A, Sokol R. Influence of *Dermanyssus gallinae* (poultry red mite) invasion on the plasma levels of corticosterone, catecholamines and proteins in layer hens. Polish Journal of Veterinary Sciences. 2009;**12**:231-235

[46] Valiente Moro C, Thioulouse J, Chauve C, Normand P, Zenner L. Bacterial taxa associated with the hematophagous mite *Dermanyssus gallinae* detected by 16S rRNA PCR amplification and TTGE fingerprinting. Research in Microbiology. 2009;**160**:63-70. DOI: 10.1016/j.resmic.2008.10.006

[47] Huong CTT, Murano T, Uno Y, Usui T, Yamaguchi T. Molecular detection of avian pathogens in poultry red mite (*Dermanyssus gallinae*) collected in chicken farms. The Journal of Veterinary Medical Science. 2014;**76**:1583-1587. DOI: 10.1292/jvms.14-0253

[48] Circella E, Pugliese N, Todisco G, Cafiero MA, Sparagano OAE, Camarda A. *Chlamydia psittaci* infection in canaries heavily infested by *Dermanyssus gallinae*. Experimental & Applied Acarology. 2011;**55**:329-338. DOI: 10.1007/s10493-011-9478-9

[49] Valiente Moro C, Fravalo P, Amelot M, Chauve C, Zenner L, Salvat G. Colonization and organ invasion in chicks experimentally infected with *Dermanyssus gallinae* contaminated by *Salmonella Enteritidis*. Avian Pathology. 2007;**36**:307-311. DOI: 10.1080/03079450701460484

[50] Zeman P, Stika V, Skalka B, Bartik M, Dusbabek F, Lavickova M. Potential role of *Dermanyssus gallinae* De Geer, 1778 in the circulation of the agent of pullorosis-typhus in hens. Folia Parasitologica. 1982;**29**:371-374

[51] Pugliese N, Circella E, Marino M, De Virgilio C, Cocciolo G, Lozito P, et al. Circulation dynamics of *Salmonella enterica* subsp. *enterica* ser. Gallinarum biovar Gallinarum in a poultry farm infested by *Dermanyssus gallinae*. Medical and Veterinary Entomology. 2019;**33**:162-170. DOI: 10.1111/mve.12333

[52] Sommer D, Heffels-Redmann U, Köhler K, Lierz M, Kaleta EF. Role of the poultry red mite (*Dermanyssus gallinae*) in the transmission of avian influenza a virus. Tierarztliche Praxis Ausgabe G: Grosstiere—Nutztiere. 2016;**1**:47-54

[53] van Emous RA. Verwachtte schade bloedluis 21 miljoen euro [Internet]. Pluimveeweb. 2017. Available from: https://www.pluimveeweb.nl/artikelen/2017/01/schade-bloedluis-21-miljoen-euro/ [cited: 05 January 2018]

[54] Van Riel J, Mul MF, Guy JH, George DR. Investigations on economics of operational control of *Dermanyssus gallinae*. In: 2nd COST Conference and Management Committee Meeting. Zagreb, Croatia. 2016. p. 39

[55] McCulloch JB, Owen JP, Hinkle NC, Mullens BA, Busch JW. Genetic structure of northern fowl mite (Mesostigmata: Macronyssidae) populations among layer chicken flocks and local house

sparrows (Passeriformes: Passeridae). Journal of Medical Entomology. 2019:tjz136. DOI: 10.1093/jme/tjz136

[56] Mul MF, Koenraadt CJM. Preventing introduction and spread of *Dermanyssus gallinae* in poultry facilities using the HACCP method. Experimental & Applied Acarology. 2009;**48**:167-181. DOI: 10.1007/s10493-009-9250-6

[57] Flechtmann CHW, Baggio D. On phoresy of hematophagous ectoparasitic Acari (Parasitiformes: Ixodidae and dermanyssidae) on coleoptera observed in Brazil. International Journal of Acarology. 1993;**19**:195-196. DOI: 10.1080/01647959308683982

[58] Reich H, Triacchini GA. Occurrence of residues of fipronil and other acaricides in chicken eggs and poultry muscle/fat. EFSA Journal. 2018;**16**:5164. DOI: 10.2903/j.efsa.2018.5164

[59] Medicines Agency E. Committee for Medicinal Products for Veterinary Use European public MRL assessment report (EPMAR) Fluralaner (Poultry). 2017. Available from: https://www.ema. europa.eu/en/documents/mrl-report/ fluralaner-poultry-european-public-maximum-residue-limit-assessment-report-epmar-cvmp_en.pdf [Accessed: 02 November 2019]

[60] Marangi M, Morelli V, Pati S, Camarda A, Cafiero MA, Giangaspero A. Acaricide residues in laying hens naturally infested by red mite *Dermanyssus gallinae*. PLoS One. 2012;77:e31795. DOI: 10.1371/journal. pone.0031795

[61] Limsuwan S, Priess B, Tansakul N, Nau H, Kietzmann K, Hamscher G. Penetration studies of Propoxur and Phoxim from eggshell into whole egg after experimental exposure and application in henhouses. Journal of Agricultural and Food Chemistry. 2007;**55**:6401-6405. DOI: 10.1021/JF070987P

[62] Gokbulut C, Ozuicli M, Aslan B, Aydin L, Cirak VY. The residue levels of spinosad and abamectin in eggs and tissues of laying hens following spray application. Avian Pathology. 2019;**48**:S44-S51. DOI: 10.1080/03079457.2019.1623380

[63] Lima-Barbero JF, Sánchez MS, Cabezas-Cruz A, Mateos-Hernández L, Contreras M, de Mera IGF, et al. Clinical gamasoidosis and antibody response in two patients infested with *Ornithonyssus bursa* (Acari: Gamasida: Macronyssidae). Experimental & Applied Acarology. 2019;**78**:555-564. DOI: 10.1007/s10493-019-00408-x

[64] Cafiero MA, Galante D, Camarda A, Giangaspero A, Sparagano O. Why dermanyssosis should be listed as an occupational hazard. Occupational and Environmental Medicine. 2011;**68**:628. DOI: 10.1136/oemed-2011-100002

[65] Pezzi M, Leis M, Chicca M, Roy L. Gamasoidosis by the special lineage L1 of *Dermanyssus gallinae* (Acarina: Dermanyssidae): A case of heavy infestation in a public place in Italy. Parasitology International. 2017;**66**:666-670. DOI: 10.1016/J. PARINT.2017.05.001

[66] Hubert J, Erban T, Kopecky J, Sopko B, Nesvorna M, Lichovnikova M, et al. Comparison of microbiomes between red poultry mite populations (*Dermanyssus gallinae*): Predominance of Bartonella-like bacteria. Microbial Ecology. 2017;**74**:947-960. DOI: 10.1007/ s00248-017-0993-z

[67] Almehmi A, Pfister AK, McCowan R, Matulis S. Implantable cardioverter-defibrillator infection caused by Tsukamurella. The West Virginia Medical Journal. 2004;**100**(5):185-186

[68] Auger P, Nantel J, Meunier N, Harrison RJ, Loiselle R, Gyorkos TW. Skin acariasis caused by *Dermanyssus gallinae*

(de Geer): An in-hospital outbreak. Canadian Medical Association Journal. 1979;**120**:700

[69] Marangi M, Cafiero MA, Capelli G, Camarda A, Sparagano OAE, Giangaspero A. Evaluation of the poultry red mite, *Dermanyssus gallinae* (Acari: Dermanyssidae) susceptibility to some acaricides in field populations from Italy. Experimental & Applied Acarology. 2009;**48**:11-18. DOI: 10.1007/s10493-008-9224-0

[70] Pugliese N, Circella E, Cocciolo G, Giangaspero A, Horvatek Tomic D, Kika TS, et al. Efficacy of λ -cyhalothrin, amitraz, and phoxim against the poultry red mite *Dermanyssus gallinae* De Geer, 1778 (Mesostigmata: Dermanyssidae): An eight-year survey. Avian Pathology. 2019;**48**:S35-S43. DOI: 10.1080/03079457.2019.1645295

[71] Thomas E, Chiquet M, Sander B, Zschiesche E, Flochlay AS. Field efficacy and safety of fluralaner solution for administration in drinking water for the treatment of poultry red mite (*Dermanyssus gallinae*) infestations in commercial flocks in Europe. Parasites & Vectors. 2017;**10**:457. DOI: 10.1186/s13071-017-2390-3

[72] Waap H, Nunes T, Mul M, Gomes J, Bartley K. Survey on the prevalence of *Dermanyssus gallinae* in commercial laying farms in Portugal. Avian Pathology. 2019;**48**:S2-S9. DOI: 10.1080/03079457.2019.1606415

[73] Mul MF, van Riel JW, Meerburg BG, Dicke M, George DR, Groot Koerkamp PWG. Validation of an automated mite counter for *Dermanyssus gallinae* in experimental laying hen cages. Experimental & Applied Acarology. 2015;**66**:589-603. DOI: 10.1007/s10493-015-9923-2

[74] Mul MF, Van Niekerk TGCM, Chirico J, Maurer V, Kilpinen O, Sparagano OAE, et al. Control methods for *Dermanyssus gallinae* in systems for laying hens: Results of an international seminar. World's Poultry Science Journal. 2009;**65**:589-600. DOI: 10.1017/S0043933909000403

[75] George DR, Finn RD, Graham KM, Sparagano OA. Present and future potential of plant-derived products to control arthropods of veterinary and medical significance. Parasites & Vectors. 2014;**7**:28. DOI: 10.1186/1756-3305-7-28

[76] El Adouzi M, Arriaga-Jiménez A, Dormont L, Nicolas B, Labalette A, Lapeyre B, et al. Modulation of feed composition is able to make hens less attractive to the poultry red mite *Dermanyssus gallinae*. Parasitology. 2019:1-43. DOI: 10.1017/S0031182019001379

[77] Camarda A, Pugliese N, Bevilacqua A, Circella E, Gradoni L, George D, et al. Efficacy of a novel neem oil formulation (RP03™) to control the poultry red mite *Dermanyssus gallinae*. Medical and Veterinary Entomology. 2018;**32**:290-297. DOI: 10.1111/mve.12296

[78] Roy L, El Adouzi M, Moraza ML, Chiron G, Villeneuve de Janti E, Le Peutrec G, et al. Arthropod communities of laying hen houses: An integrative pilot study toward conservation biocontrol of the poultry red mite *Dermanyssus gallinae*. Biological Control. 2017;**114**:176-194. DOI: 10.1016/J.BIOCONTROL.2017.08.006

[79] Lesna I, Wolfs P, Faraji F, Roy L, Komdeur J, Sabelis MW. Candidate predators for biological control of the poultry red mite *Dermanyssus gallinae*. Experimental & Applied Acarology. 2009;**48**:63-80. DOI: 10.1007/s10493-009-9239-1

[80] Lesna I, Sabelis MW, van Niekerk TGCM, Komdeur J. Laboratory tests for controlling poultry

red mites (*Dermanyssus gallinae*) with predatory mites in small 'laying hen' cages. Experimental & Applied Acarology. 2012;**58**:371-383. DOI: 10.1007/s10493-012-9596-z

[81] Van de Ven D. Q-perch, electronic control of red mite. Vencomatic Group. In: Book of Abstracts, 2nd COST Conference and Management Committee Meeting and COST Conference and Management Committee (MC) Meeting COST Action FA1404 Improving Current Understanding and Research for Sustainable Control of the Poultry Red Mite *Dermanyssus gallinae*. Zagreb, Croatia. 2016. p. 36

[82] Kilpinen O, Steenberg T. Inert dusts and their effects on the poultry red mite (*Dermanyssus gallinae*). In: Control of Poultry Mites (*Dermanyssus*). Dordrecht, The Netherlands: Springer; 2009. pp. 51-62

[83] Steenberg T, Kilpinen O. Synergistic interaction between the fungus *Beauveria bassiana* and desiccant dusts applied against poultry red mites (*Dermanyssus gallinae*). Experimental & Applied Acarology. 2014;**62**:511-524. DOI: 10.1007/s10493-013-9757-8

[84] Tavassoli M, Allymehr M, Pourseyed SH, Ownag A, Bernousi I, Mardani K, et al. Field bioassay of *Metarhizium anisopliae* strains to control the poultry red mite *Dermanyssus gallinae*. Veterinary Parasitology. 2011;**178**:374-378. DOI: 10.1016/J.VETPAR.2011.01.031

[85] de la Fuente J, Estrada-Peña A. Why new vaccines for the control of Ectoparasite vectors have not been registered and commercialized? Vaccine. 2019;**7**:75. DOI: 10.3390/vaccines7030075

[86] de la Fuente J, Contreras M. Tick vaccines: Current status and future directions. Expert Review of

Vaccines. 2015;**14**:1367-1376. DOI: 10.1586/14760584.2015.1076339

[87] de la Fuente J, Almazán C, Canales M, Pérez de la Lastra JM, Kocan KM, Willadsen P. A ten-year review of commercial vaccine performance for control of tick infestations on cattle. Animal Health Research Reviews. 2007;**8**:23-28. DOI: 10.1017/S1466252307001193

[88] de la Fuente J, Kopáček P, Lew-Tabor A, Maritz-Olivier C. Strategies for new and improved vaccines against ticks and tick-borne diseases. Parasite Immunology. 2016;**38**:754-769. DOI: 10.1111/pim.12339

[89] Schicht S, Qi W, Poveda L, Strube C. Whole transcriptome analysis of the poultry red mite *Dermanyssus gallinae* (De Geer, 1778). Parasitology. 2014;**141**:336-346. DOI: 10.1017/S0031182013001467

[90] Burgess STG, Bartley K, Nunn F, Wright HW, Hughes M, Gemmell M, et al. Draft genome assembly of the poultry red mite, *Dermanyssus gallinae*. Microbiology Resource Announcements. 2018;**7**:e01221-e01218. DOI: 10.1128/MRA.01221-18

[91] Nunn F, Bartley K, Palarea-Albaladejo J, Innocent GT, Turnbull F, Wright HW, et al. A novel, high-welfare methodology for evaluating poultry red mite interventions in vivo. Veterinary Parasitology. 2019;**267**:42-46. DOI: 10.1016/J.VETPAR.2019.01.011

[92] Arkle S, Harrington D, Kaiser P, Rothwell L, De Luna C, George D, et al. Immunological control of the poultry red mite. Annals of the New York Academy of Sciences. 2008;**1149**:36-40. DOI: 10.1196/annals.1428.057

[93] Wright HW, Bartley K, Nisbet AJ, McDevitt RM, Sparks NHC, Brocklehurst S, et al. The testing of

antibodies raised against poultry red mite antigens in an in vitro feeding assay; preliminary screen for vaccine candidates. Experimental & Applied Acarology. 2009;**48**:81-91. DOI: 10.1007/s10493-009-9243-5

[94] Bartley K, Wright HW, Huntley JF, Manson EDT, Inglis NF, McLean K, et al. Identification and evaluation of vaccine candidate antigens from the poultry red mite (*Dermanyssus gallinae*). International Journal for Parasitology. 2015;**45**:819-830. DOI: 10.1016/j.ijpara.2015.07.004

[95] Harrington DWJ, Din HM, Guy J, Robinson K, Sparagano O. Characterization of the immune response of domestic fowl following immunization with proteins extracted from *Dermanyssus gallinae*. Veterinary Parasitology. 2009;**160**:285-294. DOI: 10.1016/j.ijpara.2015.07.004

[96] Bartley K, Turnbull F, Wright HW, Huntley JF, Palarea-Albaladejo J, Nath M, et al. Field evaluation of poultry red mite (*Dermanyssus gallinae*) native and recombinant prototype vaccines. Veterinary Parasitology. 2017;**244**:25-34. DOI: 10.1016/j.vetpar.2017.06.020

[97] Harrington DWJ, Canales M, de la Fuente J, de Luna C, Robinson K, Guy J, et al. Immunisation with recombinant proteins subolesin and Bm86 for the control of *Dermanyssus gallinae* in poultry. Vaccine. 2009;**27**:4056-4063. DOI: 10.1016/j.vaccine.2009.04.014

[98] McDevitt R, Nisbet AJ, Huntley JF. Ability of a proteinase inhibitor mixture to kill poultry red mite, *Dermanyssus gallinae* in an in vitro feeding system. Veterinary Parasitology. 2006;**141**:380-385. DOI: 10.1016/J.VETPAR.2006.05.013

[99] Bartley K, Nisbet AJ, Offer JE, Sparks NHC, Wright HW, Huntley JF. Histamine release factor from

Dermanyssus gallinae (De Geer): Characterization and in vitro assessment as a protective antigen. International Journal for Parasitology. 2009;**39**:447-456. DOI: 10.1016/j.ijpara.2008.09.006

[100] Bartley K, Huntley JF, Wright HW, Nath M, Nisbet AJ. Assessment of cathepsin D and L-like proteinases of poultry red mite, *Dermanyssus gallinae* (De Geer), as potential vaccine antigens. Parasitology. 2012;**139**:755-765. DOI: 10.1017/S0031182011002356

[101] Wright HW, Bartley K, Huntley JF, Nisbet AJ. Characterisation of tropomyosin and paramyosin as vaccine candidate molecules for the poultry red mite, *Dermanyssus gallinae*. Parasites & Vectors. 2016;**9**:544. DOI: 10.1186/s13071-016-1831-8

[102] Lima-Barbero JF, Contreras M, Mateos-Hernández L, Mata-Lorenzo FM, Triguero-Ocaña R, Sparagano O, et al. A vaccinology approach to the identification and characterization of *Dermanyssus gallinae* candidate protective antigens for the control of poultry red mite infestations. Vaccines. 2019;**7**:190

[103] Lima-Barbero JF, Contreras M, Bartley K, Price DRG, Nunn F, Sanchez-Sanchez M, et al. Reduction in Oviposition of poultry red mite (*Dermanyssus gallinae*) in hens vaccinated with recombinant Akirin. Vaccine. 2019;**7**:121. DOI: 10.3390/vaccines7030121

[104] Price DRG, Küster T, Øines Ø, Oliver EM, Bartley K, Nunn F, et al. Evaluation of vaccine delivery systems for inducing long-lived antibody responses to *Dermanyssus gallinae* antigen in laying hens. Avian Pathology. 2019;**48**:S60-S74. DOI: 10.1080/03079457.2019.1612514

Chapter 14

Bronchopulmonary Lophomoniasis, Infection by Endocommensal Protozoa of Intradomiciliary Cockroaches: Presentation of a Case in an Immunocompromised Patient from Querétaro, Mexico

Maria Elena Villagrán-Herrera,

Ricardo Francisco Mercado-Curiel,

José Trinidad López-Vázquez,

Maria del Carmen Aburto-Fernández,

Nicolás Camacho-Calderón, Javier Ávila-Morales and

José Antonio De Diego-Cabrera

Abstract

Infection in humans by the intestinal protozoan of cockroaches and termites called *Lophomonas blattarum* has been diagnosed in respiratory infections of children aged 2–5 years contaminated orally or by air, with cysts or trophozoites contained in the feces of the cockroach *Periplaneta americana*. In respiratory infections of adults, it is difficult to diagnose since the cyst or trophozoite is not recognized as a human pathogen and is only related to immunosuppressed patients, transplant patients with severe lung disease and those living in poor and unhealthy sanitary conditions. Normally, its presence is manifested with fevers of 38–39°C, cough with thick expectoration, respiratory insufficiency and pulmonary abscesses. The laboratory diagnosis is mainly based on bronchoscopic cytologies and bronchoalveolar lavage biopsies. The case in question is about a 60-year-old male. Single, he lives alone, with a diagnosis of 9 baths behind non-Hodgkin lymphoma, undergoing treatment with radiotherapy and chemotherapy. For edema after treatment, thoracentesis and pericardiocentesis were performed, as well as gastrostomy, which he maintained for 1 year. He started with throat discomfort, followed by production of productive cough without blood, general weakness, and difficulty breathing, with apparent diagnosis of possible respiratory failure due to mycobacteria. It was possible to visualize the protozoan, in fresh preparations of bronchial aspirate and expectoration in wet assembly with saline solution and stained with Pap smears, Harris Hematoxylin and Eosin (H/E), and Giemsa.

IntechOpen

Keywords: American periplaneta, multiflagellated protozoan, bronchopulmonary lophomoniasis, endocommensal, immunosuppression

1. Introduction

1.1 *Lophomonas blattarum*

It is an anaerobic multiflagellated intestinal protozoan, endocommensal in the intestine of some arthropods, such as termites and cockroaches (Dictyoptera: Blattoidea), which contaminate in its path food, dust and clothes with its secretions and feces [1–11].

The genus *Lophomonas*, since 1990, has been considered among the protozoa that cause damage to the respiratory tract, especially in immunocompromised individuals (HIV/AIDS, with neoplasms, and use of corticosteroids and transplants) and in adult and pediatric asthmatic individuals [2–6].

The signs and symptoms of Lophomonas infection are similar to pneumonia and bronchitis or bronchopulmonary pathologies of various etiologies; therefore, a correct diagnosis is difficult. The above requires us to duly attend the microbiological study of expectoration, brushing, biopsy or bronchoalveolar lavage samples, whether fresh or stained preparations, especially when observing multiflagellated forms, since if you do not have enough experience trophozoites of *Lophomonas blattarum* can be confused with ciliated epithelial cell fragments (ciliocytoforia) of the bronchi [5–7].

It is important to note that conventional techniques, such as staining of Gram, Giemsa and Papanicolaou smear, do not allow adequate visualization of multiflagellating. Therefore, it is necessary that upon suspicion, a fresh preparation with saline solution is first performed on all samples of the respiratory tract that arrive at the laboratory for parasitological diagnosis, and subsequently, perfectly extended smears are stained with special dyes such as Masson's trichrome [5].

The most clinically important species are *Lophomonas blattarum* and *Lophomonas striata*. The latter was the species first identified in the intestine of the cockroach *Blatta orientalis* by S. Stein in 1860 [6]. The structure of *L. blattarum* was identified in the optical microscope in 1911 and in 1990 with a scanning and electron microscope. The shape of the Lophomonas trophozoite is usually round, oval or pyriform, ranging in size from 15 to 50 µm in diameter, with a plume of flagella that form a bunch located at the anterior end, the largest being those found far away from the apical fissure. It contains phagocytic vacuoles in its cytoplasm, with outward rhythmic movements directed to the apical end in order to eliminate excretions or trap foreign materials [1] (**Figure 1**).

The cockroaches (**Figure 2**) originate as perfectly recognized pests of closed, dark places, which abound at the beginning of the hot climate and which become visible at night when leaving their natural habitat (sewers) to look for their food in the periphery and/or inside the houses [12]. As vectors were not considered capable of transmitting pathogenic organisms to humans, however, studies were conducted by Roth and Willis in 1957, and citing evidence occurred in a pediatric hospital in Brussels, Belgium, where an epidemic of *Salmonella typhimurium* persisted in newborns, despite the rapid isolation of patients, the absence of healthy carriers and the suppression of direct or indirect contact, except for the isolation of cockroaches. However, it was discovered that at night the cockroaches walked on the clothes, blankets and bodies of the babies, and the bacteria were isolated from the body of a considerable number of insects [13]. The epidemic ceased immediately after a severe control of the cockroaches. Rueger and Olson in 1969 showed that the feces

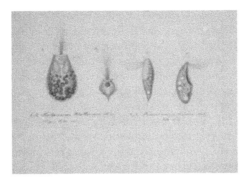

Figure 1.
In the 1860s, S. Stein discovered some multiflagellates in the cockroach's intestine. Drawings of the structures identified as Lophomonas blattarum *and* Lophomonas striata *are shown [7].*

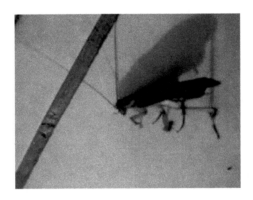

Figure 2.
Home cockroach. Photo Villagrán-Herrera.

of *Periplaneta americana* infected with *Salmonella oranienburg*, being spread over food and vessels, still contained live bacteria after 3.25–4.25 years [14]. These same authors provided a list of 18 species of domestic cockroaches; from which, it was possible to isolate the pathogenic organisms for man, due to its allergenic exposure or toxicity due to its bite [14] (**Figure 2**).

Let us consider Cornwell's paraphrase in 1968, which stated the following:

(1) Cockroaches prefer environments where both human pathogens and human food are found, freely passing from one to the other; (2) cockroaches can carry pathogens both inside and outside their bodies, which remain viable on the cuticle in the digestive tract and feces to the extent that insects can be chronic carriers and (3) the evidence is sufficient to justify the various programs of control for this insects where human health is endangered [15].

They are usually confined to buildings in cold climates, but domestic cockroaches can escape freely, and in temperate, tropical or hot weather, they can migrate to other buildings through drains, garbage dumps, septic tanks and latrines where they feed, both on human feces and on food. Isolates of intestinal diners from trapped cockroaches indicate that they are carriers of microorganisms (viruses, fungi and intestinal parasites). Among the viruses, there are 4 strains of poliovirus; and approximately 40 species of pathogenic bacteria (enterobacteria), the mycobacterium of leprosy, two pathogenic fungi (Aspergillus), and the protozoan *Entamoeba histolytica* are also mentioned. On the other hand, other pathogens that are harbored by these arthropods are mentioned under experimental conditions, such as Coxsackie virus, mouse encephalitis and yellow fever; the bacterial agents of cholera, cerebrospinal fever, pneumonia, diphtheria, undulant fever, anthrax, tetanus, tuberculosis and others; and the protozoa *Pentatrichomonas hominis*, *Giardia intestinalis* and *Balantidium coli*, agents that produce diarrhea or dysentery [13].

A protozoan that is considered important is the sporozoan *Toxoplasma gondii*, which causes human toxoplasmosis and spreads in many mammals besides birds. This disease is common in humans, although asymptomatic, but it can cause congenital defects in the fetus. It has recently been shown that the biological cycle of this coccidium is limited to domestic cats and other felines [16]. Cats can become infected by feeding on parasitized birds and rodents and subsequently transmit the parasite in their feces and a cockroach that feeds on these debris can transmit the parasite to man. Chinchilla and Ruiz in 1976 demonstrated in Costa Rica the potential transmission of *Toxoplasma gondii* by domiciliary cockroaches to humans [17] (**Figure 3**).

These species of cockroaches in urban areas have been seen mainly in nurseries, schools or hospitals, where a certain number of their population had presented lung problems of various types, and these problems were not related to the presence of these insects. It was not until the year 2015 that Dalmiro Cazorla-Perfetti found in dissected intestines of some captured insects, in addition to eggs of geohelminths, trypanosomatids, cysts and trophozoites of a multiflagellated protozoan called *Lophomonas blattarum* [18] (**Figure 4**).

On the other hand, in the city of Wuhan, in an intestinal study of 110 specimens of *Periplaneta americana* (pipe cockroach), they showed in preparations stained with Giemsa and seen at 1000 magnifications, oval, pearly shapes, from 20 to 40 μm, with a tuft of flagella extended down the central axis of the parasite and one of its trumpet-shaped ends enveloped the only nucleus shown. It also showed a thin terminal axostyle posterior to the multiflagellated part. Based on the above morphological characteristics, the parasite was identified as *L. blattarum*. Of the 110 cockroaches, 44 tested positive for *Lophomonas blattarum* (44%) [18] (**Figure 5**).

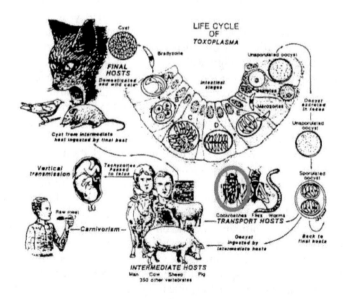

Figure 3.
Biological cycle of Toxoplasma gondii. *You can see the cockroach enclosed in a red circle, like a transporter or possible reservoir of coccidium [16].*

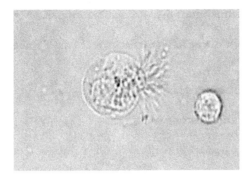

Figure 4.
Cytoplasmic and multifoflous trophozoite forms of Lophomonas blattarum *are observed 400× [19].*

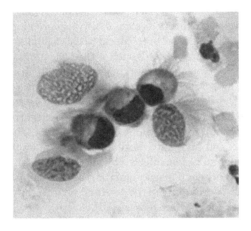

Figure 5.
Structures found in the intestinal dissections of pipe cockroaches in the city of Wuhan. Staining [18].

2. Medical importance of arthropods

The different ways in which arthropods are related to the health and well-being of man are classified into three groups:

- Arthropods as direct agents of diseases or discomfort

  ○ Entomophobia. Including illusory parasitosis

  a. Disturbances and blood loss

  ○ Accidental damage to sense organs

  a. Poisoning

  ○ Dermatosis

  a. Myiasis and associated infestations

  b. Allergies and associated conditions

- Arthropods as vectors or as intermediate hosts

- ○ Mechanical vectors (more or less casual transmission)

- ○ Mandatory vectors (including some degree of development within the arthropod)

- ○ Intermediary guests (as passive carriers)

- ○ Foretic carriers of harmful arthropods

- Arthropods as natural enemies of medically harmful insects

  - ○ Competitors

  - ○ Predatory parasites

The taxonomic scope of arthropods should be considered together with pentastomids, since the latter have always been considered as a phylum or class apart from the arthropods, however pentasthomids such as the *Linguatula serrata* whose adult forms live in the nose of dogs (and exceptionally in the human). Embryonated eggs are released via nasal mucosa or feces. If the intermediate hosts ingest the eggs, the primary four-legged larva emerges and migrates via blood vessels to the internal organs. When the final host ingests raw or undercooked meat from the infected intermediate host, the adult form develops in the nasal tract. These can be parasites of the respiratory tract and cavities of reptiles, birds and mammals. Humans can also be accidental hosts and can be infected by ingesting eggs that later develop nymphs in their tissues (visceral pentastomiasis), or ingest meat infected with nymphs in their tissues, developing in the nose and pharynx adult forms (nasopharyngeal pentastomiasis) or Halzoun disease [20].

In 1973, Lavoipierre and Rajamanickam cited cockroaches as intermediate hosts of long-necked pentasthomids [21].

2.1 Nomenclature

The modern system of naming and classifying animals dates from the 10th edition of Linnaeus Systema Naturae (1758), in which not only the first complete and ordered group of animals but also a new system of nomenclature appeared. It was Linnaeus who first devised the method of substituting specific unique names for the descriptive phrases that until then had been used in combination with the words that are now known as generic names. Linnaeus recognized six classes of animals; the fifth is the insect, whose definition allowed the inclusion of a large number of creatures that are no longer called insects, rather with their popular name, such as spiders, mites, crabs and centipedes. Its Insecta class was divided into seven orders; each of which contained several genera and each of which included numerous species [22].

2.2 Order dictyoptera

2.2.1 Cockroaches and praying mantises

The only members of this order that have any medical importance are the cockroaches (suborder Blattoidea) associated with man. These rather flattened insects, sometimes similar to beetles that move quickly, are familiar to most people; they can be easily distinguished from beetles by their very flexible, wire-like antennas [23].

Class Insecta	
Subclass Pterygota	
Division Exopterygota	
Order Dictyoptera	Cockroaches and mantids

Table 1.
Taxonomic classification of cockroaches [24].

The cockroaches form an ancient group, which goes back to the Silurian and which has few changes in its general structure since the Devonian, around 320 million years ago. They were very abundant in the Carboniferous marshes, as indicated by their fossil remains in the coal deposits of that period. They are taxonomically admitted in a separate order together with the mantids, in the Dictyoptera or as a suborder of the Orthoptera, in addition to the evidences that show a strong ancestral relationship with the termites [24] (**Table 1**).

The species associated with man attack stored food and infest premises used for storing, preparing and cooking food, such as bakehouses and kitchens, as well as sewers and rubbish dumps. They are known to carry pathogenic viruses, bacteria and helminths and to act as intermediate host for such pathogens as the nematode *Gongylonema pulchrum* Molin (gullet worm) and the Acanthocephalus *Moniliformis moniliformis* Bremser; they are also capable of causing allergic dermatitis. More than a dozen species have some degree of medical importance, but the following six species, all with worldwide distributions, are the principal vectors: the common cockroach (Blackbeetle) (*Blatta orientalis*), the American cockroach (*Periplaneta americana*), the Australian cockroach (*P. australasiae*), the German cockroach (*Blattella germanica*), the brown-banded cockroach (*Supella supellectilium**) (Serville) and the Madeira cockroach (*Leucophaea maderae*).

The following descriptions are key to identify the adults of six medically important species of cockroaches:

1. Well-developed forewings, reaching at least the tip of the abdomen.
   Front wings absent or underdeveloped, not reaching the tip of the abdomen.

2. Total length (up to the tips of the front wing) more than 18 mm.

3. Total length (up to the tips of the front wing) less than 17 mm.

4. General grayish brown color, pronotum and front wings stamped (**Figure 6F**) *Leucophaea maderae* (**Fab**).

5. Front wings with a pale yellow stripe along the basal part of the anterior margin (**Figure 6C**) *Periplaneta australasiae* (**Fab**).

6. Front wings without a pale yellow stripe along the basal part of the anterior margin (**Figure 6B**) **American Periplaneta (L.)**.

7. Pronotum with two conspicuous longitudinal dark bands. Front wings uniform color (**Figure 6D**) *Blattella germanica*.

8. Pronotum without dark bands (brown with translucent lateral margins). Forewings dark basally and pale distally in the male, and dark with pale bands in the female (**Figure 6E**) *Supella supellectilium* (**Serville**).

9. Legs from reddish brown to dark brown. Uniformly opaque pronotum. Total length greater than 15 mm (**Figure 6A**) *Blatta orientalis* **L.**

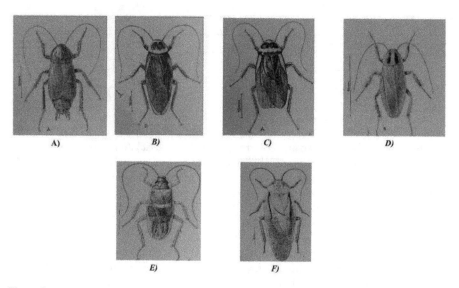

A)   B)   C)   D)

E)   F)

Figure 6.
Species of cockroaches of medical importance. A, C, D, E and F are vector agents of viruses, helminths and bacteria for both humans and animals. B is a host of the endocomponent Lophomonas blattarum, *a multifilated protozoan [23].*

Young cockroaches are similar to those of adults but lack wings [25] (**Figure 6E and F**).

The legs of insects are mainly for walking or running. The prominent antennas are filiform and multiarticulate. The mouthparts are of the generalized biting-chewing type (Orthoptera type). In most species, there are two pairs of wings; in some, the wings are vestigial, and in others, for example in *Blatta orientalis*, they are well developed in the male and short in the female. The outer pair of wings (teg-mina) is narrow, thick and coriaceous; the inner pair is membranous and folds like a fan. It is assumed that the common name in English, cockroach, is derived from the pronunciation of Cockroach name in Spanish (koo-kah-rah-chah) [24].

3. Presentation of a clinical case

This is a 60-year-old male doctor by profession, originally from Pachuca Hidalgo, who has lived in the municipality of Cadereyta for 18 years. Denies trips abroad, without physical activity, and indicates adequate personal hygiene. He refers to the diagnosis 9 years ago of non-Hodgkin lymphoma and is in treatment with radiotherapy and chemotherapy. Due to edema after treatment, thoraco-centesis and pericardiocentesis were performed, as well as gastrostomy, which he maintained for 1 year. Six months ago, he presented with respiratory symptoms, characterized by fever, malaise, cough with expectoration, and data of mild respira-tory insufficiency. It is treated with antibiotics, and salbutamol is administered; however, the symptoms reappear after 15 days.

One month ago, he presented with respiratory symptoms with the same characteristics, and he reported that a chest X-ray was performed with unspeci-fied pneumonia data. Presents 6 days ago asthenia, adynamia, hyporexia, malaise, fever of 38.5°C, self-medicated Levofloxacin 750 mg every 12 h, Ceftriaxone 1 g every 24 h, Paracetamol and Metamizol 500 mg orally. Three days

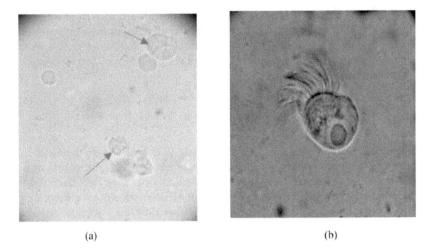

(a)   (b)

Figure 7.
(a and b) Wet assembly with saline solution, where trophozoites and cysts of Lophomonas blattarum *are observed. 400×. Photo Villagrán-Herrera.*

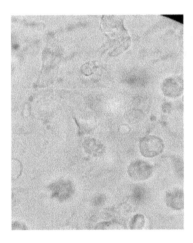

Figure 8.
Wet assembly with saline solution. Multiflagellated trophozoites and cysts were observed in a sample of unstained morning sputum. The vacuole and the many flagella in its narrow part are seen in some forms. These characteristics are compatible with Lophomonas blattarum. *Erythrocytes are seen that reveal a throat bleeding process. 400×. Photo. Villagrán-Herrera.*

later, productive cough is added, expectoration with blood streaks, and later, it becomes a uniform reddish color; likewise, the cough persists and the amount of phlegm increases. There is mild dyspnea and no predominance of hours, and salbutamol is self-medicated, showing improvement with the application of the medication. Currently fever, general malaise and mild headache persist. Freshly emitted specimens of sputum are requested and fresh observations are made with saline and several smears, which are stained with Hematoxylin and Eosin (H/E), Papanicolaou and Giemsa. The study on fresh smears reveals trophozoites and cysts of a protozoan multiflagellate identified as *Lophomonas blattarum* (**Figure 7a** and **b**).

A large amount of polymorphonuclear leukocytes was observed in the smears before staining, coinciding with an acute inflammatory process (**Figure 8**).

After the identification of the multiflagellated protozoan, treatment with met-ronidazole of 500 mg every 8 h was started orally for 7 days, improving symptoms, decreasing dyspnea and continuing with unproductive cough. Control studies are carried out 15 days after the last antiparasitic intake, and the samples were negative for the presence of this protozoan.

4. Discussion

To the cases reported in Peru, China and Spain (**Table 2**), where they found this protozoon in sputum samples, we must add 1 case recorded of a sinusitis in Iran [9], and this one that we are presenting from Mexico, since they have in common denominator deficiencies in the immune system, which makes them extremely sensitive to any infection no matter how mild. It also indicates a possible airborne transmission, with the influence of a humid environment through waste and environmental dust, and that by aspiration, the trophozoites or protozoan cysts can lodge in the bronchopulmonary epithelium, developing the infection with mani-festations similar to any bacterial or fungal pulmonary pathology, which makes diagnosis even more difficult.

Our patient presented with respiratory symptoms that indicated possible miliary tuberculosis or some acute respiratory pathology, since in the expectorant product blood threads were observed in some of the emissions, so that without the saline solution wet study, the differential diagnosis would not have been possible to reach.

The immunological commitment of the patient was a crucial and decisive factor for the development of the infection, as self-medication and the lack of an accurate diagnosis were important factors to delay his full recovery.

Autor(s) y años	Caso(s) registrados	País
Chen and Meng [26]	1	China
Dong et al. [27]	1	China
He et al. [28]	2	China
Kang et al. [29]	1	China
Liu et al. [30]	1	China
Liu et al. [31]	1	China
Martínez Girón et al. [32]	1	España
Martínez Girón & Doganci [33]	1	España
Miao et al. [34]	1	China
Shi et al. [35]	1	China
Wang [36]	26	China
Wang et al. [37]	1	China
Yang et al. [38]	1	China
Yao [39]	1	China
Yao et al. [40]	1	China
Yao et al. [41]	1	China
Yao et al. [42]	1	China
Yao et al. [43]	1	China
Yao et al. [44]	1	China

Autor(s) y años	Caso(s) registrados	País
Zerpa et al. (2010)	6	Perú
Zhang, F. et al. [45]	6	China
Zhang, R. S. et al. [46]	1	China
Zhang et al. [47]	1	China
Zhou et al. [48]	1	China
Fariba Berenji et al., 2015	1	Irán
Villagrán et al. 2016	1	México
Total	63	

Two more cases have been added. From Peru and Mexico. It is presumed that in the world, there may be many more cases that have not been reported.

Table 2.
Reported cases of bronchopulmonary diseases with Lophomonas blattarum *[5–10].*

5. Conclusions

This particular case has been the first diagnosed in the city of Querétaro and reported in the Mexican Republic and illustrates casual infection of *L. blattarum*, a rare opportunistic pathogen, probably acquired by air, developing the patient's lung infection, due to his immunocompromised state. It is essential that doctors consider *Lophomonas blattarum* in their differential clinical diagnosis. Since some dust mites are vectors of similar flagellates, whose respiratory manifestations are due to allergy, are similarly presented and are due to lack of an accurate diagnosis, they are transformed

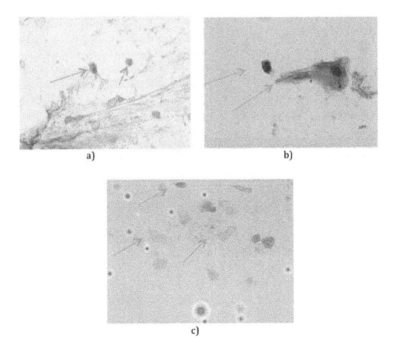

a)   b)

c)

Figure 9.
Expectoration samples stained with Papanicolaou, Hematoxylin and Eosin (H/E) and with Giemsa, respectively. Observed at 400 X. with immersion oil. Note the difference in the observation of the parasites with each of the staining procedures. Photo Villagrán-Herrera.

into chronic allergies without response to the administered treatment. Regarding the staining procedures applied to the biological sample of our patient, a great difference was observed between the multifilated structures worked in fresh and with saline solution, finding more clearly in the fresh and staining of Hematoxylin and Eosin, than with preparations with Pap smears and Giemsa (**Figure 9**).

Acknowledgements

The collaboration and support of H.T. Evelyn Flores Hernández, the Department of Pathology of the Faculty of Medicine of UAQ, are acknowledged.

Conflict of interests

The authors declare that there is no conflict of interest in relation to the publication of this clinical case.

Author details

Maria Elena Villagrán-Herrera[1]*, Ricardo Francisco Mercado-Curiel[1],
José Trinidad López-Vázquez[1], Maria del Carmen Aburto-Fernández[1],
Nicolás Camacho-Calderón[1], Javier Ávila-Morales[1] and
José Antonio De Diego-Cabrera[2]

1 Department of Biomedical Research, Faculty of Medicine, Autonomous University of Queretaro, Santiago de Querétaro, Queretaro, Mexico

2 Department of Preventive Medicine, Public Health and Microbiology, School of Medicine, Autonomous University of Madrid, Spain

*Address all correspondence to: mevh@uaq.mx

IntechOpen

© 2019 The Author(s). Licensee IntechOpen. This chapter is distributed under the terms of the Creative Commons Attribution License (http://creativecommons.org/licenses/by/3.0), which permits unrestricted use, distribution, and reproduction in any medium, provided the original work is properly cited. [cc] BY

References

[1] Gile G, Slamovits C. Phylogenetic position of *Lophomonas striata Bütschli* (*Parabasalia*) from the hindgut of the cockroach *Periplaneta americana*. Protist. 2012;**163**(2):274-283

[2] Zerpa R, Ore E, Patiño L, Espinoza Y. Hallazgo de *Lophomonas* sp. en secreciones del tracto respiratorio de niños hospitalizados con enfermedad pulmonar grave. Revista Peruana de Medicina Experimental y Salud Pública. 2010;**27**(4):575-577

[3] Martínez-Girón R, Van Woerden HC, Doganci L. Lophomonas misidentification in bronchoalveolar lavages. Internal Medicine. 2011;**50**:2721. author reply 2723

[4] Martínez-Girón R, Van Woerden HC. Clinical and immunological characteristics associated with the presence of protozoa in sputum smears. Diagnostic Cytopathology. 2013;**41**:22-27

[5] Martínez-Girón R, Van Woerden HC. Bronchopulmonary lophomoniasis: Emerging disease or unsubstantiated legend? Parasites & Vectors. 2014;**7**:284. DOI: 10.1186/1756-3305-7-284

[6] Xue J, Li Y, Yu X, Li D, Liu M, Qiu J. Bronchopulmonary infection of *Lophomonas blattarum*: A case and literature review. The Korean Journal of Parasitology. 2014;**52**(5):521-525

[7] Mu X, Shang Y, Zheng S, Zhou B, Yu B, Dong X, et al. A study on the differential diagnosis of ciliated epithelial cells from *Lophomonas blattarum* in bronchoalveolar lavage fluid. Zhonghua Jie He He Hu Xi Za Zhi. 2013;**36**(9):646-650

[8] Stein S. Vortrag über die bisher unbekannt gebliebene *Leucophyrs patula* Ehbg.und über zwei neue infusoriengattungen Gyrocorys und Lophomonas. Abh Böhmisch Ges Wiss. 1860;**1**:44-50

[9] Berenji F, Parian M, Fata A, Bakhshaee M, Fattahi F. First case report of sinusitis with *Lophomonas blattarum* from Irán. Case Reports in Infectious Diseases. 2016;**16**:Article ID 2614187. DOI: 10.1155/2016/2614187

[10] Martínez-Girón R, van Woerden C. *Lophomonas blattarum* and bronchopulmonary disease. Journal of Medical Microbiology. 2013;**62**(11):1641-1648. DOI: 10.1099/jmm.0.059311-0

[11] Li R, Gao Z-C. *Lophomonas blattarum* infection or just the movement of ciliated epithelial cells? Chinese Medical Journal. 2016;**129**:739-742

[12] Madriz EJ, Tosi J Jr. Monte espinoso tropical en: En Zonas de Vida de Venezuela. Memoria explicativa sobre el mapa ecológico. 2a edición ed. Caracas, Venezuela: Editorial Sucre; 1976. pp. 56-67

[13] Roth LM, Willis ER. The medical and veterinary importance of cockroaches. Smithsonian Miscellaneous Collections. 1957;**134**:147

[14] Rueger ME, Olson TA. Cockroaches (*Blattaria*) as vectors of food poisoning and food infection organisms. Journal of Medical Entomology. 1969;**6**:185-189

[15] Cornwell PB. The Cockroach. Vol. 1. A Laboratory Insect and Industrial Pest. London: Hutchinson; 1968. 391 pp

[16] Kean BH. Toxoplasmosis. In: Jucker E, editor. Progress in Drug Research. Vol. 18, Tropical Diseases I. Basel, Stuttgart: Birkhauser Verlag; 1974. pp. 205-210. 498 pp

[17] Chinchilla M, Ruiz A. Cockroaches as possible transport host of *Toxoplasma gondii* in Costa Rica. Journal of Parasitology. 1976;**62**:140-142

[18] Yang JX, Tang YY, Fang ZM, Tong ZZ, Li YL, Wang T. Investigation on *Lophomonas blattarum* infection in *Periplaneta americana* in Wuhan City. Zhongguo Ji Sheng Chong Xue Yu. 2014;**32**(2):161-162 (in Chinese)

[19] Cazorla-Perfetti D, Moreno PM, Yamarte PN. Identification of *Lophomonas blattarum* (Hypermastigia: Cristomonadida, Lophomonadidae), causal agent of bronchopulmonary lophomoniasis in synanthropic cockroaches from the Coro university hospital, falcon state, Venezuela. Saber. 2015;**27**(3):511-514

[20] Schmidt GD, Roberts LS. Foundations of Parasitology. San Luis: CV. Mosby; 1977. 604 pp

[21] Lavoipierre MMJ, Rajamanickam. Experimental studies on the life cycle of a lizard pentastomid. Journal of Medical Entomology. 1973;**10**:301-302

[22] Linnaeus 10ª. Edición del Sistema Nature, 1758. Available from: http://es.wikipedia.org/wiki/Carlos_Linneo

[23] Smith KGV. Insects and Other Arthropods of Medical Significance. Pub. No. 720. London: British Museum (Natural History); 1973. 561 pp.

[24] Harwood RF, James MT. Entomología Médica y Veterinaria. Editorial. México; 1987

[25] Ragge DR. Grasshoppers, crickets and cockroaches of the British Isles. London. 1965. 299 pp

[26] Chen SX, Meng ZX. Report on one case of *Lophomonas blattarum* in the respiratory tract. Zhongguo Ji Sheng Chong Xue Yu Ji Sheng Chong Bing Za Zhi. 1993;**11**:28. (in Chinese)

[27] Dong HF, Wang RF, Yang YP. One case of patients with *Lophomonas* in phlegm. Journal of Shanghai Examination. 2000;**1**:32

[28] He Q, Chen X, Lin B, Wu J, Chen J. Late oncet pulmonary *Lophomonas blattarum* infection in renal transplantation: A report of two cases. Internal Medicine Journal. 2011;**50**(9):1039-1043

[29] Kang JF, Wu ML, Zhang W, et al. Parasitic *Lophomonas* in the people cysts of lung, a case report clinical focus. 2008;**1**:63-65

[30] Liu J et al. Diagnosis and treatment of *Lophomonas blattarum* infection in 26 patients with bacterial pneumonia. Journal of Thoracic Imaging. 2009;**24**(1):49-51

[31] Liu P, Oi LY, Lei DL, Chen SM. A case of pulmonary *Lophomonas blattarum* infection. Chinese Journal of Integrative Medicine. 2007;**665**:8 (in Chinese)

[32] Martínez-Girón R, Ribas A, Astudillo-González A. Flagellated protozoa in cockroaches and sputum: The unhygienic connection? Allergy Asthma. 2007;**28**:608-609

[33] Martínez-Girón R, Doganci L. *Lophomonas blattarum*: A bronchopulmonary pathogen. Acta Cytologica. 2010;**54**(Suppl):1050-1051

[34] Miao M, Wu DP, Sun AN, Yan LZ. Pulmonary *Lophomonas blattarum* infection in a patient with allogenic hematopoietic stem cell transplantation. Chinese Journal of Integrative Medicine. 2008, 2010;**47**:837-838 (in Chinese)

[35] Shi YL, Li LH, Liao Y, Li XN, Huang XY, Liu J, et al. Diagnosis and treatment of *Lophomonas blattarum* infection in 26 patients with bacterial pneumonia. Zhonqquo Ji Sheng Chong

Xue Yu Ji Sheng Chong Bing Za Zhi.
2007;**25**:430-431 (article in Chinese)

[36] Wang K. A case of *Lophomonas blattarum* infection in lung. Zhongguo Ji Sheng Chong Xue Yu Ji Sheng Chong Bing Za Zhi. 2012;**30**:1 (in Chinese)

[37] Wang Y, Tang Z, Ji S, Zhang Z, Chen J, Cheng Z, et al. Pulmonary *Lophomonas blattarum* infection in patients with kidney allograft transplantation. Transplant International. 2006;**19**(1006):1013

[38] Yang YP, Dong HF, Wang RF. One case of *Lophomonas blattarum* in sputum. Shanghai Yi Xue Jian Yan Za Zhi. 2000;**15**:35 (in Chinese)

[39] Yao G. Bronchopulmonary infection with *Lophomonas blattarum*: Two cases report and literature review. Journal of Medical Colleges of PLA. 2008;**23**:176-182

[40] Yao G, Zhou B, Zeng L. Imaging characteristics of bronchopulmonary *Lophomonas blattarum* infection: Case report and literature review. Journal of Thoracic Imaging. 2009;**24**:49-51

[41] Yao GZ, Zeng LQ, Zhang B. Visible changes of bronchopulmonary *lophomonas blatarum* infection under bronchoscope. One case report and literature review. China Journal of Endoscopy. 2008;**10**:22 (in Chinese)

[42] Yao GZ, Zeng LQ, Zhang B, Chang ZS. Bronchopulmonary *Lophomonas blattarum* infection: Two cases report and literature review. Zhonghua Nei Ke Za Zhi. 2008b;**47**:634-637 (in Chinese)

[43] Yao GZ, Zeng LQ, Zhang B, Chi WW. The treatment of bronchopulmonary *Lophomonas blattarum* infection: One case report and literature review. Journal of Clinical Pulmonary Medicine. 2008;**12**:15 (in Chinese)

[44] Yao GZ, Cheng SK, Chang ZS. One case of bronchopulmonary infection with *Lophomonas blattarum*. Zhonghua Jie He He Hu Xi Za Zhi. 1999;**22**:507 (in Chinese)

[45] Zhang F, Li YS, Zhang HX, Cai LM, Wu ZX. Clinical treatment on two cases with bronchopulmonary *Lophomonas blattarum* infection. Journal of Clinical Medicine Practice. 2010;**14**:83-84 (in Chinese)

[46] Zhang RS, Lu L, Zhang DH, Wang X, Liu YX. Pulmonary *Lophomonas blattarum* infection in a patient with liver allograft transplantation. Chinese Journal of Organ Transplantation. 2010;**31**:767-768 (in Chinese)

[47] Zhang X, Xu L, Wang LL, Liu S, Li J, Wang X. Bronchopulmonary infection with *Lophomonas blattarum*: A case report and literature review. The Journal of International Medical Research. 2011;**39**:944-949

[48] Zhou Y, Zhu J, Li M. Report on two cases of bronchopulmonary infection with hypermastigote and review of the literature. Zhonghua Jie He He Hu Xi Za Zhi. 2006;**29**:23-25 (in Chinese)

Chapter 15

House Dust Mites: Ecology, Biology, Prevalence, Epidemiology and Elimination

Muhammad Sarwar

Abstract

House dust mites burrow cheerfully into our clothing, pillowcases, carpets, mats and furniture, and feed on human dead skin cells by breaking them into small particles for ingestion. Dust mites are most common in asthma allergens, and some people have a simple dust allergy, but others have an additional condition called atopic dermatitis, often stated to as eczema by reacting to mites with hideous itching and redness. The most common type of dust mites are *Dermatophagoides farinae* Hughes (American house dust mite) and *Dermatophagoides pteronyssinus* Trouessart (European house dust mite) of family Pyroglyphidae (Acari), which have been associated with dermatological and respiratory allergies in humans such as eczema and asthma. A typical house dust mite measures 0.2–0.3 mm and the body of mite has a striated cuticle. A mated female house dust mite can live up to 70 days and lays 60–100 eggs in the last 5 weeks of life, and an average life cycle is 65–100 days. In a 10-week life span, dust mite produces about 2000 fecal particles and an even larger number of partially digested enzyme-covered dust particles. They feed on skin flakes from animals, including humans and on some mold. Notably, mite's gut contains potent digestive enzymes peptidase 1 that persist in their feces and are major inducers of allergic reactions, but its exoskeleton can also contribute this. Allergy testing by a physician can determine respiratory or dermatological symptoms to undergo allergen immunotherapy, by exposing to dust mite extracts for "training" immune system not to overreact. The epidemiologic data on the occurrence of house dust mites convincingly associates with an increased indoor air humidity by increased occurrence of mites. The most effective way to prevent or minimize exposure to dust mites in our homes is thorough cleaning, use of high-efficiency particulate air filters and pest management. There are a number of things that can be done to get rid of dust mites, for instance, using a dehumidifier and washing bedding in hot water. Additionally, it is a noble practice to encase bedding, mattress and pillows in impermeable covers that prevent dust mites from taking up residence in beds. Owing to their everywhere presence, diversity, and wide distribution, mite species can be used as valid and reliable pieces of evidence for resolving of forensic cases.

Keywords: dust mite, allergy, itching, immunotherapy, *Dermatophagoides*

1. Introduction

The dust mites usually refer to those species of the mite family Pyroglyphidae that are known to commonly occur widely, although sometimes regionally, in the dust of human dwellings. Dust mites sometimes called dirt mites or bed mites are microscopic creatures, measuring only about one-quarter to one-third of a millimeter (250–300 microns) in length; females weigh about 5.8 μg, while males are approximately half of this weight as 3.5 μg. Nearly 72–74% of their total weight is water and they have translucent bodies with a striated cuticle. They are not insects but arthropods like spiders and ticks having eight legs, no eyes and antennae, and bear mouthpart set in front of the body [1]. Dust mites can live in mattresses, bedding, upholstered furniture, carpets, curtains and other places in homes.

Each adult person sheds about one and a half grams of skin every day. This is enough to feed one million dust mites. Dust mites are microscopic creatures that can live in bedding and carpets, and feed on this skin. They feed on flakes of dead skin or skin cells and scales commonly called dander that are shed by people and pets. They like to live indoors, where they can get plenty of food like mold spores and dead skin cells from people and pets. They cannot survive in colder and drier places, however in a warm and humid house, dust mites can survive all the year around. Dust mites thrive in temperatures of 68–77°F (20–25°C) and they also like humidity levels of 70–80% [2].

These tiny individuals (**Figure 1**) are a big source of allergens and can worsen allergies and asthma. An allergen is a substance that causes an allergic reaction. Both the body parts and the waste of dust mites are allergens for many people. Most dust mites die in low humidity level (when the humidity falls below 50%) or extreme temperature, but they leave their dead bodies and waste behind to cause allergic reactions [3].

The house dust mite species of family Pyroglyphidae, commonly occurring in dust of human dwellings, belong to six genera, the so-called *Dermatophagoides*, *Euroglyphus*, *Hirstia*, *Malayoglyphus*, *Pyroglyphus* and *Sturnophagoides*. In total, 13 species have been found in house dust and recorded from different locations throughout the world, including the United States, Hawaii, Canada, Europe, Asia, the Middle East, parts of Australia, South America, and Africa (**Table 1**).

Related species of *Dermatophagoides* have the most worldwide occurrence and are very similar, but bear differences in some physical characteristics, for example, in male ventral posterior idiosoma and the aedeagus, and in female genital opening and bursa copulatrix [4]. Additional mites occurring in house dust are the glistening mites (family Tarsonemidae), storage mites (families Acaridae, Glycyphagidae and Chortoglyphidae) and the predatory mites (family Cheyletidae); however these groups will not be examined in depth in this chapter.

Mites of family Tarsonemidae have modified legs IV (reduced, enlarged with a single tarsal claw on male, setiform on female); body with series of overlapping plates; and gnathosoma cone-like, enclosing minute palps and chelicerae. When mites are not as mentioned above, they may be with striated cuticle (family

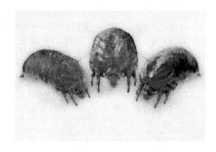

Figure 1.
House dust mites.

S. No.	Species	Locations
1	*Dermatophagoides farinae*	Commonly in the United States, not the United Kingdom
2	*D. evansi*	Europe, North America
3	*D. microceras*	Europe
4	*D. halterophilus*	Spain, Singapore, tropical regions
5	*D. pteronyssinus*	Commonly all over Europe
6	*D. siboney*	Cuba
7	*D. neotropicalis*	Tropical areas
8	*Euroglyphus maynei*	Humid geographic areas all over the world
9	*E. longior*	Holarctic, Neotropic
10	*Hirstia domicola*	United States, Canada, Europe, Asia, Middle East, parts of Australia, South Africa
11	*Malayoglyphus carmelitus*	Israel, Spain
12	*M. intermedius*	United States, Canada, Europe, Asia, Middle East, parts of Australia, South Africa
13	*Pyroglyphus africanus*	South America
14	*Sturnophagoides brasiliensis*	Brazil, France, Singapore

Table 1.
Various species of family Pyroglyphidae existing in house dust and their locations recorded (reproduced from Bronswijk [18] and Colloff [5]).

Pyroglyphidae), otherwise with smooth or papular cuticle, long serrated dorsal setae, and legs with long slim tarsi (family Glycyphagidae). Setae sci and sce are about the same length, and tegmen present in genus *Euroglyphus*, but setae sce considerably shorter than sci, and tegmen absent in *Dermatophagoides* of family Pyroglyphidae [5].

An accurate taxonomic documentation of house dust mites is very vital, simply not from a biological standpoint but about the significances of their corresponding allergenic properties as well. Numerous works on immunochemical have exposed variances among the two products hard to differentiate sibling species [6–13]. An introductory practical taxonomic identification for the most common and important house dust mites is presented at this stage. The main species, identified as *Dermatophagoides farinae* Hughes (American house dust mite), *Dermatophagoides microceras* Griffiths and Cunnington, *Dermatophagoides pteronyssinus* (Trouessart) (European house dust mite), *Euroglyphus maynei* (Cooreman) (Mayne's house dust mite), *Dermatophagoides evansi* Fain and *Euroglyphus longior* (Trouessart), are discussed here. However, three *Dermatophagoides* species, *D. pteronyssinus*, *D. farinae* and *E. maynei*, are the most common, comprising up to 90% of the house dust mite fauna of the world. Morphologically, the most conspicuous difference in these *Dermatophagoides* species is that there are no four long train hairs on the abdomen end [14].

Many aspects on the biology of house dust mites are not understood; therefore, a greater understanding of their biology may reveal new strategies for controlling of mites and their allergens in homes.

2. Family Pyroglyphidae Cunliffe 1958 acarofauna

Pyroglyphidae belongs to the order Astigmata of the subclass Acari (also known as Acarina). The order Astigmata is differentiated from other orders of Acari by the lack of stigmata on idiosoma. This order is furthermore categorized into two suborders, the Acaridia that includes free-living mites and the Psoroptidia which comprises mites parasitic in nature. The former suborder is divided into many families, including the Pyroglyphidae, to which house dust mites belong. Pyroglyphidae are minute mites (full grown adults 170–500 μm in length), cuticle excellently or crudely wrinkle, tarsi termination in a circular pulvillus and a minute claw, anus ventral in position, vestigial genital structures present in both sexual category, vulva of female reverse Y or V fashioned, oil glands existing and exposed among L2 and L3, and vertical setae lacking [15].

Pyroglyphidae is a family of nonparasitic mites, wherein a great variety of species has been observed. It includes the house dust mites that live in human dwellings, many species that live in the burrows of other animals, and some are pests of dried products stored in humid conditions. The family Pyroglyphidae contains mainly species of astigmatid mites that live in the nests of birds and mammals, where they feed on the epidermal detritus (skin, feathers) left by the host, and occurs worldwide [16].

Among the genera of the family Pyroglyphidae, the most outstanding are *Dermatophagoides* and *Euroglyphus*. Three species, *D. farinae*, *D. pteronyssinus*, and *Euroglyphus maynei*, are commonly found in homes of humans and mostly prevalent in high-use areas, where shed skin scales are collected and serve as their food. House dust mites, mostly of the genus *Dermatophagoides*, is important medically and although *D. pteronyssinus* and *D. farinae* are known as the European and American dust mites, both of these are found worldwide. Both mites *D. farinae* and *D. pteronyssinus* move steadily and slowly; however walk quickly without altering way at whatever time they are opened to an extreme light or heat. In contrary, *E. longior* and *B. evansi* express a negative phototropic response when exposed to an electric lamp of bright light [17].

The presence of house dust mites can be confirmed microscopically, which requires collecting samples from mattresses, couches, or carpets. Also, in general practice, it takes at least a 10X magnification to be able to correctly identify them. A modified Berlese funnel is commonly used for extraction of mites from stored grain and has also been successfully used for extraction of *E. longior* and *D. evansi*; however, *D. farinae* cannot be extracted from the dust in this way. A simple method to extract most house dust mites, mite fragments and debris is as follows: weigh 0.1 g of dust from the vacuum cleaner bag, filter by 0.5 and 0.125 mm mesh sieves, relocate dust on 0.125 mm sieve to a lookout glass, moist it with alcohol or ether, whirl suspension to spread out dust uniformly, let the solvent to vaporize, calculate the number of mites below a stereomicroscope, and accumulate them with a camel's hair short-bristled brush. Mites removed through these procedures can be well-maintained in 85% alcohol for an indefinite period. Short-term mounts of mites can be done in lactic acid, glycerin, mineral oil, phenol, etc. A comparatively long-lasting mounting medium is Hoyer's modified Berlese solution ringed with Canada balsam, glycerol, or glyptol. Proof of specimen identity can be done underneath a phase or interference contract microscope only [18].

Three species, *E. maynei*, *D. pteronyssinus*, and *D. farinae*, are usually observed in home environment of humans. Within homes, these mite species are at peak prevailing in high-use parts, wherever shed skin scales accumulate and assist as their diet. Hence, their highest masses are set up in carpets, nearby easy chairs and sofas, in mattresses, and in fabric-covered overstuffed furniture. But, they may also be found on clothing, in bedding, on pillows, on train and automobile seats, and from time to time in workplaces and schools. Every species is the basis of several potent allergens, which in predisposed people trigger and sensitize allergic reactions. These allergens are cause of asthma, atopic dermatitis and perennial rhinitis [19].

Dust mites are most closely related to spiders and ticks. These mites are about 25–30 millimeters in size and cannot be seen without magnification. The translucent body of a house dust mite is 300–400 μm in length and only visible under a microscope. They have eight hairy legs, a mouth-like appendage in front of the body, a tough shell and no eyes or antennae. The lifetime stages of the dust mites are eggs, larvae, protonymphs, deutonymphs, tritonymphs, and adult males and females. The duration of life cycle is dependent on temperature while relative humidity (RH) is beyond 60%. At 23°C, life cycle proceeds 36 and 34 days for *D. pteronyssinus* and *D. farinae*, respectively, to be completed. Females at 23°C create 2 or 3 eggs every day during the reproductive history. At 35 and 16°C, mite *D. pteronyssinus* ensues 15 and 23 days for complete development, respectively; however. *D. farinae* does not grow well at 35 and 16°C. A desiccation-resistant inactive protonymphal stage can occur which permits persistence during lengthy times (months) in dry (less relative humidity) environment. As soon as relative humidity circumstances turn out to be optimum, the dormancy is finished and growth carries on [20].

The female lays eggs singly or in small groups. The adult mated female can lay 40–80 eggs in its lifetime. When the egg hatches, a six-legged larva emerges. There are two nymphal stages that feed and molt before an eight-legged adult is developed. Transition from egg to adult takes about 3–4 weeks. The duration of the cycle is usually 1 month but is dependent on the climate, however 25°C and 75% relative humidity are ideal. An adult house dust mite can live for 1–3 months under favorable conditions. Normally, adult dust mites live for about a month and female dust mites live for about 8–10 weeks. It is estimated that the house dust mite can produce 20 fecal pellets/day that range from 20 to 50 μm. House dust mites are ~75% water by weight and therefore need to absorb water from the water vapor in the air, making relative humidity a critical factor for survival.

The population of *Dermatophagoides* species has been observed in hospital halls, non-carpeted patient's rooms, and carpeted patient's rooms through vacuuming of floor in winter and summer periods. As a summer control set, bedrooms in homes of workers have been checked out. Out of 141 total dust samples obtained, *D. pteronyssinus* or *D. farinae* have not been found in 60 hospital dust samples that are acquired during winter period. Even though mites have been originated in certain sites in hospital during summer dust assemblage, mite population in these localities and mean mite population for entirely samples persisted insignificant. For the period of summer dust sampling taken from bedroom carpets of altogether worker houses checked out observed positive for mites, with a number of homes having high or moderate densities (ranged 22–8340 mites/g of dirt). Prevalence of dust mite in a hospital might be retained very little even if in worker homes, mite levels are found moderate to high. The reasons accountable for little mite populations in hospital are the usage of low-pile carpets, keeping low relative humidity, and upright laundering and housekeeping practices [21].

The house dust mites *D. farinae* and *D. pteronyssinus* are cosmopolitan inhabitants of human dwellings. They are most prevalent in high-use areas in homes (e.g., beds, furniture, floors), where shed human skin scales are collected and serve as a source of food. Relative humidity is an important factor regulating the geographic prevalence and density of these mites. In humid geographic areas, most homes contain mite populations, whereas in dry (low-humidity) geographic areas, few homes contain mites. The species prevalence and density of these mites varies both geographically and between homes in the same geographic area. Although factors influencing variations in mite density between homes are not well understood, it appears that mite density is not correlated with housecleaning practices. However, carpeted floors support significantly greater mite populations than do wood or tile floors. A home may contain only one species or multiple species can coexist. Most homes are coinhabited by more than one species. In coinhabited homes, one species generally constitutes the greatest percentage of the total population, but the dominant species varies between homes within a geographic area. Knowledge of the mite species prevalence and density in a patient's home is important in evaluating the role of mites as allergens, and in selecting and assessing effective immunotherapy for individual cases. Many species of mites besides *D. farinae* and *D. pteronyssinus* may occur in homes, at times in significant numbers. Therefore, one must be careful when conducting mite surveys to differentiate between not only the primary allergy-causing species but other species as well if species, and density determinations are to be accurate and meaningful. House dust mites live in a microenvironment in which no liquid water is present. However, their bodies are 70–80% water by weight, which must be maintained above a critical lower limit in order to survive for them. Active life stages are able to survive at ambient humidity as low as 60% relative humidity because they extract sufficient water directly from unsaturated air by means of a special adaptation to compensate for water losses. A desiccation-resistant protonymph can survive prolonged periods at low relative humidity, and this stage probably serves as a source of mites for breeding during optimal conditions [22, 23].

An understanding of the life cycle of house dust mites, as well as environmental factors influencing mite populations, can be exploited in mite control. Experiments have been carried out to observe the influences of specific relative humidity maintained at 20°C on population dynamics of mixed and single species of *E. maynei*, *D. pteronyssinus*, and *D. farina*, with indefinite diet. The population density of mixed and single species (*D. pteronyssinus* and *D. farinae*) exponentially increased when reared at 65, 70, and 75% RH. The average population growth amounts are 32.5 ± 4.7 and 17.3 ± 4.4 per week for *D. pteronyssinus* and *D. farina*, respectively. Average populations doubling up periods are 4.2 ± 1.3 and 2.2 ± 0.3 weeks for *D. farinae* and *D. pteronyssinus*, respectively. Diversified cultures of species, initiated with identical numbers of *D. pteronyssinus* and *D. farina*, caused greater percentages of *D. pteronyssinus* and *D. farina*. In cultures taking place with 25% of one species and 75% of the other, the more frequent species throughout the experiment continued prevailing and in similar ratios. Population densities of *D. pteronyssinus* and *D. farina* both kept at 85% RH dropped over a period of 12-week culturing owing to growth of mold. At 65, 70, 75 and 85% RH, mite *E. maynei* is not capable to stay alive which indicates that its requirements of climate are dissimilar from those of *D. pteronyssinus* and *D. farina*. When held at 21–22°C and relative humidity of ≤50%, population densities of *D. pteronyssinus* and *D. farina* cultures dropped; on the other hand, noteworthy amounts of populations lasted for 10 weeks at 50% RH. At 45% RH, half-life for dryness of *D. pteronyssinus* and *D. farina* is 11.5 and 1.2 weeks, respectively, however, 4.0 and 86.3 weeks, respectively, at 50% RH. The information indicates that a ≤50% RH would have to be retained for longer times to decrease *D. pteronyssinus* and *D. farina* both through drying processes. The outcomes of this work express that *D. pteronyssinus* and *D. farina* have great population growth and reproductive potential rates, which designate that mite decline processes must be thoroughgoing otherwise densities of mite will reappear to great points rapidly following remediation if suitable diet and appropriate microclimatic situations occur [24, 25].

Mites are complex organisms, which produce thousands of different proteins and other macromolecules. Allergens from dust mites are connected to body secretions (chitinase), fecal material (enzymes) and body anatomy (muscle tropomyosin). Twenty diverse sets of mite allergens have been categorized. The incidence of reactivity to the majority of these allergens between patients sensitive to dust mites is beyond 50%. Sensitivity to allergens differs equally within and between persons.

Generally, the prevalence of sensitivity to house dust mites is about 27.5% in the few populations. Allergens from one species may be species specific, or they may cross-react with allergens from another mite species. Most patients with mite sensitivities are allergic to multiple allergens of a species and to multiple mite species.

Allergies to dust mites are associated with allergic rhinitis and asthma. Systemic anaphylaxis may take place after eating of unheated or heated mite-polluted diets. This problem can be more widespread in subtropical and tropical states than earlier documented. The greatly common signs resulting after the consumption of mite-polluted flour are breathlessness, wheezing, angioedema and rhinorrhea, and these start in the middle of 10 and 240 minutes later after eating of contaminated foods [26].

3. Dust mite habitat

House dust mites primarily feed on organic detritus such as flakes of shed skin. Other nutrients are provided by animal dander, pollen, bacteria and mold. House dust mites reproduce and survive the greatest in soft stuffs (like carpets with lengthy pile, bedclothes and plush toys) that contain a big source of their diet source. The unchanging environmental circumstances are best provided inside homes. Internal domestic humidity is very vital, when moisture is less than 50%; house dust mites are incapable to sustain their water balance and become more vulnerable to desiccation. The house dust mites select diet which has been pre-decomposed by fungi that decrease fat content of skin cells. The fungi in turn usage house dust mite skin cells and feces as nitrogen source, which form a minute ecosystem in their environment [27].

The maximum vital limiting cause for house dust mite population densities is air humidity. House dust mite osmoregulation is through cuticle and for that purpose, they need a great ambient air humidity to avoid extreme water loss. Additionally, supracoxal glands take up ambient water vapor actively and protonymph stage in the life cycle is desiccation resistant. Greater house dust mite population densities are created when indoor absolute air humidity is beyond 7 g/kg (45% relative humidity at 20°C). As a result, aeration by air-conditioning structures is being established as a resource of mite control. In an integrated approach, a number of other features of home atmosphere are likewise being operated to render the habitation less fit for mites. The prospective occurs for evolving models of house dust mite populations, environmental features and influences of several tactics to control [28].

4. House dust mite fauna of prominence

Pyroglyphidae is divided into subfamily Pyroglyphinae wherein anterior extremity of the body is prolonged by a pointed or forked tegmen, which covers the base of the gnathosoma in both male and female, while tegmen absent in the second subfamily Dermatophagoidinae.

4.1 Subfamily Dermatophagoidinae Fain, 1963

Males in *Dermatophagoides* Bogdanov are with hairs sce much longer and thicker than sci and tarsus III without spines. Perianal ring is simple (not denticulate) and with a hysteronotal shield. Females have hairs sce much longer and thicker than sci. Legs III and IV are equal or subequal in length, and hysteronotal shield is absent. However, *Malayoglyphus*, *Hirstia* and *Sturnophagoides* do not have this combination of characters.

4.1.1 Dermatophagoides farinae *Hughes (American house dust mite)*

American house dust mite *D. farinae* (**Figure 2**) is found in flour, poultry and pig feeds, safflower seed meal, and albumin tannate in the drugstore. Differential diagnosis in females are the following: idiosoma is 395–435 µm in length; propodonotal shield about 1.4 times as lengthy as broad; vestibule of bursa sclerotized well and designed similar to a calabash pipe; bursa is not extended further than this vestibule; generally tarsus I with well-built curled progression (ongle); and epigynum crescent fashioned. In males, idiosoma is 285–345 µm long; males either homeomorphic with epimera I free (and normal first legs) or heteromorphic with epimera I fused to form a V or Y (and enlarged I legs).

Females of *D. farinae* tarsi I and II are with prominent, pointed apical spine (s); bursa copulatrix broad and strongly sclerotized in region adjacent to external opening (arrow); and sclerotized section pointed. Females: tarsus I with short, straight, blunted spine (s); and tarsus II lacking spine. Bursa copulatrix is narrow and weakly sclerotized in region adjacent to external opening anteriorly. Female is with central area of dorsum among hairs d2-d2-d3-d3 with crosswise striations in the frontal half and with oblique or convex striations in the latter half. Bursa copulatrix proximal portion is without sclerifications and distal portion widened into a minute, sclerified, and triangular sack. Male hysteronotal shield is short (broader than long) and not reaching the base of hairs d2. Epimera I either free or fused to form a sternum and legs I generally swollen. Male tarsus I is with small apical protuberance (process S) and curved apical spine (f), and tarsus II with process S and no spine.

Duration of the life cycle at 16, 23, 30 and 35°C, and fecundity at 23°C and 75% RH have been determined for *D. farinae*. Durations of the life cycles at 30 and 23°C are 17.5 ± 1.2 and 35.6 ± 4.4 days, respectively. At 16 and 35°C, only a small number of eggs finalized growth to the adult stage. At 75% RH and 23°C, following development of female from tritonymph, the preoviposition period is 3.7 ± 1.1 days. The mean reproductive duration is 34.0 ± 10.7 days with an average of total 65.5 ± 17.4 eggs laid per female. Longevity of female is 63.3 ± 64.6 days after termination of egg production. The females weigh approximately 5.8 ± 0.2 µg (fresh weight), while males are approximately half of this weight 3.5 ± 0.2 µg [29].

Studies of the life cycle of cultured *D. farinae* found that after initial mating, *D. farinae* females lived for 63.3 days after their egg production period ended. The long period after cessation of egg production for *D. farinae* suggested that *D. farinae* females could mate multiple times and produce eggs continuously for a longer period. This study revealed that *D. farinae* females are capable of more than one successful mating that results in an increased egg production than that of a single mating. Females actively attract males during the reproductive period, but not

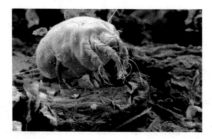

Figure 2.
Dermatophagoides farinae.

afterward even though it continues to live a long time. These females have 11 days longer reproductive period and produced 30.7% more eggs than in females that only mated one time after they emerged from the tritonymphal stage. However, the post-reproductive period is still long (58.6 days) [30].

Adopting the separate culturing technique, under a continuous temperature at 25°C, the effects of relative humidities of 86, 76, 61 and 36% on the life cycle of *D. farinae* and *D. pteronyssinus* have been detected. At 76% RH, the development of eggs to adults takes place in the shortest period of 39.6 ± 6.6 (29–60) days, for egg 8.1 ± 0.1 days, for larva 8.2 ± 0.3 days, for protonymph 17.0 ± 5.7 days and for tritonymph 6.6 ± 0.4 days. The number of eggs laid is generally 1 or 2 per day by a female, but, certain females in a day sometimes laid 5 or 6 eggs. The biggest total number of eggs (80.6 ± 8.2) laid per female is observed at 86% RH, while nu-mated female at 76% RH showed longest longevity of 188.8 ± 60.9 days ranging from 92 to 378 days. The longevity of the female is usually longer than that of the male [31].

4.1.2 Dermatophagoides pteronyssinus *(Trouessart) (European house dust mite)*

This particular species of mite has been found in all dust samples from many different countries in varying numbers. Hysteronotal shield of *D. pteronyssinus* (**Figure 3**), in males, is lengthy (lengthier than wide), and spreading further front-ward than hairs d2, epimera I diverging or parallel and legs I are usual. Females are only with central area of dorsum among hairs d2-d2-d3-d3 having longitudinal patterns. Bursa copulatrix has proximal portion with a sclerite in the form of a daisy and distal portion expanded very slightly. Base of receptaculum seminis are U-shaped in cross section, broader apically than basally, circular with 10–13 lobes when viewed from above and ductus bursae of uniform thickness.

The life cycle of *D. pteronyssinus* has been studied at 25°C and 80% relative humidity. Observations made on freshly laid eggs until they develop into adults and periods between different stages are recorded. The life cycle of *D. pteronyssinus* consists of five stages: egg, larva, protonymph, tritonymph and adult. Adult females lay up to 40–80 eggs singly or in small groups of 3–5. After eggs hatch, a six-legged larva emerges and after two nymphal stages occur, an eight-legged nymph appears. The life cycle from egg to adult is about 1 month with the adult living an additional 1–3 months. The average life cycle for a house dust mite is 65–100 days. A mated female house dust mite can last up to 70 days, laying 60–100 eggs in the last 5 weeks of her life. The eggs required an average of 11.26 days to develop into adults.

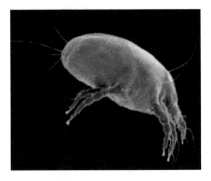

Figure 3.
Dermatophagoides pteronyssinus.

The ranges of life longevity of mated males and females are 18–64 and 20–54 days, respectively. At 76% RH, mite *D. pteronyssinus* exhibited the shortest duration of development. It took a total duration of 37.1 ± 2.5 days with a range from 30 to 54 days, for egg 6.2 ± 0.3 days, for larva 10.7 ± 0.3 days, for protonymph 8.6 ± 1.0 days and for tritonymph 11.4 ± 2.2 days. The largest total number of eggs, 76.2+22.2, is laid by a female of *D. pteronyssinus*. In a 10-week life span, a house dust mite will produce approximately 2000 fecal particles and an even larger number of partially digested enzyme-covered dust particles. The conditions used in the rearing experiments may be considered optimal for maintaining culture of *D. pteronyssinus* [32].

4.1.3 Dermatophagoides microceras *Griffiths and Cunnington (House dust mite, dust mite)*

House dust mite *Dermatophagoides microceras* Griffiths and Cunnington (**Figure 4**) is a species first described in 1971 and part of the Pyroglyphidae family of mites. This mite has been identified in house dust in various geographic regions, including Great Britain, Scandinavia, the Netherlands, Spain and United States; however its distribution in the rest of the world has not been explored well. Morphologically, males tarsus I is without small apical protuberance (process S), but with curved spine and tarsus II without process S or spine. Females tarsus I with short, straight, blunted spine, tarsus II lacking spine and bursa copulatrix narrow as well as weakly sclerotized in region adjacent to external opening. In females, propodonotal shield is about 1.4 times as lengthy as wide; idiosoma 395–435 μm in length; vestibule of bursa absent, bursa unfastens at the bottom of a non-sclerotized depression of tegmen; first portion of bursa proper is a little dilated and clearly sclerotized; and apical progression of tarsus I mostly very minor or absent. In males, idiosoma is 285–345 μm in length; males either heteromorphic with epimera I joined to form a V or Y shape (and first legs enlarged) or homeomorphic with epimera I free (and first legs normal) [33].

D. microceras is more closely related to *D. farinae*, and the biological and immunochemical identification of these two species are argued. Using an enzyme-linked immunosorbent assay (ELISA) technique, the response of mite material from different stock cultures demonstrated that *D. farinae* and *D. microceras* are discrete entities, and also at the major allergen level, with no apparent subspecies or strain variation. Females of *D. farinae* and *D. microceras* receptaculum seminis not U-shaped in cross section, while males with hysteronotal shield as long as broad and extending anteriorly to point between setae d1 and e or slightly anterior of d1 [34].

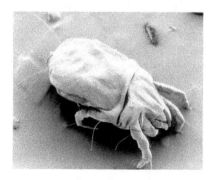

Figure 4.
Dermatophagoides microceras.

4.1.4 Dermatophagoides evansi *Fain, Hughes and Johnston*

Specifically, *Dermatophagoides evansi* Fain (**Figure 5**) Hughes and Johnston mites are found in the poultry dust samples and also in bird's nests. Hen poultry farmers and their families, but also other professionals working in the poultry industry, such as veterinarians, may be exposed to house dust mites. In females, bursa copulatrix is strongly enlarged in its distal third and very narrow in proximal two thirds (internal); and spermatheca sclerotized and tulip-like. In males, hysteronotal shield markedly spread frontward away from bases of setae d1; adanal suckers 12 μm in span; coxae II shut; legs III 1.8 times denser (at level of femur) and 1.6 times lengthier (length of 4 distal segments) than legs IV; tarsus I with 2 uneven apical progressions (ongles); tarsus II with a slight apical progression; setae cp 110 μm in length; setae d2 located at 55–65 μm from opening of fat gland; setae h2 and h3 with bases intensely sclerotized; epimera I free; and males are homeomorphic. The males differ from males of *D. pteronyssinus* primarily through dorsal hysterosomal shield that is longer and narrower; ratio width (at level of setae d1):length = 1:2.5 [whereas in *D. pteronyssinus* this ratio is 1.8–1.9]; while legs III and IV are much more unequal than in *D. pteronyssinus* [35].

The life cycle of *D. evansi* has been studied and reared at a relative humidity of 75–80% and temperature 25–27°C in a medium consisted of human skin or chicken skin scales plus baker's yeast powder. The average period of mite life cycle for each stage in days is the following: egg 8.3; larva and protonymph 5.4; tritonymph 6.6; female 52.9; and male 28.9. The mean time necessary for accomplishment of one generation is 28.7 days. The female is oviparous, parthenogenesis not detected, and lays 35.5 mean eggs during its life span. The adults copulate repeatedly and the female-male ratio is 1:1.2 [36].

4.2 Subfamily Pyroglyphinae Cunliffe, 1958

Female with the distal part of the bursa copulatrix in the form of a small, oval and strongly sclerotized pocket, while male is with anal suckers (*Euroglyphus* Fain), but male and female are without this combination of characters in *Pyroglyphus*. In *Euroglyphus maynei* (Cooreman), male trochanters I–III without hairs and is with a large oval anal plate spreading near to posterior edge of body, while female hairs ga, ae and those of trochanters I–III missing, and have a small posterior vulval lip that does not shelter to anterior of vulva. In case of *Euroglyphus longior* (Trouessart), male trochanters I–III with one hair and is with a minute hexagonal anal plate distant from posterior edge of the body. Female hairs ga, ae and those on trochanters I–III present, and posterior vulval lip is long nearly completely casing to vulva.

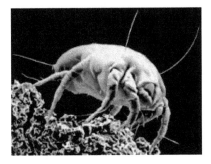

Figure 5.
Dermatophagoides evansi.

4.2.1 Euroglyphus maynei *(Mayne's house dust mite) (Cooreman)*

The house dust mite *Euroglyphus maynei* (Cooreman) (**Figure 6**) infests stored products and is considered pests in cottonseed meal, bean curd, Chinese medicines, crabmeat and shrimps. This occurs in homes worldwide and is an important source of many allergens. Differential diagnosis in both sexes; setae sci and sce about the same length and tegmen (t) present. Length of idiosoma 195–225 μm; posterior edge of idiosoma with 2 minute lobes without hairs; tegmen well developed, triangular with rounded apex (not bifid in the male); cuticle somewhat sclerotized with rather fine formed markings or creases; hysteronotum within a median shield with margins poorly distinct; anterior legs missing chitinous membranes; chaetotaxy condensed; tibials IV, trochanterals I–III, anal external setae and genital anterior setae are absent; tarsi IV with 3 setae; tarsi III with 5 setae; dorsal setae very short and thin; setae h3 very short (maximum length 50 μm) and thin; setae h2 very thin and short (not more than 30 μm); and genu I with one solenidion. In males, tegmen with unforked, rounded apex; dorsal setae variable; opisthosoma slightly but narrowed backwards regularly; anus more posterior (anal suckers situated at 25 μm from posterior body margin); posterior body margin wide and straight with 2 small paramedian lobes; adanal suckers well developed; and tarsi IV lacking suckers. In females, setae sce short (maximum 50 μm) and thin; at bases of legs II no chitinous pouches; tegmen either prominent and triangular but with apex rounded and not forked or poorly developed and rounded with a small median notch; posterior lip of vulva short and punctate, not covering vulvar slit; or anterior angle of posterior vulvar lip not incised; vulva uncovered; tegmen triangular with rounded, not incised apex; hysteronotum striated with a median shield; copulatory vestibule ovoid, strongly sclerotized and opaque; and tarsi I–IV without apical processes nor spines [37].

The reproductive biology of house dust mite *E. maynei* is not studied well. This mite is generally less common than *D. pteronyssinus* and *D. farinae* in homes. While it is present, it commonly coinhabits with species of *Dermatophagoides* and in geographic distribution, is more restricted. The period of life cycle (egg to adult) for *E. maynei* at 75% relative humidity as well as 23 and 30°C and fecundity at 75% RH and 23°C have been concluded, and data compared similar to data for *D. pteronyssinus* and *D. farinae*. Adults hatched from eggs at 23°C after 28 days and at 30°C in 20 days. At 23°C, females during a reproductive period of 24 days produced 1.4 eggs/day. At 23°C, mite *E. maynei* has a smaller life cycle than *D. pteronyssinus* and *D. farinae*; however, at 30°C, this have a lengthier life cycle and produced fewer eggs than both mites [38].

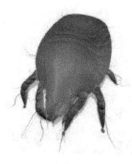

Figure 6.
Euroglyphus maynei.

4.2.2 Euroglyphus longior *(Trouessart)*

This species infests stored products, and is considered pests in granary debris, wheat, bean, oat, barley, rice, dried clover and hide dust [39]. Data used for identification of this mite are the following: length of idiosoma is 245–265 μm and posterior edge of idiosoma with 2 distinct lobes each having 3 hairs. Male (darker, smaller) internal and external scapular setae and II pair of legs in line, a small hexagonal anal plate distant from posterior edge of body, anal suckers present, while trochanters I–III with one hair. Female (paler, larger) internal base of seminal receptacle simple, while posterior vulval lip or membrane long and almost entirely covering the vulva (on genital plate external genital opening). Hairs go, ae and those on trochanters I–III present.

The determination of the life cycle of the mite species has provided vital information on its biology showing that pre-reproductive period from mating to birth of first eggs is 12.78 ± 1.06 days and reproductive period between production of first and last eggs 39.78 ± 4.99 days. Fecundity, the total number of eggs laid per female is 48.00 ± 3.89 and rate of reproduction calculated as the number of eggs laid per of female's reproductive period 1.33 ± 0.18. Finally, the development of immatures is completed in 30.14 ± 3.4 days [40].

The house dust mites *D. farinae*, *D. pteronyssinus* and *E. maynei* are cosmopolitan inhabitants of human dwellings. They are most prevalent in high-use areas in homes (e.g., beds, furniture, floors), where shed human skin scales are collected and serve as a source of food. Relative humidity is an important factor regulating the geographic prevalence and density of these mites. In humid geographic areas, most homes contain mite populations, whereas in dry (low-humidity) geographic areas, few homes contain mites. The species prevalence and density of these mites varies both geographically and between homes in the same geographic area. Although factors influencing variation in mite density between homes are not well understood, it appears that mite density is not correlated with housecleaning practices. However, carpeted floors support significantly greater mite populations than do wood or tile floors. A home may contain only one species or multiple species may coexist. Most homes are coinhabited by more than one species. In coinhabited homes, one species generally constitutes the greatest percentage of the total population, but the dominant species varies between homes within a geographic area [41].

Knowledge of the mite species prevalence and density in a patient's home is important in evaluating the role of mites as allergens, and in selecting and assessing effective immunotherapy for individual cases. Many species of mites besides *D. farinae*, *D. pteronyssinus* and *E. maynei* may occur in homes, at times in significant numbers. Therefore, one must be careful when conducting mite surveys to differentiate between not only the primary allergy-causing species but other species as well if species and density determinations are to be accurate and meaningful. House dust mites live in a microenvironment in which no liquid water is present. However, their bodies are 70–80% water by weight, which must be maintained above a critical lower limit in order to survive. Active life stages are able to survive at ambient humidities as low as 60% relative humidity because they extract sufficient water directly from unsaturated air by means of a special adaptation to compensate for water losses. A desiccation-resistant protonymph can survive prolonged periods at low relative humidity and this stage probably serves as a source of mites for breeding during optimal conditions [42].

There are 47 different species of house dust mites, and dust mites *D. farinae*, *D. pteronyssinus* and *E. maynei* are sources of multiple potent allergens in the indoor environment. An ambient RH is a key factor in determining where these mites are found. Bedding, carpeting, and furniture cushions all trap and hold moisture, allowing these tiny creatures to flourish. Dust mites settle down in carpet, draperies, stuffed animals and upholstered furniture. Mattresses, pillows and soft bedding are favorite hangouts [43]. These same symptoms can be caused by a variety of other allergens as well, so consultancy to an allergist is needed for their testing. To diagnose a dust mite allergy, a physician may suggest a skin test [skin prick test (SPT)] or blood test (specific IgE blood test).

5. Epidemiology of house dust mites

For a lot of years, it has been advocated that allergens resulting from house dust mite show a foremost part in pathogenesis of eczema, asthma and certain circumstances of allergic rhinitis. In recent times, allergens by house dust mite have been refined and precise immunoassays established with which acquaintance to allergens and house dust mites can be more simply determined. By means of these tools, epidemiological homework have delivered positive confirmation that not merely house dust mite acquaintance has been linked with the majority of asthma cases in young adults and children but then again that it is causally connected to asthma development. Two main allergenic dust mite species, *D. pteronyssinus* and *D. farina*e, are important components in the development of asthma [44].

Epidemiologic data available on incidence of house dust mites in residences demonstrate a perfect relationship among increased interior air humidity and increased existence of dust mites in house dust. Moreover, in temperate climates, there is threshold level of indoor air humidity 7 g/kg (45% relative humidity at normal indoor air temperature). Interior air humidity under this level for prolonged times will eliminate house dust mites from residences. A decrease in residents involvement to house dust mites is executed by lessening of indoor air humidity through organized mechanical air circulation. Individually, ventilation levels are assessed from actual house size, inhabitant numbers and mean outdoor air humidity in winter. In divergence, more moist zones of the world with mean outdoor humidity beyond 6–7 g/kg in winter will keep up great densities of house dust mites uniformly and a decrease in indoor air humidity will have a relatively slight effect on existence of house dust mites. Modern construction of energy-efficient houses by better fastening of building envelope, paralleled by an alike makeover of older houses, has increased indoor air humidity and is perhaps the cause of nearly fourfold rise in incidence of house dust mites in residences [45].

There are up to 2 million dust mites living in a standard mattress. Dust mites produce mite feces, which add up to 200 times of their own body weight within their lives of 2 months [46]. Although exposure to house dust mite allergen is a major risk factor for allergic sensitization and asthma, the percentages of homes with dust mite allergen concentrations at or greater than detection, 2.0 µg bed dust and 10.0 µg bed dust, have been estimated to be 46.2, and 24.2%, respectively. Independent predictors of higher levels have been lower household income, older homes, no resident children, single-family homes, musty or mildew odor, heating sources other than forced air and higher humidity in bedroom. Most of homes in a bed have measurable levels of dust mite allergen. Levels earlier allied to allergic asthma and sensitization in bedrooms are common. Predictors can be utilized to detect situations under which homes are more possibly to have greater levels of dust mite allergen [47].

Epidemiologic works [48] studying the relationship among house dust mite distribution and outdoor humidity level have revealed that: (1) Outdoor humidity level that is reliant on climate of region and altitude is linked to house dust mite distribution, and peak number of mites is originated in the most moist regions. (2)

Indoor humidity level that is reliant upon seasonal difference in outdoor humidity is connected to number of mites and the greatest number of mites is originated during the months wherever indoor humidity level is at peak. (3) Pronounced variances in the number of mites in diverse residences at the same time of year and in same area can be attributed owing to changes in indoor air humidity among residences.

Additional studies [49] recommend that there is a lesser edge of absolute humidity of 7.0 g water vapor/kg dry air, equivalent to 45% relative humidity at 20–23°C, under that house dust mites will not multiply. In residences with less than 7.0 g/kg, vapour house dust mites will arise as background contamination only and in numbers commonly below 100 mites/g dust.

For geographic regions with a temperate environment, it can be identified rather exactly that in order to stop buildup of hazardous levels of house dust mites in residences, indoor air humidity might be kept under a level of 7.0 g/kg or 45% relative humidity at usual indoor air temperature for a small number of winter months for every year. This extreme absolute humidity level in air indoor once more can be altered into a tiniest ventilation level stated in ACH (air changes per hour that strips with geographical locality (average outdoor air humidity in three dry winter months)) and inhabitants mass in the residence. As a whole, if (1) average outdoor air humidity in three winter months is recognized, (2) it is expected that each occupant of family creates a mean of 3000 g water vapor/24 hour in the residence, (3) water vapor is rapidly disseminated similarly to all air in construction, (4) rooms have a 2.0 m ceiling height, (5) a security margin of 30% is added to the minimum ventilation level, and steady-state situation can be calculated (production of water vapor divided by elimination equals 1):

$$1 = N \times 3000 \times 1.3/m^2 \times 2 \times (\text{indoor AH} - \text{outdoor AH}) \times \text{ach} \times 24 \quad (1)$$

where N = absolute number of inhabitants in household, m^2 = area of dwelling in square meters, indoor AH = maximum wanted indoor air absolute humidity (usually set to 7.0 g/kg), outdoor AH = average 3-month outdoor absolute humidity (three most dry winter months), and ACH = air changes per hour (ACH of 1.0 means that all air is exchanged once every hour).

From these calculations, figures can be made that the lowest ventilation desired may without difficulty be assessed with variable family size and space of the residence. Climate analysis with controlled and improved building ventilation is presently used to eradicate house dust mites from residences occupied by patients with asthma caused by allergy due to house dust mites [45].

6. Prevalence of house dust mites

The precise nature of dust mite density or the seasonal populations of house mites in homes are of paramount importance to reduce their development and in clarifying the role they play in dust allergy. A surrounding relative humidity is an important feature that controls prevalence and geographic spreading of these mites. This is for the reason that in humid air water vapors are key source of liquid for their existence. They thrive and survive fine at relative humidity exceeding 50%, however dry and decease at relative humidity less than this. As a result, dust mites and allergens they produce are an important problem merely for persons who live in moist temperate and tropical geographic regions. Mites D. pteronyssinus and/or D. farinae are prevalent in homes in Asia, Europe, the United States, and South America. However, most home environment are coinhabited by several species, but then again the greatest species prevalence differs both between homes in a geographic region and between geographic regions. For instance, in the United States, both *D. pteronyssinus* and *D. farinae* are prevalent in homes; however *D. farinae* is more prevalent in homes than *D. pteronyssinus* within northern moist environments. However, in South America, *D. pteronyssinus* is prevalent in homes, whereas *D. farinae* is not. In temperate type of weather, densities of *D. pteronyssinus* and *D. farinae* display distinct periodic variations that are equivalent to seasonal instabilities in indoor relative humidity. Their great densities arise for the duration of moist summer months and little densities in winter, while relative humidity in homes is low [50].

Significantly, higher abundance levels of the house dust mites *D. farinae* and *D. pteronyssinus* arise on the most greatly used carpeted floor areas and fabric-upholstered furniture by the family living in bedrooms and room. Mattresses do not originate to be the key foci for occurrence of mites. There is no major positive correlation known among frequency or thoroughness of cleaning and mite abundance, as well as age of furnishings or dwelling and amount of dust. Considerably, greater mite levels arise on carpeted floorings than on non-carpeted grounds. A continuous vacuuming does not considerably decrease abundance of mites. Density of mites demonstrated a seasonal variability, with the lowermost mass during dryer along with late heating season and the uppermost mass arising in humid summer months. Alive mites are more plentiful than deceased mites for the period when overall abundance is great. In homes occupied by both mite species, *D. farinae* is more prevailing, excluding in one home that has considerably a greater relative humidity [51].

Of the systematically isolated mites from house dust samples, 90% are pyro-glyphids, with 75% of these *D. pteronyssinus*, 10.5% *D. farinae* and 3.6% *E. maynei*, while Cheyletidae constituted 5.7% of the house dust mites. The maximum number of house dust mites recorded is 6500/g of house dust and the highest numbers are isolated in samples from humid areas (Feldman-Muhsam et al. 1985). Mites are present in 97% of the house dust samples and the maximum number of mites (7440/g dust) is found in the carpet. Most of the mites are isolated from the carpets and sofas (37.0 and 33.7%, respectively) and less from the beds (29.3%) [52].

It is well known that mite prevalence is greater in more humid geographic areas than in dry ones. Outdoor climatic conditions and indoor ambient RH are essentially the same for all homes in similar vicinity. Therefore, differences in mite abundance must be associated with other features of the homes (RH in mite micro-habitat) and persons residing in these. A very important factor that correlates with the level of mite prevalence is the presence or absence of carpeting. Carpeted floors contain significantly more mites than tile or wood floors and none or very few mites are found on wood or vinyl-covered floors. Apparently, long-pile carpets reduce the efficiency of vacuuming and provide an excellent microhabitat for accumulation of food material and moisture for mites survival and breeding. From homes of house dust-sensitive patients, removing of fitted carpet would decrease the level of mites contact making from floors. Anywhere this cannot be undertaken or is not desir-able; usage of short-pile carpets rather than large rough pile types would deal with important decline in levels of mites [53].

7. Phylogenetic relationships of family Pyroglyphidae

The pyroglyphids presently consist of 47 species and 20 genera, whose species are parasites associated with birds and mammals that contribute to house dust allergy problem. There has been no detailed phylogenetic analysis of the family

Pyroglyphidae. However, in essence, pyroglyphids are initially bird's-nest inhabitants; however they experienced an alteration in habitation to human nest and bed around the time of the first human settlement and are linked with agrarian production, specifically 10,000 years before. The glycyphagoid and acaroid mites of human residences made habitat transference from nests of small mammals and also come across habitat correspondences within homes, with diets in the form of cereals, seeds and other plant resources. By giving the similarity of trophic niches of human residences to those existing naturally, it is not astonishing that a number of mite species have become allied to human dwellings. Most importantly, many species of pyroglyphoid, glycyphagoid and acaroid appeared to have retained the ancestral ability to feed on fungi [54]. The "host" relationships with birds point out that both subfamilies of pyroglyphids that comprise species found in house dust, Dermatophagoidinae and Pyroglyphinae, are geographically the most widespread and species-rich, and connected with a greater variety of avian taxa than those subfamilies which do not comprise species that are found in house dust. This has a tendency to advocate that Dermatophagoidinae and Pyroglyphinae might denote ancestral taxa within family.

8. Dust mites management

The most effective way to treat dust mite allergies is to eliminate as many dust mites as possible from homes. Dust mites cannot be completely eliminated from home; however, they can be reduced. Reducing dust mites in houses can eliminate or lessen dust mite allergies. Having great physician care and sublingual treatment of dust mite allergies along with cleanup and prevention can be the keys in controlling of dust mite allergies.

8.1 Dust mite allergy treatment

Generally, people who have dust allergies are familiar with sneezing (act of expelling a sudden and uncontrollable burst of air through the nose and mouth), but sneezing is not the only uncomfortable symptom. Typically, sneezing occurs after external elements, or an adequate outside stimulating substance moves across nasal hairs to touch the nasal mucosa. This activates the discharge of histamines that irritate the nerve cells in the nose, causing signals being sent to the brain to start sneezing through the trigeminal nerve complex. The function of sneezing is to expel mucus containing irritants from the nasal cavity [55, 56].

Dust allergies also give to many people a stuffy or runny nose or cause their eyes to itch or become red and watery. A house is thought to be a cheering shelter; however for people having dust allergies, a home can generate painful indications. Strangely sufficient, allergy signs frequently get worse for the period of vacuuming or immediately after it, sweeping and dusting at a place. The practice of dusting can bring dirt particles up by creating these easier to breathe inside. If a person thinks he or she may have an allergy to any of the components of house dust, then see an allergist to pinpoint the cause of symptoms. Often an allergist will need to conduct a skin test and may order a blood test to determine exactly what is triggering an allergic reaction. After a dust allergy is identified, an allergist may recommend one or more of the treatments such as medications, allergy shots (subcutaneous immunotherapy), tablets (oral immunotherapy) and changes to personal household routine. A person may be prescribed by antihistamines to relieve sneezing, runny and stuffed nose, and itching in the nose and eyes; nasal corticosteroids to reduce swelling in nose and block allergic reactions; commonly sodium nose spray to block the release of chemicals that cause allergy symptoms, including histamine and leukotrienes; leukotriene antagonists, pills which can improve both allergy and asthma symptoms; decongestant pills, liquids and allergy shots; and dust mite sublingual immunotherapy in which tablets of dust mite purified protein are placed under the tongue that may prevent and decrease symptoms of dust mite allergies [57].

8.2 Dust mite prevention strategies

No matter how much clean a home is, dust mites cannot be completely eliminated. However, as a first line of defense, dust mite mass can be condensed by exploiting the subsequent practices. Practice a dehumidifier or an air conditioner to keep humidity intensities at or lower than 50%. Enclose pillows and mattress in dustproof protections or allergen-resistant shelters. Wash down all blankets and bedding in hot water at 130–140°F to kill dust mites, once a week, and non-washable bedclothes can be kept cold overnight. Change feathered or wool bedding articles with synthetic materials and traditional animal stuffed products by washable ones. Within bedrooms, change wall-to-wall fitted carpet by naked floors, and get rid of fabric curtains and covered furniture, at whatever time imaginable. Practice a moist cleaner or duster to get rid of dust and at no time use a dry cloth, as it rises allergens up. Utilize a double-layered microfilter sack or a high-efficiency particulate air filter in a vacuum cleaner. Wear a mask while vacuuming, and stay out of the vacuumed area for 20 minutes after vacuuming, to allow dust and allergens to settle. The dust mite prevalence could be kept very low, and the factors responsible for the low mite density are maintenance of low relative humidity, use of low-pile carpets, and good housekeeping and laundering practices [58].

8.3 Control of house dust mites

An abstract of the study identifies that air conditioning can lessen relative humidity and population of dust mite in home environment in comparison to homes without dehumidification or air conditioning. However, humidity lessening does not stop populations of mites from developing further than the threshold of inducing allergies. An air-conditioning usage in combination with an efficient dehumidifier is effective in dropping of relative humidity in these homes lower than the threshold needed for mite population development, reproduction and growth. Subsequent to fourth week of study, 75% of dehumidifiers fitted homes have zero amount of live mites. House dust mites in clothing and bedding are the source of major allergens, and an average threshold before developing allergies is 100 mites/g of dust [59, 60].

Based upon studies of only *D. pteronyssinus*, weekly washing of clothing and bedding in hot water is suggested to remove allergens and destroy dust mites. But, most often washing is done in cold or warm water and other species of mites are also involved. A study has investigated the fatal influence of different temperatures of hot water alone and hot, warm, and cold water comprising chlorine bleach and detergents on *D. farinae*, *E. maynei*, and *D. pteronyssinus*. Mites have been dipped in test solutions for various lengths of time and at various temperatures, permitted time to recover, and then examined for existence. Mite *D. farinae* has been noted to be the most sensitive to temperature and chlorine bleach among the other two species. In 50°C water alone, 100% death of *D. farinae* has been found within 10 minutes, while most *E. maynei* and *D. pteronyssinus* stayed alive. But, soaking for 5 and 12 minutes at 53°C has been required to destroy all *E. maynei* and *D. pteronyssinus*, respectively. Washing with cleansing agents at suggested and doubled concentrations and chlorine bleach mostly increased mortalities of three mite species compared to water alone. Soaking in warm water comprising different detergents alone for 4 hours made mortalities of 2–35%, 14–46% and 19–50% for *D. pteronyssinus*, *E. maynei* and *D. farinae*, respectively. Weekly washing of bed linens in warm water comprising bleach and most detergents presoaked for 4 hours can kill maximum number of *D. farinae*, and depending on detergent brand destroy adequate numbers of *D. pteronyssinus*. With warm water comprising the suggested concentrations of different detergents, soaking alone for 4-hour also killed enough numbers of *E. maynei*, *D. farinae* and *D. pteronyssinus*. So, accumulative influence of weekly washing with long presoaks of bed linens must considerably decrease mite levels over time, mainly when pillows and mattresses are sealed to stop reinfestation [61].

People can use mite killers (a number of powders and sprays are available) on mite-infested materials and reapply these occasionally as per manufacturer's directions. Furthermore, antibiotics have been tested, aiming at the control of *D. pteronyssinus* house dust mite. In culture medium, sulfaquinoxaline 30% within 3 weeks killed all the mites, whereas 30 mg/100 mg of culture medium of declomycin, oxytetracycline, tetracycline HCl, and aureomycin in 3 weeks killed 52, .058.9 and 94.6%, respectively, of mites. Cessations of nourishing and reduced coordination have been detected in mite cultures after 24 hours following the use of sulfaquinoxaline, and a week later, no eggs have been found [62–65].

Copper oxide (CuO) has broad-spectrum antimicrobial and antifungal properties and a study taken on common *D. farinae* house dust mite has tested the acaricidal efficiency of CuO-impregnated fabrics. The general mobility or vitality of mites has been reduced when they are exposed to CuO-impregnated fabrics and when possible, dust mites transferred to fabrics where no CuO existed. The mortality of mites exposed for 10 days to fabrics containing 0.2% (w/w) CuO remained significantly higher than the mortality of mites on control fabrics (72 ± 4 and 18.9 ± 0.3%, respectively). The death rate reached to 95.4 and 100% after 47 and 5 days with fabrics comprising 0.4 and 2% CuO, respectively. The acaricidal influence of copper oxide appears because of direct toxicity, and usage of fabrics comprising copper oxide might therefore be a significant opportunity for decreasing populations of house dust mites and the burden of dust mite allergens [66].

9. Domestic mites and forensic science

In fact, mites can be found in all habitats, even in the pores of our skin and almost every single person carries mites. Thus, they may even proof useful, for instance, in forensics. More than 100 species of mites from over 60 families are collected from animal carcasses and approximately 75 mite species from over 20 families gathered from human corpses [67], also including the astigmatid mite taxa. Domestic mites and other dust mites are present globally; however composition of species can be different between seasons, dwellings and even within places of a same indoor atmosphere (floors vs. stuffing furniture, floors vs. beds, or dust from a library desk vs. bookshelves). Distinguished variances in acarofauna of house dust mites among locations can provide valuable facts, for example, as an indicator of time and statuses of a death [68].

Surveys of dust samples have been taken from dwellings, hospitals, libraries, research laboratories, drugstores, offices and other workplaces. More than 30 mite species are found of which the most abundant and common include dust mites especially *D. farinae*. The highest mite densities (g $(-^1)$ dust) are noted in dwellings [69]. Thus, this knowledge may be useful in the field of forensic medicine.

Since dust mites feed on the flakes of shed human skin, so human genetic material is expected to be present in these creatures. A study has been conducted to find out if house dust mites can carry the DNA of the house occupants. If this is true, human DNA isolated from the mites, obtained from a crime scene, could be used as evidence in court. The DNA profiles of people (10.25%) from homes (96.3%) showed an exact match with those found in the mite samples from the same house [70]. So, identified human DNA in house dust mites suggests that one can investigate a crime by analyzing DNA samples from house dust mites found in a crime scene and by comparing them with the DNA profiles obtained from victims and suspects.

The blowflies or flesh flies might carry out their life cycle around and in dead body, whereas mites may well forage on young stages of flies. The mites might breed more quickly than their fly carriers, posing themselves as appreciated timeline markers [71]. There are atmospheres at someplace where insects are either rare or absent, or the ecological situations hinder in their contact to carcass. At this point, mites that are previously present and mites which reach through air currents, by walking, or with material transfer come to be vital. There are eight different waves of arthropods colonizing carcasses of human. The first wave comprises flies and mites, whereas sixth wave is exclusively made up of mites. The scope of forensic acarology goes further in forensic investigations as mites compete with insects for food (dead body), slowing their development, or may even feed on insects. Observing mites can improve estimations of postmortem intervals that rely on timeline of when various species usually reach on a carcass and in whatever way long they proceed to grow, thus letting for more precise estimates in murder case. Mites are specific to microhabitat and might deliver evidential data on relocation or movement of bodies or finding a doubt at a crime scene [72]. Therefore, dust mites can be used as evidence in fields of forensic sciences.

10. Conclusion

House dust mites got their names from habitat of household dust and feed on any protein that comes in their way and find easy pickings in the dead skin scales that humans shed every day. House dust mites are not insects but arachnids and relate to spiders and ticks by having lengthy legs. Thirteen important house dust mite species have been identified; but two species that are the greatly common and key cause of allergen include *D. pteronyssinus* and *D. farinae* within Pyroglyphidae family. Unlike scabies mites or skin follicle mites, house dust mites do not burrow under skin and are not parasitic. Severe dust mites infestation in the home has been linked to atopic dermatitis, and epidermal barrier damage documented. Allergenic products of the common species of house dust mites are incompletely cross-reacting, carrying both common and species-specific determinants. It is because of this a correct identification of the mite species is important. It is important to remember that as droppings of dead dust mites continue to provoke allergic reactions, it must be needed not only to reduce their populations but also take steps to remove their dead bodies and feces from homes. Allergy testing of a person can determine whether house dust mites trigger respiratory or dermatological symptoms. If tests show allergic to house dust mites, then reduce immune system response by undergoing allergen immunotherapy. A healthcare provider may recommend medicine to lessen the symptoms of dust mite allergies.

Strategies to reduce dust mites in homes include to cover mattresses, pillows, and quilts with dust mite-resistant covers; wash sheets and pillowcases weekly in water hotter than 55°C; hot tumble dry (for half an hour after dry) or dry clean household items; wash blankets every 2 months; use synthetic rather than feather pillows; remove sheepskin or woolen underlays; remove all soft toys from bedroom and replace with wooden or plastic toys; damp dust or use electrostatic cloths to clean hard surfaces weekly; reduce humidity to have a dry and well-ventilated house; avoid upholstered furniture; avoid heavy curtains; wash clothing before use if stored for a long time; as well as remove carpets and vacuum home weekly. The truth is that the utility of mites especially in cases where conditions such as the environment of the corpse it is found and the manner of death are not suitable for the presence or arrival of insects, mite populations on corpses can become an important evidence for elucidating of forensic cases.

Author details

Muhammad Sarwar
National Institute for Biotechnology and Genetic Engineering (NIBGE), Faisalabad, Pakistan

*Address all correspondence to: drmsarwar64@gmail.com

IntechOpen

© 2020 The Author(s). Licensee IntechOpen. This chapter is distributed under the terms of the Creative Commons Attribution License (http://creativecommons.org/licenses/by/3.0), which permits unrestricted use, distribution, and reproduction in any medium, provided the original work is properly cited. (cc) BY

References

[1] Sarwar M. Biology and ecology of some predaceous and herbivorous mites important from the agricultural perception. In: Haouas D, Hufnagel L, editors. Pests Control and Acarology. London, UK: IntechOpen; 2019. p. 29

[2] Sarwar M. Mites (Arachnida: Acarina) affecting humans and steps taking for the solution of problematics. International Journal for Research in Mechanical Engineering. 2016;1(7):1-14

[3] Sarwar M. Diseases transmitted by blood sucking mites and integrated mite management for their prevention. American Journal of Food Science and Health. 2016;2(6):169-175

[4] Sarwar M. Feasibility for development of comparative life histories and predation of predatory mites in Phytoseiidae complex and their experimental manipulations for pests control. International Journal of Animal Biology. 2015;1(5):150-157

[5] Colloff MJ. Taxonomy and identification of dust mites. Allergy. 1998;53(48S):7-12

[6] Sarwar M, Kongming W, Xuenong X. Evaluation of biological aspects of the predacious mite, *Neoseiulus cucumeris* (Oudemans) (Acari: Phytoseiidae) due to prey changes using some selected arthropods. International Journal of Acarology. 2009;35(6):503-509

[7] Sarwar M, Xuenong X, Wang E, Kongming W. The potential of four mite species (Acari: Phytoseiidae) as predators of sucking pests on protected cucumber (*Cucumis sativus* L.) crop. African Journal of Agricultural Research. 2011;6(1):73-78

[8] Sarwar M, Kongming W, Xuenong X, Wang E. Evaluations of four mite predators (Acari: Phytoseiidae)

released for suppression of spider mite infesting protected crop of sweet pepper (*Capsicum annuum* L.). African Journal of Agricultural Research. 2011;6(15):3509-3514

[9] Sarwar M, Xuenong X, Kongming W. Suitability of webworm *Loxostege sticticalis* L. (Lepidoptera: Crambidae) eggs for consumption by immature and adults of the predatory mite *Neoseiulus pseudolongispinosus* (Xin, Liang and Ke) (Acarina: Phytoseiidae). Spanish Journal of Agricultural Research. 2012;10(3):786-793

[10] Sarwar M. Comparing abundance of predacious and phytophagous mites (Acarina) in conjunction with resistance identification between Bt and non-Bt cotton cultivars. African Entomology: Journal of the Entomological Society of Southern Africa. 2013;21(1):108-118

[11] Sarwar M. Management of spider mite *Tetranychus cinnabarinus* (Boisduval) (Tetranychidae) infestation in cotton by releasing the predatory mite *Neoseiulus pseudolongispinosus* (Xin, Liang and Ke) (Phytoseiidae). Biological Control. 2013;65(1):37-42

[12] Sarwar M. Influence of host plant species on the development, fecundity and population density of pest *Tetranychus urticae* Koch (Acari: Tetranychidae) and predator *Neoseiulus pseudolongispinosus* (Xin, Liang and Ke) (Acari: Phytoseiidae). New Zealand Journal of Crop and Horticultural Science. 2014;42(1):10-20

[13] Sarwar M. Comparative life history characteristics of the mite predator *Neoseiulus cucumeris* (Oudemans) (Acari: Phytoseiidae) on mite and pollen diets. International Journal of Pest Management. 2016;62:140-148

[14] Arlian LG. Chiggers and other disease-causing mites. In: Encyclopedia

of Insects. 2nd ed. London, UK: Academic Press; 2009. p. 1168

[15] Samsinak K, Vobrazkova E, Dubinina V. Contribution to the taxonomic status of *Del'matophagoides schel'emetell'skyi* Bogdanoff, 1864. Folia Parasitologica. 1982;**29**:375-376

[16] Suggars AL. House dust mites: A review. Journal of Entomological Science. 1987;**1**(S):3-15

[17] Motavalli-Haghi F, Sharif M, Esmaeli R, Rafinejad G, Parsi B. Identification of different species of mites in dust, collected from residents of Sari Township in 1999-2000. Journal of Mazandaran University of Medical Sciences. 2003;**13**(38):54-58

[18] Bronswijk JEMH. House Dust Biology for Allergists, Acarologists and Mycologists. The Netherlands: NIB Publishers; 1981. p. 316

[19] Service MW. Medical Entomology for Students. 3rd ed. Cambridge: Cambridge University Press; 2004

[20] Spieksma FTM. Identification of house-dust mites. Aerobiologia. 1998;**6**(2):187-192

[21] Hart BJ. Biology and ecology of house dust mites, *Dermatophagoides* spp. and *Euroglyphus* spp. Immunology and Allergy Clinics of North America. 1989;**9**(2):339-356

[22] Arlian L, Confer P, Rapp C, VyszenskiMoher D, Chang JCS. Population dynamics of the house dust mites *Dermatophagoides farinae, D. pteronyssinus*, and *Euroglyphus maynei* (Acari: Pyroglyphidae) at specific relative humidities. Journal of Medical Entomology. 1998;**35**(1):46-53

[23] Calvo M, Fernandez-Caldas E, Arollano P, Marin F, Carnes J, Hormaechea A. Mite allergen exposure, sensitisation and clinical symptoms

in Valdivia, Chile. Journal of Investigational Allergology and Clinical Immunology. 2005;**15**:189-196

[24] Hart BJ, Fain A. Morphological and biological studies of medically important house-dust mites. Acarologia. 1988;**29**:285-295

[25] Hart BJ. Life cycle and reproduction of house-dust mites: Environmental factors influencing mite populations. Allergy. 1998;**53**(48 S):13-17

[26] Sanchez-Borges M, Capriles-Hulett A, Fernandez-Caldas E, Suarez-Chacon R, Caballero F, Castillo S, et al. Mite contaminated foods as a cause of anaphylaxis. Journal of Allergy and Clinical Immunology. 1997;**99**(6 Pt 1):738-743

[27] Denning DW, O'Driscoll BR, Hogaboam CM, Bowyer P, Niven RM. The link between fungi and severe asthma: A summary of the evidence. European Respiratory Journal. 2006;**27**:615-626

[28] Sarwar M. Stored grain and stored product mites from Pakistan and Azad Kashmir. Pakistan and Gulf Economists. 2004;**23**(10):30-31

[29] Arlian LG, Dippold JS. Development and fecundity of *Dermatophagoides farinae* (Acari: Pyroglyphidae). Journal of Medical Entomology. 1996, 1986;**33**(2):257-260

[30] Alexander A, Fall N, Arlian L. Mating and fecundity of *Dermatophagoides farinae*. Experimental and Applied Acarology. 2002;**26**(1-2):79-86

[31] Matsumoto K, Okamoto M, Wada Y. Effect of relative humidity on life cycle of the house dust mites, *Dermatophagoides farinae* and *D. pteronyssinus*. Japanese Journal of Sanitary zoology. 1986;**37**(1):79-90

[32] Podder S, Biswas H, Gupta SK, Saha GK. Life-cycle of house dust mite *Dermatophagoides pteronyssinus* (Acari: Pyrogylphidae) under laboratory conditions in Kolkata metropolis. Acarina. 2009;**17**(2):239-242

[33] Griffiths DA, Cunnington AM. *Dermatophagoides microceras* sp. n.: A description and comparison with its sibling species, *D. farinae* Hughes, 1961. Journal of Stored Products Research. 1971;**7**(1):1-14

[34] Cunnington AM, Lind P, Spieksma FTM. Taxonomic and immunochemical identification of two house dust mites *Dermatophagoides farina* and *Dermatophagoides microceras*. Journal of Allergy and Clinical Immunology. 1987;**79**(2):410-411

[35] Solarz K. House Dust Mites, Other Domestic Mites and Forensic Medicine. Rijeka: IntechOpen; 2011. pp. 327-358

[36] Mumcuoglu KY, Lutzky I. The life-cycle of *Dermatophagoides evansi* Fain, 1967 (Acari: Pyroglyphidae), a mite associated with poultry. Acarologia. 1990;**31**(2):191-194

[37] Morgan MS, Vyszenski-Moher DL, Arlian LG. Population growth and allergen content of cultured *Euroglyphus maynei* house dust mites. International Archives of Allergy and Immunology. 2015;**166**:267-272

[38] Arlian LG, Morgan MS. Reproductive biology of *Euroglyphus maynei* with comparisons to *Dermatophagoides farinae* and *D. pteronyssinus*. Experimental and Applied Acarology. 2015;**66**(1):1-9

[39] Siddiqui QH, Sarwar M. Pre and post-harvest losses in wheat. Pakistan and Gulf Economist. 2002;**21**(6):30-32

[40] Arlian LG. Biology and ecology of house dust mites, *Dermatophagoides* spp. and *Euroglyphus* spp. Immunology and Allergy Clinics of North America. 1989;**9**(2):339-356

[41] Arlian LG, Morgan MS. Biology, ecology, and prevalence of dust mites. Immunology and Allergy Clinics of North America. 2003;**23**(3):443-468

[42] Mahakittikun V, Boitano JJ, Ninsanit P, Wangapai T, Ralukruedej K. Effects of high and low temperatures on development time and mortality of house dust mite eggs. Experimental and Applied Acarology. 2011;**55**(4):339-347

[43] Colloff MJ. Dust mites. Experimental and Applied Acarology. 2010;**52**(4):449-450

[44] Platts-Mills TA, Ward GW Jr, Sporik R, Gelber LE, Chapman MD, Heymann PW. Epidemiology of the relationship between exposure to indoor allergens and asthma. International Archives of Allergy and Immunology. 1991;**94**:339-345

[45] Korsgaard J. Epidemiology of house-dust mites. Allergy. 1998;**53**(48 S):36-40

[46] El-Dib NA. House dust mites—What might a mite do? Encyclopedia of life support systems, UNISCO. Medical Sciences. 2007;**1**:182-193

[47] Arbes SJJ, Cohn RD, Yin M, Muilenberg ML, Burge HA, Friedman W, et al. House dust mite allergen in US beds: Results from the first National Survey of Lead and Allergens in Housing. Journal of Allergy and Clinical Immunology. 2003;**111**(2):408-414

[48] Platts-Mills TAE, Heyden ML, Chapman MD, Wilkins SR. Seasonal variation in dust mite and grass pollen allergens in dust from the houses of patients with asthma. Journal of Allergy and Clinical Immunology. 1987;**79**:781-791

[49] Munir AK, Bjorksten B, Emarson R, Ekstrand-Tobin A, Warner A, Nim K. Mite allergens in relation to home conditions and sensitization of asthmatic children from three climatic regions. Allergy. 1995;**50**:55-64

[50] Feldman-Muhsam B, Mumcuoglu KY, Osterovich T. A survey of house dust mites (Acari: Pyroglyphidae and Cheyletidae) in Israel. Journal of Medical Entomology. 1985;**22**:663-669

[51] Arlian LG, Bernstein IL, Gallagher JS. The prevalence of house dust mites, *Dermatophagoides* spp. and associated environmental conditions in homes in Ohio. Journal of Allergy and Clinical Immunology. 1982;**69**(6):527-532

[52] Mumcuoglu KY, Gat Z, Horowitz T, Miller J, Bar-Tana R, Ben-Zvi A, et al. Abundance of house dust mites in relation to climate in contrasting agricultural settlements in Israel. Medical and Veterinary Entomology. 1999;**13**:252-258

[53] Lang JD, Mulla MS. Seasonal dynamics of house dust mites. *Dermafophagoides* spp. in homes in Southern California. Environmental Entomology. 1978;7:281-286

[54] Oconnor BM. Evolutionary ecology of astigmatic mites. Annual Review of Entomology. 1982;**27**:385-409

[55] Nonaka S, Unno T, Ohta Y, Mori S. Sneeze-evoking region within the brainstem. Brain Research. 1990;**11**(2):265-270

[56] Breitenbach RA, Swisher PK, Kim MK, Patel BS. The photic sneeze reflex as a risk factor to combat pilots. Military Medicine. 1993;**158**(12):806-809

[57] Cole EC, Cook CE. Characterization of infectious aerosols in health care facilities: An aid to effective engineering controls and preventive strategies. American Journal of Infection Control. 1998;**26**(4):453-464

[58] Babe KS Jr, Arlian LG, Confer PD, Kim R. House dust mite (*Dermatophagoides farinae* and *Dermatophagoides pteronyssinus*) prevalence in the rooms and hallways of a tertiary care hospital. Journal of Allergy and Clinical Immunology. 1995;**95**(4):801-805

[59] Sarwar M. Mites—The tiny killers to push honeybee colonies into collapse and integrated pest management. International Journal for Research in Applied Physics. 2016;**1**(7):12-21

[60] Sarwar M. Mite culprits for causing mortality and reduction in population of honey bee colonies and measures for pests control. International Journal for Research in Applied Chemistry. 2016;**1**(7):10-22

[61] Vyszenski-Moher DL, Arlian LG, Neal JS. Effects of laundry detergents on *Dermatophagoides farinae*, *Dermatophagoides pteronyssinus*, and *Euroglyphus maynei*. Annals of Allergy, Asthma & Immunology. 2002;**88**(6):578-583

[62] Sarwar M. Frequency of insect and mite Fauna in chilies *Capsicum annum* L., onion *Allium cepa* L. and garlic *Allium sativum* L. cultivated areas, and their integrated management. International Journal of Agronomy and Plant Production. 2012;**3**(5):173-178

[63] Sarwar M. Mite pests (Acari) in mango (*Mangifera indica* L.) plantations and implementation of control strategy. Bioscience and Bioengineering. 2015;**1**(3):41-47

[64] Sarwar M. Biological control to maintain natural densities of insects and mites by field releases of lady beetles (Coleoptera: Coccinellidae).

International Journal of Entomology and Nematology. 2016;**2**(1):21-26

[65] Mumcuoglu KY, Schlein Y. Sulfaquinoxaline, a possible means for the control of the house dust mite *Dermatophagoides pteronyssinus*. Revue Suisse de Zoologie. 1978;**85**:635-640

[66] Mumcuoglu KY, Gabbay J, Borkow G. Copper oxide impregnated fabrics for the control of house dust mites. International Journal of Pest Management. 2008;**54**:235-240

[67] Braig HR, Perotti MA. Carcasses and mites. Experimental and Applied Acarology. 2009;**49**(1-2):45-84

[68] Perotti MA. Megnin re-analysed: The case of the newborn baby girl, Paris, 1878. Experimental and Applied Acarology. 2009;**49**(1-2):37-44

[69] Solarz K. Indoor mites and forensic acarology. Experimental and Applied Acarology. 2009;**49**(1-2):135-142

[70] Çakan H, Güven K, Çevik F, Demirci M, Kocazeybek B. Investigation of human DNA profiles in house dust mites: Implications in forensic acarology. Romanian Journal of Legal Medicine. 2015;**23**(3):187-192

[71] Sarwar M. Typical flies: Natural history, lifestyle and diversity of Diptera. In: Sarwar M, editor. Life Cycle and Development of Diptera. London, UK: IntechOpen; 2020. p. 50

[72] Perotti MA, Goff M, Baker AS, Turner BD, Braig HR. Forensic acarology: An introduction. Experimental and Applied Acarology. 2009;**49**(1-2):3-13

Chapter 16

Leishmaniasis

Salwa S. Sheikh, Amaar A. Amir, Baraa A. Amir and Abdulrazack A. Amir

Abstract

Leishmaniasis is a vector-borne tropical/subtropical disease caused by an intracellular parasite transmitted to humans by sand fly bite. It is endemic in Asia, Africa, the Americas, and the Mediterranean region. Worldwide reports include 1.5–2 million new cases each year, more than 300 million at risk of acquiring the disease, and 70,000 deaths per year. Clinical features depend on the *Leishmania* species and immune response of the host, varying from localized cutaneous disease to visceral form with potentially fatal outcome; however, the common presentation is either cutaneous, mucocutaneous, or visceral leishmaniasis. Many therapeutic agents are being used in *Leishmania* treatment, but the only effective treatment is achieved with current pentavalent antimonials. WHO considers Leishmaniasis as one of the "Neglected Tropical Diseases" that continues to be prevalent despite international, national, and local efforts towards its control and elimination over the last decade. This chapter reviews the global perspective of Leishmaniasis with increasing recognition of emerging "Atypical forms" and new surge of disease across the world mainly due to increasing conflicts in endemic areas leading to forced migration among other causes. All these challenges related to environment, disease, and vector pose major implications on WHO's leishmaniasis control and elimination plan.

Keywords: *Leishmania*, sand fly, vector, parasite, protozoa, phlebotomine

1. Introduction

Leishmaniasis is a vector-borne disease caused by an obligate intracellular protozoa of genus *Leishmania* and is transmitted by the bite of a female phlebotomine sand fly (**Figure 1**). It is a poverty-related disease with an estimated 0.7–1 million new cases reported per year from approximately 100 endemic countries. It is reported from all continents except Australia and Antarctica.

The disease is primarily zoonotic with exception of *L. donovani* and *L. tropica*, although some evidence exists that animal reservoir exists for these species too. There are about 53 species of *Leishmania* described with more than 20 species pathogenic to humans and each distinct species causing different clinical manifestations ranging from self-resolving cutaneous ulcers to disfiguring mucocutaneous lesions to life-threatening systemic visceral disease [1–3]. The outcome depends on multiple factors including parasite characteristics, vector itself, and host factors in a particular patient's immune status. The World Health Organization (WHO) considers leishmaniasis as not only one of the neglected tropical diseases but also a

IntechOpen

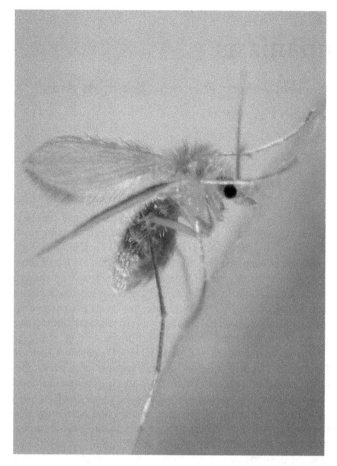

Figure 1.
This photograph depicts a right lateral view of a Phlebotomus papatasi *sand fly which had landed atop the skin surface of a human volunteer. This specimen had just completed its ingestion of its blood meal, which is visible through its distended transparent abdomen. Sand flies like this* P. papatasi *are responsible for the spread of the vector-borne, parasitic disease, leishmaniasis (courtesy of Centers for Disease Control and Prevention/ prof. Frank Hadley Collins and James Gathany) (https://phil.cdc.gov/Details.aspx?pid=10276).*

public health problem that requires elimination by developing effective therapeutic regimens and prevention/control plans.

2. Epidemiology

The disease classification is complex and can be characterized by either its *clinical presentation* into cutaneous (localized or disseminated), mucocutaneous, and visceral or *geographic location* into *Old World leishmaniasis* mainly including Africa, Asia, the Middle East, the Mediterranean, and India or *New World leishmaniasis* including Central and South America (**Table 1**) [4–6].

More than 90% of the cases of visceral leishmaniasis (VL) cases worldwide were reported from 7 countries in 2015 including Brazil, Ethiopia, Kenya, India, Somalia, Sudan, and South Sudan; however, the disease remains endemic in more than 60 countries [1]. The Indian subcontinent accounts for almost 70% of the world's anthroponotic visceral leishmaniasis cases, India having the highest incidence

Genus	Division	Subgenera	Species	Disease	Geographic Area
Leishmania	Euleishmania	*L. (Sauroleishmania)*	*L. tarentolae*		Old world
			L. adleri		
			L. hoogstraali		
		L. (Leishmania)	*L. enriettii*		
			L. major	Cutaneous leishmaniasis	
			L. gerbilli		
			L. turanica		
			L. arabica		
			L. tropica	Cutaneous leishmaniasis	
			L. aethiopica	Cutaneous leishmaniasis	
			L. donovani	Visceral leishmaniasis	
			L. infantum	Visceral leishmaniasis	
			L. martiniquences		New world
			L. mexicana	Cutaneous leishmaniasis	
			L. amazonensis	Cutaneous leishmaniasis	
			L. aristidesi		
			L. venezualenesis	Cutaneous leishmaniasis	
			L. forattinii		
		L. (Viannia)	*L. braziliensis*	Cutaneous & mucocutaneous leishmaniasis	
			L. peruviana	Cutaneous leishmaniasis	
			L. guyanensis	Cutaneous leishmaniasis	
			L. panamensis	Cutaneous leishmaniasis	
			L. lainsoni		
			L. naiffi		
			L. lindenbergi		
			L. utingensis		
	Paraleishmania		*L. colombiensis*		
			L. equatorensis		
			L. hertigi		
			L. herreri		
			L. deanei		

Table 1.
Leishmania *taxonomy showing most of the clinically significant Leishmania species [1, 5, 6, 14].*

followed by Nepal and Bangladesh. In immunocompromised patients, *Leishmania* parasites can persist for decades after management and may reappear exhibiting fulminant reactivation when immunity is compromised. Between 5 and 50% of treated VL cases may develop post-kala-azar dermal leishmaniasis (PKDL), depending on geographic location, secondary to the interferon gamma-driven immune response against dermal parasite [7–9].

More than 90% of cutaneous leishmaniasis (CL) and mucocutaneous leishmaniasis (ML) cases are reported from Pakistan, Afghanistan, Syria, Saudi Arabia, Iran, Brazil, Algeria, and Peru. The number of reported VL cases has decreased substantially in the past decade most likely due to early diagnosis and better access to treatment. In East Africa, however, the fatal disease case number continues to be sustained. However there is a surge in endemic CL across the world predominantly due to increased conflicts with forced displacement of population and living in poor sanitary conditions. In addition, there is also an increase in the number of overall *Leishmania* cases reported worldwide and increased new cases reported from nonendemic areas [10–12]. A renaissance of CL is seen in conflict areas of Middle East in particular Syria mainly due to collapse of public health systems, exposure of nonimmune population, and poor living conditions.

2.1 Risk factors

Population migration of susceptible individuals in endemic areas as well as into nonendemic areas, malnutrition, poverty, and immune status of the host play a major role. Temperature is another important factor as *Leishmania* species for cutaneous disease grow best at lower temperature, while species causing VL grow better at core temperatures.

The pathogenesis appears related to T-cell cytotoxicity. The promastigotes activate complement system through alternate pathway with suppression of cell-mediated immunity against the organism. In self-resolving and asymptomatic patients, T helper type 1 cells (Th1) predominate with interleukin-2 (IL-2), interferon gamma, and IL-12 as important cytokines helping with disease resolution. In visceral and diffuse cutaneous forms, T helper type 2 cells (TH2) predominate with patients exhibiting anergy to the organism. These cells secrete IL-4, IL-5, IL-9, IL-13, and IL-17E/IL-25.

A susceptibility gene in band 22q12 is identified in parts of Sudan with high prevalence of VL [13].

Coinfection of VL with HIV is a major challenge. Both infections share a common immunopathologic mechanism involving macrophages and dendritic cells of reticuloendothelial system, therefore leading to an accelerated progression of both diseases in coinfection.

3. Life cycle

Leishmania is scientifically classified as a "genus" that belongs to the "order" of Trypanosomatidae family, under the "class" of Kinetoplastea, under the "phylum" of Euglenozoa. The parasite *Leishmania* exists in two forms: flagellated promastigote form in sandflies and cultures and nonflagellated amastigote form in animals and humans (**Figure 2**) [14, 15]. The sandflies acquire infection when they bite an animal or human host. The parasite develops over 4–25 days in the sandflies and transforms into a promastigote form where they multiply by binary fission in the midgut and move upwards to the pharynx. Infection is transmitted mainly during days 6–9 after ingestion when there is heavy pharyngeal infection and promastigotes are regurgitated via a bite to the host. The sand fly can regurgitate more than 1000 parasites per bite. In the host some of the flagellates are destroyed, whereas others enter intracellular lysosomal organelles of macrophages of

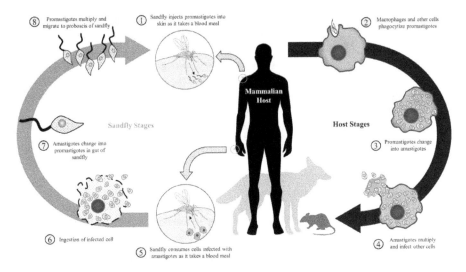

Figure 2.
Leishmania life cycle.

reticuloendothelial system. The flagella of the organisms are lost, and amastigotes are formed that continue to multiply until the infected host cells get filled with organisms and rupture releasing free amastigotes that invade new cells, thus continuing the vicious cycle of *Leishmania* infection (**Figure 2**). The incubation period depends on the individual parasite species. In certain geographic areas, the transmission cycle can be maintained by the infected animals and does not require infected humans. In other areas where disease transmission has the anthroponotic cycle via humans, the disease transmission can be controlled by effective treatment of infected patients [16].

3.1 Mode of transmission

The disease is mainly transmitted by the bite of a 2–3 mm in size female "*Phlebotomus* sand fly" in Old World leishmaniasis and *Lutzomyia* in the New World disease. There are approximately 20 pathogenic *Leishmania* species and up to 500 known phlebotomine sand fly species identified as vectors of disease [17, 18]. The disease is mostly zoonotic with humans being incidental hosts infected by sand fly bite.

4. Clinical presentation

In addition to the known classic disease spectrum and clinical presentations, new unusual and atypical forms are emerging which is adding to the complexity of achieving control and disease eradication goal [19].

4.1 Cutaneous leishmaniasis

CL causing *Leishmania* parasites are divided into New world and Old world species. The New World species affect mainly Central and South America and include *L. amazonensis*, *L. braziliensis*, *L. mexicana*, and *L. guyaensis*, among others. The Old World species examples include *L. tropica*, *L. major*, and *L. aethiopica* that are common in the Indian subcontinent, the Middle East, the Mediterranean basin, and East

Africa. CL is usually a limited cutaneous disease. The lesions develop as papules at the sand fly bite site and progress over weeks to months to develop larger nodules that eventually ulcerate (**Figure 3**). Lesions are often itchy and may have a hyperkeratotic wart-like appearance. These lesions often self-heal in 2–18 months, leaving a permanent, often disfiguring, scar, leading to major cosmetic concern and social stigma.

Approximately 10% of CL cases may progress to severe disease such as diffuse CL, ML, disseminated CL, and/or *L. recidivans* [1, 20].

4.1.1 Uncommon variants of CL

Uncommonly, CL variants are encountered that are associated with various underlying immune responses.

L. recidivans typically follows a healed *L. tropica* cutaneous infection and presents as new lesions encircling the old scar. The lesions show predominantly

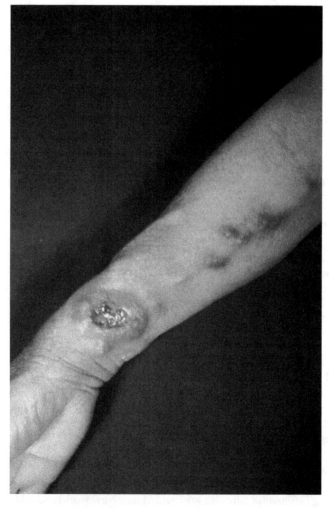

Figure 3.
This photograph depicts the volar surface of a patient's extended right arm, who had been ill with leishmaniasis, having been infected with Leishmania *sp. protozoa, which had manifested itself as a cutaneous form of the disease (courtesy of Centers for Disease Control and Prevention/Dr. martins Castro and Dr. Lucille K. Georg) (https://phil.cdc.gov/Details.aspx?pid=12161).*

increased number of lymphocytes making it difficult to histologically distinguish from tuberculosis.

Diffuse cutaneous leishmaniasis presents with multiple widespread nontender, non-ulcerating lesions, resembling lepromatous leprosy, and a negative leishmanin skin test (LST). The skin is heavily infiltrated by organisms and the patients lack a cellular immune response. These are caused *by L. amazonensis, L. aethiopica, and L. mexicana.*

Disseminated cutaneous leishmaniasis presents with 10 or more mixed-type lesions in multiple body parts and is mostly seen in Latin America with frequent involvement of the mucosa. Histologically, the organisms are scant in the skin lesions, and patients show positive antibodies against *Leishmania* and positive LST test.

Most cases of diffuse cutaneous leishmaniasis and *L. recidivans* are chronic and resistant to treatment, may be exceedingly disfiguring, and can be associated with low mortality rates.

L. infantum/L. chagasi predominantly causes VL; however, it may lead to atypical cutaneous disease. Reported cases are autochthonous, seen in immunocompetent hosts, and diagnosed in different regions [19].

L. donovani is also mainly responsible for VL; however, some atypical autochthonous CL cases by *L. donovani* are reported [19].

4.2 Mucocutaneous leishmaniasis

ML presents as destructive lesions involving oronasal mucosa with involvement of the nasal septum, lips, and palate. Ninety percent of ML cases show a previous CL scar. The disease is often chronic and progressive with destructive, disfiguring midfacial lesions leading to extensive mutilation. Secondary infection and respiratory tract invasion may lead to patient's demise. It is frequently seen in immunocompromised individuals and being a potentially life-threatening disease requires immediate/early diagnosis and treatment [21, 22]. Less than 5% of patients infected by *L. braziliensis* and a small percent of those infected by *L. panamensis* and *L. guyanensis* can develop mucosal involvement months to years after cutaneous disease resolution [13].

4.3 Visceral leishmaniasis

L. donovani is the main species causing VL and humans are the main reservoir for it. *L. infantum* also causes visceral disease; however, it is zoonotic. VL is characterized by a "pentad" of persistent irregular fever, hepatosplenomegaly, weight loss, pancytopenia, and hypergammaglobulinemia. The fever characteristically shows a double rise in 24 hours with spikes of fever and afebrile intervals in between. It is the most devastating and fatal forms of leishmaniasis. The spectrum ranges from asymptomatic infection to fulminant life-threatening disease. The disease may present with an acute or insidious onset, however the typical presentation is that of wasted, thin, cachectic appearance with prominent abdominal distention due to hepatosplenomegaly. Jaundice is considered to be a bad prognostic sign. The incubation period is 2 weeks–8 months. High parasite burden is often associated with malnutrition and wasting in particular in children [23, 24]. VL is often associated with hyperpigmentation of the skin most likely secondary to production of adrenocorticotropic hormones. In such cases it is referred to as kala-azar/black fever [25]. VL, if untreated, is fatal within 2 years; mortality is mostly due to secondary bacterial infection, immunosuppression, hemorrhage due to hematopoietic infiltration, and severe anemia [13].

4.3.1 Uncommon variants of VL

Gulf War soldiers: An uncommon form of VL is described in some US veterans who were infected while participating in Gulf war. These patients had only mild symptoms and light parasitic burden. *L. tropica* was identified as the causative agent in some of these cases [19, 26].

Viscerotropic leishmaniasis: This is an indolent form of disease that has a distinct clinical presentation; however it does not progress to or develop classic VL.

VL-HIV coinfection: HIV is considered to be responsible for the re-emergence of the VL. Both organisms share common pathologic immunologic system involving the reticular endothelial system, therefore leading to accelerated progression of the disease. VL in an HIV-infected person should be considered an acquired immune deficiency syndrome (AIDS)-defining illness, and HIV testing should be mandatory in all patients presenting with VL [1, 27]. Atypical disseminated leishmaniasis can be seen in these patients with lesions involving the gastrointestinal tract and the respiratory tract [21, 28].

L. tropica, *L. amazonensis, and* L. major generally associated with CL are reported to be viscerotropic and uncommonly may lead to visceral disease [19].

4.4 Post-kala-azar dermal leishmaniasis

PKDL was commonly seen in India and Africa as a late complication of VL secondary to *L. donovani* and rarely *L. infantum,* the latter typically in immuno-compromised patients [29]. Patients often present months to as many as 20 years after VL with hypopigmented or erythematous skin lesions which over time progress to develop plaques and nodules over the face and trunk. These lesions are often nontender and have preserved sensation, a feature distinguishing this from lepromatous leprosy. The lesions often resolves spontaneously; however, relapse is common, and resistant forms to antimonial treatment have been reported [1, 13].

5. Diagnosis

Centers for Disease Control and Prevention (CDC) has a practical guide for laboratory diagnosis of leishmaniasis at http://www.cdc.gov/parasites/leishmania sis/health_professionals/index [18].

Cutaneous and mucocutaneous lesions usually show normal values in routine laboratory testing. VL, on the other hand, may exhibit normocytic normochromic anemia, leukopenia, and/or thrombocytopenia due to bone marrow or spleen involvement. In addition there may be involvement of other organs leading to their respective abnormal functions such as abnormal liver function test in patients with significant hepatic disease.

Characteristically the diagnosis is confirmed by visualizing the amastigote form of the protozoa from infected tissue by performing invasive procedure such as dermal scraping or biopsies for cutaneous lesions and/or fine-needle aspirates/ biopsies for visceral disease (**Figure 4**). The smears are often stained with Giemsa, Leishman, and/or Wright's stain and slides reviewed under oil immersion. Histori-cally, splenic puncture was considered the most sensitive method and golden stan-dard procedure; however it is potentially life-threatening, carries a high risk of complications such as hemorrhage, and therefore currently is considered unneces-sary. In endemic areas with high clinical suspicion, clinical history and physical examination is often sufficient to reach the diagnosis. Since the localized disease has

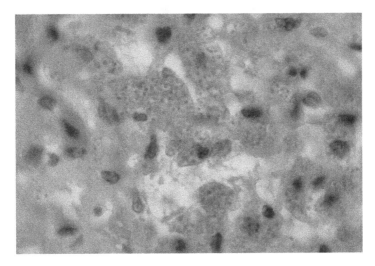

Figure 4.
This photomicrograph of a subcutaneous tissue sample reveals the presence of numerous Leishmania donovani *parasites (courtesy of Centers for Disease Control and Prevention/Dr. Martin D. Hicklin) (https://phil.cdc.gov/Details.aspx?pid=330).*

prominent cell-mediated immunity to the organism, especially when long-standing, isolation, identification, and culture of these organisms can be extremely challenging. In cutaneous disease the organism may be visualized in samples obtained by biopsy, scraping, or FNA in approximately 70% of cases, while the culture from the skin shows only 40% sensitivity [13, 30].

A skin punch biopsy is recommended for the CL to be taken from the raised edge of an active lesion where parasites exist. In addition to the formalin-fixed sections, touch preparations/tissue impression slides can also be prepared and examined. The diagnostic finding is to identify the amastigotes with their eosinophilic rod-like cytoplasmic kinetoplast (**Figures 5** and **6**). In long-standing lesions, biopsy of the necrotic center of the lesion, and cases with low burden disease, the biopsy may show false-negative results.

Mucosal biopsies and/or dental scrapings are used for mucocutaneous lesions to look for organisms.

Invasive procedures such as aspirates or biopsies from the spleen, bone marrow, lymph node, and/or liver were used to diagnose VL. However, technology advancement and development of rapid diagnostic tests (RDT) such as recombinant K39 assay with its high sensitivity and specificity made the above invasive procedures unnecessary. In general, the positivity rate for identification of amastigotes in splenic aspirate is 98% and in bone marrow aspirate/biopsy is 54–86% [31, 32]. Blood samples, except in HIV-infected patients, and lymph nodes have lower sensitivity.

Leishmanin skin test/Montenegro skin test, similar to purified protein derivative (PPD) test used for *Mycobacterium tuberculosis*, is a marker of cellular immune response and tests for delayed-type hypersensitivity reaction. The test uses injection of killed promastigotes in the skin. If there is a skin induration of at least 5 mm after 48–72 hours, the test is considered positive. The test is negative in acute infection as it shows positive results after 2–3 months of infection. In addition the test is negative in active VL and immunosuppressed patients due to anergic response. In the United States, no skin tests for leishmaniasis are approved because of lack of standardization; however, it is used in developing countries and is useful in epidemiological surveys as a marker of previous exposure [1].

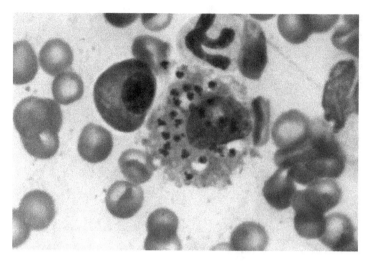

Figure 5.
This photomicrograph depicts some of the histopathologic details seen in a canine bone marrow smear, processed using Giemsa stain, in the case of leishmaniasis. This particular view displays Leishmania donovani *parasites contained within one of the bone marrow histiocytes (courtesy of Centers for Disease Control and Prevention/Dr. Francis W. Chandler) (https://phil.cdc.gov/Details.aspx?pid=30).*

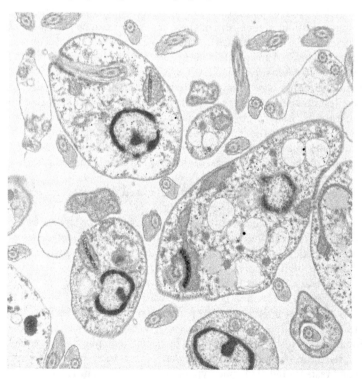

Figure 6.
This is a transmission electron microscopic image of Leishmania major *amastigotes, which had been grown in a cell culture. Note the dense kinetoplasts in the cytoplasm (courtesy of Centers for Disease Control and Prevention/Cynthia goldsmith and Luciana Flannery) (https://phil.cdc.gov/Details.aspx?pid=22001).*

Several serological assays for detection of antibodies against leishmaniasis have been developed using various techniques such as direct agglutination (DAT), immunofluorescence assay (IFA), enzyme-linked immunosorbent assay (ELISA), and western blot. Although these tests show high sensitivity for acute VL, they are not specific for this disease and may show false positivity with other organisms.

Detection of antibodies to recombinant K 39 antigen appears to correlate with active VL disease in species such as *L. donovani, L. chagasi*, and *L. infantum*. These RDTs however are not useful in cutaneous and mucocutaneous infection. Based on a Cochrane review of RDTs, the sensitivity for rK39 RDT assay is excellent at 97% in Indian subcontinent but low in East Africa and Sudan at 85%. More recently, an rK28 antigen-based RDT shows better sensitivity in Sudan [33, 34]. Recent efforts in developing tests that detect antigens show promising results but still with certain limitations; latex agglutination test has moderate sensitivity of 64% and higher specificity of 93%, while most recent ELISA test shows more than 90% sensitivity [1, 35].

Molecular techniques including polymerase chain reaction (PCR), with significant advances in technology, show higher sensitivity; however, due to the higher cost and complexity of the procedure, they are not available in resource-limited settings. This is particularly true in VL. These tests have a higher sensitivity for cutaneous lesions: reverse transcriptase loop-mediated isothermal amplification (LAMP) technology exhibiting a sensitivity of 98% in CL.

6. Treatment

Multiple factors play a role in treatment decision-making for *Leishmania* that include the specific species, geographic location, comorbidities, and the type of disease whether CL, ML, PKLD, or VL. On most part, it is considered as a treatable and curable disease; however it requires an immunocompetent system. Despite multiple efforts and after all these years, the treatment of *Leishmania* still remains a problem. This is mostly because of indiscriminate treatment leading to frequent emergence of parasite resistance, and the side effects of antileishmanial therapeutic agents call for a search for alternative treatment including the use of natural products such as plants and herbs [36]. Traditionally, medicinal plants have been used throughout the history and are still being used as an alternative therapy to conventional health care, in particular in developing countries and mainly in rural areas that are often deprived of public health resources [37]. This science of using medicinal plants as therapeutic agents is referred to as phytotherapy [38]. The alternate therapies, when studied, show different mechanisms of action. Plants have several secondary metabolites, for example, flavonoids, polysaccharides, lactones, alkaloids, diterpenoids, and glycosides that may activate the immunological system [39]. As an example, a combination of miltefosine and nanoparticles of curcumin, a component of turmeric, displayed lymphocyte proliferation and increased the phagocytic capacity of peritoneal macrophages [40]. Another example is tricin which is isolated from *Casearia arborea*, an evergreen tea, that was reported to modulate the respiratory burst, thus helping in parasite elimination.

Other mechanisms reported as possible mechanisms of action include reactive oxygen species generation and apoptosis-inducing potential. Examples of the latter include ethanolic extract of seeds and leaves of *Azadirachta indica* and essentials oils of *Artemisia campestris* and *Artemisia herba-alba* that act as an apoptosis inductor in promastigotes of *L. donovani* and *L. infantum* [36].

Several studies have been carried out to assess the efficacy of such alternate treatment; however, the results have not been very encouraging. Most of the plants show immunomodulatory effect, but no leishmanicidal effect has been validated, supporting the notion that substances obtained from plants may complement the treatment of leishmaniasis because of their immunomodulatory effects, but there is no direct effect against the parasite.

There are recommended guidelines for *Leishmania* treatment by the WHO [16]. In addition, a panel of the Infectious Diseases Society of America (IDSA) and the American Society of Tropical Medicine and Hygiene (ASTMH) have developed management guidelines for *Leishmania* patients. These guidelines are mainly for physicians practicing in North America and are based, whenever possible, on randomized clinical trials and a systematic method of grading the quality of evidence and strength of recommendation [41].

6.1 Cutaneous leishmaniasis

Most CL cases spontaneously regress in immunocompetent hosts over 2–18 months, and therefore conservative approach can be used in particular for those caused by *L. major* and *L. mexicana*. On the other hand, *L. braziliensis* has a low spontaneous cure rate. The decision to treat CL and ML is often to reach a goal of reducing the risk of disfigurement, scarring, dissemination, accelerating cure, and subsequent progression to mucocutaneous disease in cases of CL. In addition it is important to classify cutaneous lesions into simple or complex cutaneous lesions based on certain criteria that are then used for treatment decision-making process. These include immunocompetent versus immunocompromised host status, regional lymphadenopathy, multiplicity of lesions (>4), lesions of >5 cm in size, lesions on sensitive areas (such as face, ears, eyelids, lips, fingers/toes, genitalia, or joints), more than 6 months duration, and *Leishmania* species that are more likely to be associated with ML, unusual presentations such as diffuse or disseminated CL, and *L. recidivans*. Traditional treatment for CL has been intralesional injections mostly sodium stibogluconate, thermotherapy, cryotherapy, and topical agents such as paromomycin. The combination of intralesional antimonials and cryotherapy is often the first-line treatment option for CL, resulting in higher cure rates. There has been lack of standardization and poor trial designs for therapeutic regimens in the past. Recently efforts are being carried out to develop unified criteria to define measurable endpoints for different treatment regimens. The treatment regimen decision regarding whether to give local or systemic therapy or choice of therapeutic modality is based on the geographic location and the infecting *Leishmania* species.

Local treatment includes a combination of intralesional antimonials and cryotherapy, paromomycin ointment containing methylbenzethonium chloride, paromomycin containing 0.5% gentamicin, and paromomycin with allopurinol for *L. recidivans*.

Systemic regimens include oral fluconazole, pentavalent antimonials with or without pentoxifylline, ketoconazole, miltefosine, liposomal amphotericin B (LAMB), and pentamidine isethionate.

Systemic treatment for CL is usually used for immunosuppressed patients, mucocutaneous lesions, diffuse/extensive lesions, and refractory disease. In addition infection by *L. braziliensis* and *L. infantum* should be considered for systemic treatment (**Tables 2** and **3**) [1, 17, 18].

6.2 Mucocutaneous leishmaniasis

For mucocutaneous disease systemic regimens include pentamidine isethionate, pentavalent antimonials + pentoxyfilline, and LAMB (**Table 4**) [17, 18].

Leishmania species	Local therapy	Systemic therapy	Relapse treatment
L. Mexicana	1. 15% paromomycin and 12% methylbenzethonium chloride ointment twice daily for 20 days (B) 2. Thermotherapy: 1–3 sessions with localized heat (50 °C for 30 s) (A) 3. Intralesional antimonials: 1–5 ml per session every 3–7 days (1–5 infiltrations) (B)	1. Ketoconazole: adult dose, 600 mg oral daily for 28 days (B) 2. Miltefosine: 2.5 mg/kg per day orally for 28 days (B)	1. Amphotericin B deoxycholate, as above 2. Pentavalent antimonials: as above plus topical imiquimod every other day for 20 days (A) 3. Liposomal amphotericin B: 3 mg/kg per day, by infusion, up to 20–40 mg/kg total dose may be considered
L. guyanensis and L. panamensis	(same treatment regimen as L. mexicana)	1. Pentamidine isethionate, intramuscular injections or brief infusions of 4 mg salt/kg per dose every other day for 3 doses (C) 2. Pentavalent antimonials: 20 mg Sb5+/kg per day intramuscularly or intravenously for 20 days (C) 3. Miltefosine: 2.5 mg/kg per day orally for 28 days (B)	(same treatment regimen as L. mexicana)
L. braziliensis	(same treatment regimen as L. mexicana)	1. Pentavalent antimonials: 20 mg Sb5+/kg per day intramuscularly or intravenously for 20 days (A) 2. Amphotericin B deoxycholate: 0.7 mg/kg per day, by infusion, for 25–30 doses (C) 3. Liposomal amphotericin B: 2–3 mg/kg per day, by infusion, up to 20–40 mg/kg total dose (C)	(same treatment regimen as L. mexicana)
L. amazonensis, L. peruviana, and L. venezuelensis	(same treatment regimen as L. mexicana)	1. Pentavalent antimonials: 20 mg Sb5+/kg per day intramuscularly or intravenously for 20 days	(same treatment regimen as L. mexicana)

Table 2.
Treatment regimens for cutaneous leishmaniasis, New World species, as per WHO recommendations (adopted from WHO) (https://www.who.int/leishmaniasis/research/978924129496_pp67_71.pdf?ua=1) [8].

Leishmania species	Local therapy	Systemic therapy
L. major	**1.** 15% paromomycin/12% methylbenzethonium chloride ointment twice daily for 20 days (A) **2.** Intralesional antimonials, 1–5 ml per session plus cryotherapy (liquid nitrogen: – 195 °C), both every 3–7 days (1–5 sessions) (A) **3.** Thermotherapy, 1–2 sessions with localized heat (50 °C for 30 s) (A) **4.** Intralesional antimonials or cryotherapy independently, as above (D)	**1.** Fluconazole, 200 mg oral daily for 6 weeks (A) **2.** Pentavalent antimonials, 20 mg Sb5+/kg per day intramuscularly or intravenously for 10–20 days (D) **3.** Pentavalent antimonials, 20 mg Sb5+/kg per day intramuscularly or intravenously plus pentoxyfylline, 400 mg three times a day for 10–20 days (A)
L. tropica and L. infantum	**1.** 15% paromomycin/12% methylbenzethonium chloride ointment, as above (D) **2.** Intralesional antimonials plus cryotherapy, as above (D) **3.** Thermotherapy, as above (A) **4.** intralesional antimonials, alone, as above (B) **5.** Cryotherapy, alone, as above (C)	**1.** Pentavalent antimonials, 20 mg Sb5+/kg per day intramuscularly or intravenously for 10–20 days (D) **2.** Pentavalent antimonials, 15–20 mg Sb5+/kg per day intramuscularly or intravenously for 15 days plus oral allopurinol 20 mg/kg for 30 days, to treat leishmaniasis recidivans caused by L. tropica (C)
L. aethiopica	(same treatment regimen as *L. tropica* and *L. infantum*)	**1.** Pentavalent antimonials 20 mg Sb5+/kg per day intramuscularly or intravenously plus paromomycin, 15 mg (11 mg base)/ kg per day intramuscularly for 60 days or longer to treat diffuse cutaneous leishmaniasis (C)

Table 3.
Treatment regimens for cutaneous leishmaniasis, Old World species, as per WHO recommendations (adopted from WHO) (https://www.who.int/leishmaniasis/research/978924129496_pp67_71.pdf?ua=1) [8].

6.3 Post-kala-azar dermal leishmaniasis

Treatment regimens for PKDL are scant. In general, majority of cases from East Africa are self-healing and therefore do not require treatment. In contrast, in the Indian subcontinent, these patients are treated. Since vast majority of these patients are healthy and the risk is cosmetic, the risk benefit should be weighed before initiating therapy. Selected treatment regimens are recommended by the WHO,

Recommended treatment regimens for all cases of mucocutaneous leishmaniasis
1. Pentavalent antimonials: 20 mg/kg per day intramuscularly or intravenously for 30 days (C)
2. Pentavalent antimonials: as above plus oral pentoxifylline at 400 mg/8 h for 30 days (A)
3. Amphotericin B deoxycholate: 0.7–1 mg/kg by infusion every other day up to 25–45 doses (C)
4. Liposomal amphotericin B: 2–3 mg/kg daily by infusion up to a total dose of 40–60 mg/kg (C)
5. In Bolivia: miltefosine at 2.5–3.3 mg/kg per day orally for 28 days (B)

Table 4.
Treatment regimens for mucocutaneous leishmaniasis as per WHO recommendations (adopted from WHO) (https://www.who.int/leishmaniasis/research/978924129496_pp67_71.pdf?ua=1) [8].

when patients require treatment, that include miltefosine, amphotericin B deoxycholate, and LAMB mainly for Indian subcontinent. As for East Africa, the WHO based on evidence grading recommends pentavalent antimonial, LAMB, miltefosine, and combination treatment (pentavalent antimonial with paromomycin) (**Table 5**) [17, 18].

6.4 Visceral leishmaniasis

Traditionally VL has been treated by pentavalent antimonials. Recently there is emergence of resistance in the Indian subcontinent. Current recommendations for VL in East Africa include pentavalent antimonials, LAMB, or combination treatment (including pentavalent antimonials with paromomycin). As for the Indian subcontinent, the recommendations include LAMB, amphotericin B deoxycholate, miltefosine, and one of the combination therapies: LAMB with miltefosine, LAMB with paromomycin, or miltefosine with paromomycin [1]. As for complicated VL, elderly patients, and pregnant patients in East Africa, it is recommended to have LAMB treatment because of its better safety. LAMB monotherapy is not recommended in patients with less severe disease in Asia due to lack of proven efficacy in that region [42]. In Asia, sodium stibogluconate, rather than LAMB, is considered the first-line treatment for *L. infantum* and *L. donovani*. The WHO recommended LAMB therapy in the initial elimination phase for *L. donovani* in

Geographic areas affected by post-kala-azar dermal leishmaniasis	Recommended treatment regimens ranked by preference
East Africa	1. Pentavalent antimonials: 20 mg Sb5+/kg per day intramuscularly or intravenously for 30–60 days, when indicated (C)
	2. Liposomal amphotericin B: 2.5 mg/kg per day by infusion for 20 days, when indicated (C)
Bangladesh, India, and Nepal	1. Amphotericin B deoxycholate: 1 mg/kg per day by infusion, up to 60–80 doses over 4 months (C)
	2. Miltefosine orally for 12 weeks at dosage as above in visceral leishmaniasis (A)

Table 5.
Treatment regimens for post-kala-azar dermal leishmaniasis as per WHO recommendations (adopted from WHO) (https://www.who.int/leishmaniasis/research/978924129496_pp67_71.pdf?ua=1) [8].

Geographic areas affected by visceral leishmaniasis	Leishmania species	Recommended treatment regimens ranked by preference
Bangladesh, Bhutan, India and Nepal	*L. donovani*	**1.** Liposomal amphotericin B: 3–5 mg/kg per daily dose by infusion given over 3–5 days period up to a total dose of 15 mg/kg (A) by infusion or 10 mg/kg as a single dose by infusion (A) **2.** Combinations (co-administered) (A): • Liposomal amphotericin B (5 mg/kg by infusion, single dose) plus miltefosine (daily for 7 days, as below) • Liposomal amphotericin B (5 mg/kg by infusion, single dose) plus paromomycin (daily for 10 days, as below) • Miltefosine plus paromomycin, both daily for 10 days, as below **3.** Amphotericin B deoxycholate: 0.75–1.0 mg/kg per day by infusion, daily or on alternate days for 15–20 doses (A) **4.** Miltefosine: for children aged 2–11 years, 2.5 mg/kg per day; for people aged ≥ 12 years and < 25 kg body weight, 50 mg/day; 25–50 kg body weight, 100 mg/day; > 50 kg body weight, 150 mg/day; orally for 28 days (A) **OR** Paromomycin: 15 mg (11 mg base) per kg body weight per day intramuscularly for 21 days (A) **5.** Pentavalent antimonials: 20 mg Sb5+/kg per day intramuscularly or intravenously for 30 days in areas where they remain effective: Bangladesh, Nepal and the Indian states of Jharkhand, West Bengal and Uttar Pradesh (A)
East Africa (Ethiopia, Eritrea, Kenya, Somalia, Sudan and Uganda) and Yemen	*L. donovani*	**1.** Combination: pentavalent antimonials (20 mg Sb5+/kg per day intramuscularly or intravenously) plus paromomycin (15 mg [11 mg base] per kg body weight per day intramuscularly) for 17 days (A) **2.** Pentavalent antimonials: 20 mg Sb5+/kg per day intramuscularly or intravenously for 30 days (A) **3.** Liposomal amphotericin B: 3–5 mg/kg per daily dose by infusion given over 6–10 days up to a total dose of 30 mg/kg (B) **4.** Amphotericin B deoxycholate: 0.75–1 mg/kg per day by infusion, daily or on alternate days, for 15–20 doses (A) **5.** Miltefosine orally for 28 days at dosage as above (A)
Mediterranean Basin, Middle East, Central Asia, South America	*L. infantum*	**1.** Liposomal amphotericin B: 3–5 mg/kg per daily dose by infusion given over a 3–6 days period, up to a total dose of 18–21 mg/kg (B) **2.** Pentavalent antimonials: 20 mg Sb5+/kg per day intramuscularly or intravenously for 28 days (B) **3.** Amphotericin B deoxycholate: 0.75–1.0 mg/kg per day by infusion, daily or on alternate days for 20–30 doses, for a total dose of 2–3 g (C)

Table 6.
Treatment regimens for visceral leishmaniasis as per WHO recommendations (adopted from WHO) (https://www.who.int/leishmaniasis/research/9789241294969_pp67_71.pdf?ua=1) [8].

the Indian subcontinent; however currently several combination regimens are available which will alleviate the risk of resistance development to LAMB therapy (**Table 6**) [17, 18].

6.5 Human immunodeficiency virus (HIV): Visceral leishmaniasis coinfection

VL should be treated as an opportunistic infection if diagnosed in patients with HIV, warranting lifelong antiretroviral therapy regardless of CD4 count [27]. The core infected patients require longer treatment with higher doses since they are at a higher risk for disease relapse, poor outcome, and increased mortality. In addition, developing VL disease in HIV patients adversely affects their response to antiretroviral therapy [43]. Current WHO recommendation, so far, is LAMB for all regions. Some cases may require combination treatment including LAMB with mitefosine, pentavalent antimonials, and/or amphotericin B deoxycholate. Randomized control trials are ongoing in both Ethiopia and India comparing combination of LAMB and miltefosine with LAMB monotherapy [44, 45].

6.6 Surgical intervention

Surgical intervention is not the recommended modality of treatment in majority of leishmaniasis cases; however, surgery may be required in certain cases such as splenectomy in resistant disease, orofacial surgery for severely debilitating ML, and cosmetic surgery for disfiguring cutaneous lesions.

7. Prevention and control

L. donovani is perhaps one of the most virulent *Leishmania* species and is present in South Asian region, one of the highest incidence areas of VL. Between 2005 and 2013, *Leishmania* ranked the second worst next only to malaria among the 16 categories of "neglected tropical diseases" [46]. In 2005 the WHO and the government representatives of India, Nepal, and Bangladesh signed a memorandum of understanding with commitment to mutually cooperate in order to achieve VL elimination from these countries by 2015. The objective was to reduce the annual incidence of VL to below 1/10,000 inhabitants by 2015 using detection and treatment of VL cases and vector control measures [47]. The target was not achieved by the expected date of 2015 due to high cost and limited availability of treatment, lack of effectiveness of vector control measures, emergence of parasite resistance, and low community coverage of health services in all areas. A second target was set for 2017; however, the WHO has recently reset the target of VL elimination from the Indian subcontinent to year 2020 [48]. In the Eastern Mediterranean region, a specific target was set for CL to detect 70% of all cases and at least treat 90% of them. There is crucial gap in planning elimination of VL in Asia and VL and CL in other regions. These elimination campaigns will require more intense work and better strategic planning in addition to the high cost required. Currently, there is increased global awareness about the disease and the dire need for its elimination, in particular, after Asian elimination initiative of VL and 2012 London declaration on neglected tropical diseases. Having said that, many challenges still exist that counteract these efforts. These include poor sanitary conditions, conflict zones leading to forced migration, emerging atypical variants, poor public awareness especially in nonendemic areas, suboptimal diagnostic modalities, and limited treatment options [1, 49].

7.1 Mass treatment

The VL elimination initiative in the Indian subcontinent in collaboration with the WHO was based on diagnosis and treatment of VL patients using mass treatment to reach the target of reducing the annual VL incidence to below 1/10,000. This plan was dependent on actively looking for and diagnosing *Leishmania* patients. However, the target date was missed because of several factors including limitations of diagnostic tools to diagnose patients actively, lack of health-care coverage in certain areas in developing countries in particular rural regions, lack of proper vector control, and high cost and limited availability of treatment [46–48].

7.2 Vector control strategies

Including insecticide-treated nets and indoor insecticide sprays are used for areas where sandflies bite indoor. Recently resistance to dichlorodiphenyltrichloroethane (DDT) is reported to emerge, and therefore other synthetic products such as pyrethroids started to be used [50]. In areas like Africa where the vector mainly bites outdoor, selective outdoor spraying might be effective in reducing vector density. In addition alternative vector control measures have been proposed and used such as plastering of walls and floors using mud and lime. However these environmental management methods need further evaluation and validation. The KALANET project was the only trial that evaluated the impact of "long-lasting insecticidal nets" on *L. donovani* and concluded that these nets have beneficial effects against *L. donovani* as they provide some degree of personal protection against infection as compared to those using untreated nets or no nets. Further prospective studies are needed to evaluate integrated vector management measures on VL and other vector-borne diseases [47].

7.3 Reservoir eradication/control

In areas of zoonotic transmission should be effectively targeted to reduce the human infection rate from infected animal reservoir. Several reservoir control measures have been used including animal elimination in certain areas, canine vaccines, and insecticides used on dogs such as spot-on insecticide which are drops applied on skin under the hair in the neck region, insecticide-impregnated dog collars, and whole body insecticide use. Studies on efficacy of animal reservoir intervention programs are limited and show lack of generalizability of intervention measures as well as mixed results [17]. In addition there are also conflicting results on the impact of dogs in transmission of leishmaniasis since not all infected dogs become infectious. All the above factors point towards a fundamental gap in our knowledge of disease biology and its transmission.

7.4 Minimizing outdoor exposure

At dawn to dusk which are the peak bite times and use of insecticide-treated nets and/or fine-mesh nets since the sandflies are small in size and can pass through standard mosquito nets.

7.5 Transmission via blood

Infected patients should not donate blood or organs since the parasite can be transmitted through blood.

7.6 Immunization/vaccination

Several candidate vaccines are in preclinical development, and at least three are currently in clinical studies; however, no effective vaccine has been identified to date to effectively prevent human leishmaniasis [51]. Some studies show vaccination by killed *Leishmania* promastigotes, and live BCG can develop protection against CL, but no protection is seen against VL. Approximately 90–98% of leishmaniasis patients recover after disease and develop natural acquired immunity mainly due to Th1 lymphocyte activation and its reaction towards the infecting parasite. This strongly supports the ongoing vaccination development efforts, hopefully looking forward for a clinically efficient vaccine to be available in the near future.

All the above measures have shown some success; however, they are costly and require extensive coordination efforts globally. Early diagnosis and treatment remain the main control strategy since untreated patients serve as reservoirs of parasites. In most countries majority of patients present themselves to the health care, suggesting that many cases will remain in the community for long periods before seeking health care due to reduced awareness. Strategy for eradication would require surveillance with early detection and prompt treatment measures applied globally, mostly in heavily infested areas.

7.7 Postinfection immunity

Successfully treated patients who receive full course of therapy by effective agents and self-resolving infections generally acquire immunity from the infecting species in 97–98% of the cases.

7.8 Long-term monitoring

Prolonged monitoring and follow-up evaluations of patients after successful treatment are recommended for relapse or recurrence of the disease. Yearly follow-up is recommended for patients infected with *L. braziliensis* for up to a decade for early detection of any progression to mucocutaneous disease. Certain complex cases of ML, diffuse CL, *L. recidivans*, and PKDL can be difficult to treat and may require prolonged therapy. In addition, retreatment and/or second-line medications may be required for patients with resistant disease.

8. Conclusion

There has been increasing global awareness about leishmaniasis and the need for its eradication. However, there are many challenges that hinder this global initiative and maintain leishmaniasis as one of the neglected tropical diseases. These challenges include but are not limited to high cost, variability of clinical spectrum, cyclic transmission patterns, changing disease foci, emerging atypical and resistant forms, suboptimal diagnostics, limited treatment options/availability, and suboptimal community awareness and health-care coverage, in particular in nonendemic areas. Several preventive measures using various strategies are needed to tackle personal human protection against infection, interventions targeting vector and animal reservoir control. With the current known challenges and limitations of resources, perhaps integrated approach to control this infection and focus on development of effective vaccine for protection may be a strategic way to use the limited resources available to reach the WHO's set target of leishmaniasis reduction/elimination [17].

For WHO to reach its leishmaniasis elimination target, seriously committed global efforts with substantial funding will be required. However, the question whether complete accomplishment of this goal is technically achievable, given the abovementioned challenges, remains to be answered.

Author details

Salwa S. Sheikh[1*], Amaar A. Amir[2], Baraa A. Amir[2] and Abdulrazack A. Amir[3]

1 Pathology Services, Johns Hopkins Aramco Healthcare, Dhahran, Saudi Arabia

2 Imam Abdulrahman Bin Faisal University, Dammam, Saudi Arabia

3 Office of Academic Affairs, Johns Hopkins Aramco Healthcare, Dhahran, Saudi Arabia

*Address all correspondence to: salwa.sheikh@jhah.com; sheikhss28@gmail.com

IntechOpen

© 2020 The Author(s). Licensee IntechOpen. This chapter is distributed under the terms of the Creative Commons Attribution License (http://creativecommons.org/licenses/by/3.0), which permits unrestricted use, distribution, and reproduction in any medium, provided the original work is properly cited. (cc) BY

References

[1] Burza S, Croft SL, Boelaert M. Leishmaniasis. The Lancet. 2018; **392**(10151):951-970. Available from: https://www.thelancet.com/journals/lancet/article/PIIS0140-6736(18)31204-2/fulltext

[2] Alvar J, Vélez ID, Bern C, Herrero M, Desjeux P, Cano J, et al. Leishmaniasis worldwide and global estimates of its incidence. PLoS One. 2012;7(5):e35671. Available from: https://journals.plos.org/plosone/article?id=10.1371/journal.pone.0035671

[3] Gramiccia M, Gradoni L. The current status of zoonotic leishmaniases and approaches to disease control. International Journal for Parasitology. 2005;**35**(11-12):1169-1180. Available from: https://www.sciencedirect.com/science/article/abs/pii/S0020751905002420?via=ihub

[4] Auwera GVD, Dujardin J-C. Species typing in dermal leishmaniasis. Clinical Microbiology Reviews. 2015;**28**(2):265-294. Available from: https://cmr.asm.org/content/28/2/265

[5] Aronson N. Cutaneous leishmaniasis: Clinical manifestations and diagnosis. UpToDate. Available from: https://www.uptodate.com/contents/cutaneous-leishmaniasis-clinical-manifestations-and-diagnosis [Accessed: 12-08-2019]

[6] Bern C. Visceral leishmaniasis: Clinical manifestations and diagnosis. UpToDate. Available from: https://www.uptodate.com/contents/visceral-leishmaniasis-clinical-manifestations-and-diagnosis [Accessed: 12-08-2019]

[7] Zijlstra EE. The immunology of post-kala-azar dermal leishmaniasis (PKDL). Parasites & Vectors. 2016;**9**(1):464. Available from: https://parasitesandvectors.biomedcentral.com/articles/10.1186/s13071-016-1721-0

[8] Burza S, Sinha PK, Mahajan R, Sanz MG, Lima MA, Mitra G, et al. Post Kala-Azar dermal leishmaniasis following treatment with 20 mg/kg liposomal amphotericin B (Ambisome) for primary visceral leishmaniasis in Bihar, India. PLoS Neglected Tropical Diseases. 2014;**8**(1):e2611. Available from: https://journals.plos.org/plosntds/article?id=10.1371/journal.pntd.0002611

[9] Uranw S, Ostyn B, Rijal A, Devkota S, Khanal B, Menten J, et al. Post-Kala-azar dermal leishmaniasis in Nepal: A retrospective cohort study (2000–2010). PLoS Neglected Tropical Diseases. 2011;**5**(12):e1433. Available from: https://journals.plos.org/plosntds/article?id=10.1371/journal.pntd.0001433

[10] Desjeux P. Leishmaniasis: Current situation and new perspectives. Comparative Immunology, Microbiology and Infectious Diseases. 2004;**27**(5):305-318. Available from: https://www.sciencedirect.com/science/article/pii/S0147957104000232?via=ihub

[11] Pavli A, Maltezou HC. Leishmaniasis, an emerging infection in travelers. International Journal of Infectious Diseases. 2010;**14**(12):e1032-e1039. Available from: https://www.ijidonline.com/article/S1201-9712(10)02485-9/fulltext

[12] Wall EC, Lockwood DN, Armstrong M, Chiodini PL, Watson J. Epidemiology of imported cutaneous leishmaniasis at the hospital for Tropical Diseases, London, United Kingdom: Use of polymerase chain reaction to identify the species. The American Journal of Tropical Medicine and Hygiene. 2012;**86**(1):115-118. Available from: http://www.ajtmh.org/content/journals/10.4269/ajtmh.2012.10-0558

[13] Stark CG. Leishmaniasis. Medscape. 2019 Available from: https://emedicine.

medscape.com/article/220298-overview [Accessed 08-08-2019]

[14] Sunter J, Gull K. Shape, form, function and leishmania pathogenicity: From textbook descriptions to biological understanding. Open Biology. 2017; 7(9):170165. Available from: https://royalsocietypublishing.org/doi/10.1098/rsob.170165

[15] Hide M, Bucheton B, Kamhawi S, Bras-Gonalves R, Sundar S, Lemesre J-L, et al. Understanding human leishmaniasis: The need for an integrated approach. In: Encyclopedia of Infectious Diseases. Wiley-Liss. John Wiley & sons, Inc, Publication; 2007. pp. 87-123. Available from: https://www.mivegec.ird.fr/images/stories/PDF_files/0012.pdf

[16] Stockdale L, Newton R. A review of preventative methods against human leishmaniasis infection. PLoS Neglected Tropical Diseases. 2013;7(6):e2278. Available from: https://journals.plos.org/plosntds/article?id=10.1371/journal.pntd.0002278

[17] WHO Report on Global Surveillance of Epidemic-prone Infectious Diseases - Leishmaniasis. WHO. World Health Organization; 2015. Available from: https://www.who.int/csr/resources/publications/CSR_ISR_2000_1leish/en/ [Accessed 12-08-2019]

[18] CDC - Leishmaniasis. CDC. Centers for Disease Control and Prevention. Available from: https://www.cdc.gov/parasites/leishmaniasis/ [Accessed 12 August 2019]

[19] Thakur L, Singh KK, Shanker V, Negi A, Jain A, Matlashewski G, et al. Atypical leishmaniasis: A global perspective with emphasis on the Indian subcontinent. PLoS Neglected Tropical Diseases. 2018;12(9):e0006659. Available from: https://journals.plos.org/plosntds/article?id=10.1371/journal.pntd.0006659

[20] Scott P, Novais FO. Cutaneous leishmaniasis: Immune responses in protection and pathogenesis. Nature Reviews Immunology. 2016;16(9): 581-592. Available from: https://www.nature.com/articles/nri.2016.72

[21] Zijlstra EE. PKDL and other dermal lesions in HIV Co-infected patients with leishmaniasis: Review of clinical presentation in relation to immune responses. PLoS Neglected Tropical Diseases. 2014;8(11):e3258. Available from: https://journals.plos.org/plosntds/article?id=10.1371/journal.pntd.0003258

[22] Cincurá C, Lessa MM, Machado PRL, Glesby MJ, Carvalho EM, Oliveira-Filho J, et al. Mucosal leishmaniasis: A retrospective study of 327 cases from an endemic area of leishmania (Viannia) braziliensis. The American Journal of Tropical Medicine and Hygiene. 2017;97(3):761-766. Available from: http://www.ajtmh.org/content/journals/10.4269/ajtmh.16-0349

[23] Zacarias DA, Rolão N, Pinho FAD, Sene I, Silva JC, Pereira TC, et al. Causes and consequences of higher leishmania infantum burden in patients with kala-azar: A study of 625 patients. Tropical Medicine & International Health. 2017; 22(6):679-687. Available from: https://onlinelibrary.wiley.com/doi/full/10.1111/tmi.12877

[24] Malafaia G. Protein-energy malnutrition as a risk factor for visceral leishmaniasis: A review. Parasite Immunology. 2009;31(10):587-596. Available from: https://onlinelibrary.wiley.com/doi/abs/10.1111/j.1365-3024.2009.01117.x

[25] ELkhair EB. Elevated cortisol level due to visceral leishmaniasis and skin hyper-pigmentation are causally related. International Journal of Science, Commerce and Humanities. 2014;2: 86-92

[26] Magill AJ, Grogl M, Gasser RA, Sun W, Oster CN. Visceral infection caused by leishmania tropica in veterans of operation desert storm. New England Journal of Medicine. 1993;**328**(19): 1383-1387. Available from: https://www. nejm.org/doi/full/10.1056/ NEJM199305133281904

[27] Control of the leishmaniases: Report of a meeting of the WHO Expert Commitee on the Control of Leishmaniases, Geneva, 22-26 March 2010. WHO. World Health Organization; 1970. Available from: https://apps.who.int/iris/handle/10665/ 44412 [Accessed 08-08-2019]

[28] Ejara ED, Lynen L, Boelaert M, Griensven JV. Challenges in HIV and visceral leishmania co-infection: Future research directions. Tropical Medicine & International Health. 2010;**15**(10): 1266-1267. Available from: https:// onlinelibrary.wiley.com/doi/full/ 10.1111/j.1365-3156.2010.02612.x

[29] Stark D, Pett S, Marriott D, Harkness J. Post-Kala-Azar dermal leishmaniasis due to leishmania infantum in a human immunodeficiency virus type 1-infected patient. Journal of Clinical Microbiology. 2006 Mar;**44**(3): 1178-1180. Available from: https://jcm. asm.org/content/44/3/1178

[30] Sundar S, Rai M. Laboratory diagnosis of visceral leishmaniasis. Clinical and Vaccine Immunology. 2002;**9**(5):951-958. Available from: https://cvi.asm.org/content/9/5/ 951/article-info

[31] Zijlstra EE, Nur Y, Desjeux P, Khalil EAG, El-Hassan AM, Groen J. Diagnosing visceral leishmaniasis with the recombinant K39 strip test: Experience from the Sudan. Tropical Medicine and International Health. 2008;**6**(2):108-113. Available from: https://onlinelibrary.wiley.com/doi/abs/ 10.1046/j.1365-3156.2001.00680.x

[32] Wortmann G, Sweeney C, Houng H-H, Weina P, Zapor M, Hochberg L, et al. Rapid identification of leishmania complexes by a real-time Pcr assay. The American Journal of Tropical Medicine and Hygiene. 2005;**73**(6):999-1004. Available from: http://www.ajtmh.org/ content/journals/10.4269/ajtmh. 2005.73.999

[33] Boelaert M, Verdonck K, Menten J, Sunyoto T, Griensven JV, Chappuis F, et al. Rapid tests for the diagnosis of visceral leishmaniasis in patients with suspected disease. Cochrane Database of Systematic Reviews. 2014;**2014**: CD009135. Available from: https:// www.cochranelibrary.com/cdsr/doi/ 10.1002/14651858.CD009135.pub2/full

[34] Mukhtar M, Abdoun A, Ahmed AE, Ghalib H, Reed SG, Boelaert M, et al. Diagnostic accuracy of rK28-based immunochromatographic rapid diagnostic tests for visceral leishmaniasis: A prospective clinical cohort study in Sudan. Transactions of the Royal Society of Tropical Medicine and Hygiene. 2015;**109**(9):594-600. Available from: https://academic.oup. com/trstmh/article-abstract/109/9/594/ 1913629?redirectedFrom=fulltext

[35] Vallur AC, Tutterrow YL, Mohamath R, Pattabhi S, Hailu A, Abdoun AO, et al. Development and comparative evaluation of two antigen detection tests for visceral leishmaniasis. BMC Infectious Diseases. 2015;**15**(1): 384. Available from: https://bmcinfectd is.biomedcentral.com/articles/10.1186/ s12879-015-1125-3

[36] Oliveira RMD, Melo SDA, Penha-Silva TAD, Almeida-Souza F, Abreu-Silva AL. Alternative treatment for leishmaniasis. In: Leishmaniases as Re-emerging Diseases. IntechOpen. 2018. Available from: https://www.intechopen. com/books/leishmaniases-as-re-emerg ing-diseases/alternative-treatment-for-leishmaniasis

[37] Cragg GM, Grothaus PG, Newman DJ. Impact of natural products on developing new anti-cancer agents. Chemical Reviews. 2009;**109**(7): 3012-3043. Available from: https://pubs.acs.org/doi/10.1021/cr900019j

[38] Almassy Júnior AA. Folhas de chá: Plantas medicinais na terapêutica humana. Vol. 233. Vicosa: UFV; 2005. Available from: https://www.editoraufv.com.br/produto/folhas-de-cha-plantas-medicinais-na-terapeutica-humana/1111246

[39] Jantan I, Ahmad W, Bukhari SNA. Plant-derived immunomodulators: An insight on their preclinical evaluation and clinical trials. Frontiers in Plant Science. 2015;**6**:655. Available from: https://www.frontiersin.org/articles/10.3389/fpls.2015.00655/full

[40] Tiwari B, Pahuja R, Kumar P, Rath SK, Gupta KC, Goyal N. Nanotized curcumin and miltefosine, a potential combination for treatment of experimental visceral leishmaniasis. Antimicrobial Agents and Chemotherapy. 2017;**61**(3):e01169-16. Available from: https://aac.asm.org/content/61/3/e01169-16

[41] Aronson N, Herwaldt BL, Libman M, Pearson R, Lopez-Velez R, Weina P, et al. Diagnosis and treatment of leishmaniasis: Clinical practice guidelines by the Infectious Diseases Society of America (IDSA) and the American Society of Tropical Medicine and Hygiene (ASTMH). The American Journal of Tropical Medicine and Hygiene. 2016;**96**(1):24-45. Available from: http://www.ajtmh.org/content/journals/10.4269/ajtmh.16-84256

[42] Balasegaram M, Ritmeijer K, Lima MA, Burza S, Genovese GO, Milani B, et al. Liposomal amphotericin B as a treatment for human leishmaniasis. Expert Opinion on Emerging Drugs. 2012;**17**(4):493-510. Available from: https://www.tandf online.com/doi/full/10.1517/14728214.2012.748036

[43] Jarvis JN, Lockwood DN. Clinical aspects of visceral leishmaniasis in HIV infection. Current Opinion in Infectious Diseases. 2013;**26**(1):1-9. Available from: https://insights.ovid.com/article/00001432-201302000-00002

[44] Ritmeijer K. Old and new treatments for HIV/VL co-infection. In: Proceedings of the Fifth World Leishmaniasis Congress. Brazil: Porto de Galhinas; 2013

[45] Mahajan R, Das P, Isaakidis P, Sunyoto T, Sagili KD, Lima MA, et al. Combination treatment for visceral leishmaniasis patients Coinfected with human immunodeficiency virus in India. Clinical Infectious Diseases. 2015; **61**(8):1255-1262. Available from: https://academic.oup.com/cid/article/61/8/1255/377023

[46] Karunaweera ND, Ferreira MU. Leishmaniasis: Current challenges and prospects for elimination with special focus on the South Asian region. Parasitology. 2018;**145**(4):425-429. Available from: https://www.cambridge.org/core/journals/parasitology/article/leishmaniasis-current-challenges-and-prospects-for-elimination-with-special-focus-on-the-south-asian-region/F91C2C42B2C5B1C000193C50949502A6

[47] Picado A, Dash A, Bhattacharya S, Boelaert M. Vector control interventions for visceral leishmaniasis elimination initiative in South Asia, 2005–2010. Indian Journal of Medical Research. 2012;**136**(1):22-31. Available from: https://www.ncbi.nlm.nih.gov/pmc/articles/PMC3461713/

[48] Selvapandiyan A, Croft SL, Rijal S, Nakhasi HL, Ganguly NK. Innovations for the elimination and control of visceral leishmaniasis. PLoS Neglected Tropical Diseases. 2019;**13**(9):e0007616.

Available from: https://journals.plos.
org/plosntds/article?id=10.1371/journal.
pntd.0007616

[49] London Declaration on Neglected
Tropical Diseases. Uniting to Combat
NTDs; 2012. Available from: https://
unitingtocombatntds.org/london-
declaration-neglected-tropical-diseases/
[Accessed: 08 August 2019]

[50] Coleman M, Foster GM, Deb R,
Singh RP, Ismail HM, Shivam P, et al.
DDT-based indoor residual spraying
suboptimal for visceral leishmaniasis
elimination in India. Proceedings of the
National Academy of Sciences. 2015;
112(28):8573-8578 Available from:
https://www.pnas.org/content/112/28/
8573

[51] Alvar J, Croft SL, Kaye P,
Khamesipour A, Sundar S, Reed SG.
Case study for a vaccine against
leishmaniasis. Vaccine. 2013;**31**:B244-
B249. Available from: https://www.
sciencedirect.com/science/article/pii/
S0264410X12017318?via=ihub

Chapter 17

A New Outlook in Lymphatic Filariasis Elimination in India

Susanta Kumar Ghosh and Pradeep Kumar Srivastava

Abstract

In India, human lymphatic filariasis (LF) is the most common vector-borne disease after malaria. It is a roundworm nematode parasitic helminthiases group of diseases under Filarioidea type of infection. The parasites are found in the lymphatic system, damage the system leading to deformities of body organs. Of the eight human filarial parasites, *Wuchereria bancrofti*, *Brugia malayi* and *B. timori* are involved with the lymphatic system. Globally *W. bancrofti* is the most predominant species sharing 90% of the burden. In India, *W. bancrofti* and *B. malayi* are present. The revised control strategy was aimed at a single-dose mass drug administration (MDA) and home-based morbidity management. The Elimination of LF (ELF) was initiated in 2004 in 202 districts which were expanded later in 256 districts after a pilot study in LF endemic districts initiated in 1997. The initial start of ELF campaign was with a single drug, i.e. diethylcarbamazine (DEC), but later in 2007, a combination of two drugs DEC and albendazole (ALB) were given through MDA. Now a third drug ivermectin (IVM) has been added to accelerate the elimination process by 2020 which is the global goal of elimination under Global Programme to Eliminate Lymphatic Filariasis (GPELF).

Keywords: lymphatic filariasis, elimination, *Wuchereria bancrofti*, *Brugia malayi*, diethylcarbamazine, albendazole, ivermectin, DEC-medicated salt, transmission assessment survey, xenomonitoring

1. Introduction

There are eight parasites responsible for filarial infections. Three parasites *Wuchereria bancrofti* (Cobbold 1877), *Brugia malayi* (Brug 1927) and *B. timori* (Partono et al. 1977) are responsible for lymphatic filariasis (LF) that impairs the lymphatic system leading to severe organ deformities leading to social stigma [1–3]. In India, the first two species *W. bancrofti* and *B. malayi* are present. *W. bancrofti* contributes 99.4% of the total burden. It is a roundworm nematode parasitic helminthiasis group of diseases under the Filarioidea type of infection. The main affected organs are legs and genitals causing 'elephantiasis' and hydrocele in males and breast filariasis in females followed by relentless disability causing social stigma. In Indian local language the disease is known as 'Hathipaon'. In India, LF is the second most vector-borne disease after malaria and globally ranks third after malaria and tuberculosis. The World Health Organization (WHO) estimated that LF is found in 81 tropical and subtropical countries with 120 million infected cases and with one billion people at risk; 947 million people are threatened, whereas 40 million people are disfigured by this infection. Four countries India, Indonesia,

Bangladesh (all Asian countries) and Nigeria (Africa) contribute about 70% of the LF infection in the world [4].

In the sixth century BC in his book, *Susruta Samhita*, Susruta mentioned this disease. In the seventh century AD in his memoir, *Madhava Nidhana*, Madhavarakara first described the signs and symptoms of this disease. In 1709, Clarke described 'Malabar legs' from Cochin which is synonymous with elephantiasis. In 1872 in Calcutta (now Kolkata), Lewis first described the microfilariae (Mf) in human blood [5].

LF is distributed in economically challenged countries. *W. bancrofti* is the most predominant species of human filariasis. It was recognized primarily as an urban disease which does not have animal reservoirs. Later it is reported from rural areas also. The parasites develop only in humans and in mosquitoes. But the adult worms may survive for 8–10 years and produce huge numbers of Mf from time to time. This is actually the real challenge in containing the disease.

2. Search methods

We have searched MEDLINE (PubMed) and CAB Abstracts, checked the reference lists of all studies identified by the search, also performed Google Search on specific topics and examined references listed in review articles and previously compiled bibliographies.

3. Genesis and evolution of the elimination of lymphatic filariasis

LF is responsible for deformities and disfigures of potential organs caused by this disease which make social stigma leading to hardship on normal life. Many marriageable persons undergo physical and psychological distress throughout their lives. LF is one of the six infectious diseases identified by the International Task Force for Disease Eradication of the WHO as 'eradicable' or 'potentially eradicable' in 1993 [6]. In 1997, the World Health Assembly resolved to eliminate LF as a public health problem globally [7]. In 2000, the WHO launched Global Programme to Eliminate Lymphatic Filariasis (GPELF). Following the London declaration on neglected tropical diseases (NTDs) in 2012, and consequent on several recent advances on the new knowledge of the pathogenesis, the biology of the parasite, development of better diagnostic tools and treatment strategies of LF, GPELF has an aim to eliminate this disease globally by 2020. India, a signatory to the World Health Assembly resolution, had initially set the target for elimination of filariasis by the year 2015 [4] but later aligned with global target of 2020 which is again to be reset. This programme is based on two components consisting of (i) interruption of transmission to prevent the disease by mass drug administration (MDA) and (ii) alleviation of the morbidity (lymphedema and hydrocele) associated with the disease [8]. Of the two strategies, preventive chemotherapy delivered through MDA has gained prominence as interruption of transmission after the implementation of the GPELF.

4. Mass drug administration: scientific background

Before the concept of MDA, the main strategy of LF management was selective treatment by identifying Mf carriers microscopically and/or clinically manifested cases and their treatment with diethylcarbamazine (DEC) for 12 days for individual cure. This strategy was focused on individual level where the people with low parasitaemia and asymptomatic were left and therefore infection persisted in the community. In the subsequent years, there were significant improvements of LF diagnosis and treatment. Combination of double to triple drugs in single doses has been found to be efficacious than monotherapy. Albendazole (ALB) and more recent ivermectin (IVM) have been added to DEC. Now DEC + ALB is used in the MDA programme, and additionally IVM has been advocated for treating the entire population at high risk [5].

Human pharmacokinetic studies on the two regimens of single-dose drugs have shown that all the three drugs when administered singly or as a partner were well tolerated and safe in both microfilaraemic and non-microfilaraemic cases. Efficacy studies of repeated annual MDAs on different combination drugs of ALB + DEC, ALB + IVM and DEC + IVM indicated significant reductions on Mf rate for long periods [9]. Microsimulation models based on drug coverage, its efficacy and endemicity level of LF have indicated the effectiveness of MDA on ELF. This enabled to assess the number of MDA rounds necessary to achieve elimination [10, 11].

5. Filariasis control initiatives in India

LF is considered one of the NTDs that cause huge deformities and disabilities on the society. India contributes the major burden globally. The initial effort was to establish the concept of controlling the disease. In the concept of its elimination on the line of global initiative, India has made significant progress. In India, LF is caused by two roundworm nematode parasites *W. bancrofti* and *B. malayi* and is transmitted by the mosquito vectors *Culex quinquefasciatus*, *Mansonia annulifera* and *M. uniformis*. *B. malayi* which contributes to a negligible proportion is present in Kerala, Andhra Pradesh, Odisha, Madhya Pradesh, Assam and West Bengal. In general, Bihar state has the highest endemicity while Goa the lowest [12]. Here a detailed recent account has been enumerated.

5.1 National filaria control programme

After the pilot project in Orissa from 1949 to 1954 and based on its assessment, In India, the National Filaria Control Programme (NFCP) was launched in 1955. The main objective was to control the problem, have effective planning for control measures in endemic areas and also to train health personnel to strengthen the programme. The immediate control measures were mass drug administration of DEC, antilarval measures in urban areas and indoor residual spray in the rural areas. The programme was assessed four times by the assessment committees in 1961, 1971, 1982 and 1995, respectively. In 1961, the assessment revealed the failure of mass DEC administration due to community reluctance and ineffectiveness of insecticidal indoor spray due to the high resistance in the vector, and therefore as per recommendation of assessment committee, recurrent antilarval measures, establishment of new control units in endemic urban areas and provision of disposal of sewage and sullage were instituted. In 1971, the assessment committee recommended the detection and treatment of Mf cases with DEC at a dose of 6 mg/kg per day for 12 days and antilarval measures. Again in 1982, the assessment committee recommended extension of NFCP to rural areas through primary health-care system with 100% central assistance [5]. The fourth assessment in 1995 recommended to launch a project on the eradication of *B. malayi*, integrated vector control for all vector borne diseases, adoption of model bye-laws for effective control of vectors in domestic situation and fresh delimitation survey in rural areas.

5.2 Diethylcarbamazine-medicated salt

Mass treatment with DEC-medicated salt at community level has been used in a number of places as a control measure for lymphatic filariasis. In India this regimen was initiated as pilot projects in 1968–1969 in Uttar Pradesh and Andhra Pradesh. This showed very encouraging results. A recent review from 11 communities from China, India, Taiwan, Tanzania and Haiti on DEC-medicated salt in high-endemic districts and also in *B. malayi* areas opined high impact of this strategy which may be an end game for LF elimination. In 1976–1977 the distribution of 0.1% DEC-medicated salt was distributed in a population of 25,000 in Lakshadweep Island. There was an 80% reduction on Mf rate and 90% on circulating Mf after 1 year. Similarly, 0.2% salt conducted in Karaikal, Puducherry, showed 98% reduction on Mf [13]. A recent study on DEC-fortified salt (0.2%) and iodine for the elimination of diurnally sub-periodic *W. bancrofti* in Andaman and Nicobar Island showed encouraging results. Community coverage of >90% resulted in the reduction of Mf rate from 2.27 to 0.14% in the DEC-salt-arm (<1% in all the villages) and 1.26 to 0.74% (>1% in 4 out of 14 villages) in the MDA-arm. Antigen prevalence reduced to zero from 1.0 (DEC-salt + MDA-arm) to 6.3% (MDA-arm) in 2–3 years old, 1.2 to 3.6% from 2.9 in the DEC-salt-arm and 4.5% in the MDA-arm among 6–7 years old [14]. However, studies have indicated that it has to be used in specific situations [15].

5.3 Improved diagnosis of lymphatic filariasis

There are several methods for the diagnosis of LF. The microfilariae can be detected directly through blood smear examination, membrane filtration method, DEC-provocative test and quantitative buffy coat methods. Other methods are polymerase chain reaction (PCR), ultrasonography, lymphoscintigraphy (LSG), X-ray diagnosis and also hematology [16].

Circulating microfilariae can be detected by examining thick smears (20–60 μl) of finger-prick blood. Based on the periodicity of the microfilariae, blood samples are collected either at night hours or during daytime (in Andaman Nicobar Islands where *W. bancrofti* is transmitted by Aedes). The method is cheap and feasible at individual and community levels for mapping the endemicity of lymphatic filariasis and monitoring of MDA activities [17]. It has been observed that blood smear preparation on the micro-slides is a cumbersome process. Alternatively though not recommended in the programme, the finger-pricked whole blood (50 μl) can be collected in citrate–phosphate-dextrose (CPD) solution charged (25 μl) in 1.5 ml microfuge tubes. The tubes can be kept in +4°C freezer and can be examined within 48 hours. CPD-mixed whole blood (20 μl) are drawn by micropipette and placed in a micro-slide. The blood is smeared on the micro-slide and examined under10× microscope when the blood is wet. In positive samples, live moving parasites can be seen easily. This is a very simple method and can be easily executed. If needed, the dry smears can be stained for future reference.

The Filariasis Test Strip (FTS) of Alere (now Abbott Diagnostics) is a rapid diagnostic test recommended for mapping, monitoring and transmission assessment surveys (TAS) for the qualitative detection of *W. bancrofti* antigen in human blood samples. Now, the FTS has replaced the Binax Now filariasis immunochromatographic test (ICT), which also detects the same antigen in blood samples. The Brugia Rapid point-of-care cassette test (BRT) manufactured by Reszon Diagnostics is recommended for use during TAS to detect IgG4 antibody against *Brugia spp.* in human blood samples [17].

5.4 Mass drug administration its coverage and impact

In India, in the initial process of ELF, a district-level survey in 2000 revealed that of the 289 districts, 257 were endemic for LF [18]. In 2002, the National Health Policy had set the interim goal for the elimination of this disease in India by the year 2015 [19]. To support GPELF by raising funds and helping in various other ways, a global coalition was forged among 43 different donors constituting the Global Alliance to Eliminate Lymphatic Filariasis (GAELF). One of the partners GlaxoSmithKline has volunteered to supply the total quantity of albendazole tablets required to eliminate LF globally, free of cost [20]. The DEC tablets needed for the programme in India is being supplied by the central government [19].

In 2004, the elimination of LF programme was launched on June 5 in 202 districts of 15 states and 5 union territories. However, based on the experience of MDA in June 2004 when high temperature prevailed in most of the places, the date of 'National Filaria Day' was changed to November 11 in consultation with the states. To promote and create awareness on LF, this date was observed as 'National Filaria Day' since then. In the beginning, DEC was introduced under the MDA programme and, in 2007 ALB, was added with DEC as a global strategy. Gradually 255 districts were brought under MDA, and the assessment in 2013 indicated that 203 districts out of 255 had reported microfilaria rate <1% [21–24]. The number of districts reporting Mf rate below 1% increased to 222 and in 53 districts where MDA was withdrawn as halt in transmission was indicated. A transmission assessment survey (TAS) was qualified for 68 districts. The remaining districts were struggling to achieve the goal, making the MDA twice in a year [25].

5.5 Transmission assessment survey

TAS is a tool designed to know whether or not transmission is interrupted by MDA. In case, the transmission has been interrupted; the prevalence of circulating antegenaemia among children born after initiation of MDA should be below critical threshold, so that the transmission of disease is no longer sustainable and future generation will be free from this disease. Before TAS, it should be ensured that all implementation units (IUs) have had at least five effective MDAs with >65% of population coverage and each of sentinel, spot and additional spot sites had achieved <1% Mf rate [26].

China and the Republic of Korea have declared to have eliminated lymphatic filariasis as a public health problem in 2007 and 2008, respectively. According to the WHO, 81 endemic countries were reduced to 72 requiring MDA. Out of the 72 countries, 15 have been declared to have eliminated LF as a public health problem. These countries are Togo, Egypt, Maldives, Sri Lanka, Thailand, American Samoa, Cambodia, Cook Islands, Marshall Islands, Niue, Palau, Tonga, Vanuatu, Viet Nam and Wallis and Futuna [26].

Another six countries, namely, Malawi, Brazil, Bangladesh, Kiribati and Lao PDR have stopped MDA and are under post-MDA surveillance. Recent report indicates that two countries Kiribati and Yemen have eliminated LF [17]. Out of the remaining, 5 have not yet started MDA, 32 have fully scaled up MDA and 14 thought to be started and MDA is yet to be scaled up fully [26].

6. Discussion

Now India is on a critical phase for ELF facing serious challenges. The main challenge is the implementation of MDA with improved actual drug compliance so as to cover >80% at-risk population. It is required to have continued IEC activities, community engagement and all-round support [27]. It is really a huge operational and logistical challenge to cover about 650 million populations for the MDA programme.

In June 2018, in the 10th GPELF meeting at New Delhi, India, the government of India launched Accelerated Plan for Lymphatic Filariasis Elimination (APELF). A triple-drug therapy or IDA (IVM, DEC and ALB) along with community engagement has been planned for accelerating the LF elimination in India [28, 29]. As a pilot project, IDA has been rolled out successfully across four districts in India. These districts are Arwal in Bihar (20 December 2018), Simdega in Jharkhand (10 January 2019), Nagpur in Maharashtra (20 January 2019) and Varanasi in Uttar Pradesh (20 February 2019). A total of 8.07 million people out of 10.7 million vulnerable people (75.4%) were benefitted with the IDA medicines. The IDA approach is to be scaled up in all endemic districts to eliminate LF by 2021. It is expected that with triple-drug combination, if effective, actual drug compliance is achieved; the MDA districts may qualify for TAS and also clear the TAS successfully.

Another important issue is asymptomatic cases in children age group. In some endemic areas, about 30% of children have acquired LF by the age of 4 years either with the presence of Mf or *W. bancrofti* antigen in their blood [30]. Similarly, in a *B. malayi* area in Kerala, asymptomatic Mf has been demonstrated in children through LSG [31]. LF parasites in human do not have animal reservoirs. But human dirofilariasis, i.e. zoonotic transmission to human, cannot be ruled out. This thing should be kept in mind after successful ELF in human [32]. There are other issues of management of acute and chronic filariasis cases and treatment of adenolymphangitis (ADL) cases with antibiotics since the majority of acute episodes are bacterial origin. The APELF provides free morbidity management and disability prevention services through kits and corrective surgeries [28].

Vector surveillance is another important tool to facilitate in instituting vector control measures as well as to assess the infection in vectors in the areas. Xenomonitoring, in other words, the presence of Mf larvae in vector mosquitoes, is a method to assess the effectiveness of the post-MDA and TAS. Specific PCR technique is applied [33]. Recently Khatri et al. screened the presence of *W. bancrofti* L3-specific *Ssp1* gene in trapped mosquitoes by PCR in certain districts in Maharashtra and Karnataka. This indicated that MDA needed to be strengthened [33]. Scaling up xenomonitoring is a big challenge in existing infrastructure with weak strength of skilled entomologists. At present IVM has been planned to introduce in all LF endemic districts in India covering many districts endemic for malaria also. IVM introduction in context of malaria control is towards targeting their vector populations [34]. It is important to assess the impact of other coexistent diseases in the same eco-endemic regions [35].

7. Conclusion

India is on a very strong ground to achieve lymphatic elimination [19]. Several efforts are now in place. The total disability-adjusted life years (DALYs) lost due to LF is around 2.06 million, resulting in an annual wage loss of US $811 million [36]. A special emphasis has been given on the general hygiene and environmental management of mosquito vectors under the *Swachh Bharat Mission* (Clean India Movement) and also to provide special incentive under the *Ayushman Bharat* to make the programme effective and successful [37].

Conflict of interest

The authors declare no conflict of interest.

Author details

Susanta Kumar Ghosh[1*] and Pradeep Kumar Srivastava[2]

1 ICMR-National Institute of Malaria Research, Bengaluru, India

2 National Vector Borne Disease Control Programme, Delhi, India

*Address all correspondence to: ghoshnimr@gmail.com

IntechOpen

© 2020 The Author(s). Licensee IntechOpen. This chapter is distributed under the terms of the Creative Commons Attribution License (http://creativecommons.org/licenses/by/3.0), which permits unrestricted use, distribution, and reproduction in any medium, provided the original work is properly cited. [cc] BY

References

[1] Cobbold TS. Discovery of the adult representative of microscopic filariae. Lancet. 1877;2:70-71

[2] Brug SL. Filaria malayi, new species. Parasitic in man in the Malay Archipelago. Transactions of the 7th Congress of the Far Eastern Association of Tropical Medicine. 1927;iii:279

[3] Partono F, Aennis DT, Atmosoedjono S, et al. *Brugia timori* sp.n. (nematode: Filarioidea) from Flores Island, Indonesia. Journal of Parasitology. 1977;63:540-546

[4] WHO. Lymphatic Filariasis. Geneva: WHO; 2020. Available from: https://www.who.int/news-room/fact-sheets/detail/lymphatic-filariasis

[5] Aggarwal VK, Sashindran VK. Lymphatic filariasis in India: Problems, challenges and new initiatives. Medical Journal, Armed Forces India. 2006;62:359-362

[6] Centers for Disease Control and Prevention (CDC), Atlanta, USA. Recommendations of the International Task Force for Disease Eradication. MMWR. 1993;42:1-38

[7] Ottesen EA. Towards elimination of lymphatic filariasis. In: Angelico M, Rocchi G, editors. Infectious Diseases and Public Health. Tel Aviv: Balaban Publishers; 1998. pp. 58-64

[8] Seim AR, Dreyer G, Addiss DG. Controlling morbidity and interrupting transmission: twin pillars of lymphatic filariasis elimination. Revista da Sociedade Brasileira de Medicina Tropical. 1999;32:325-328

[9] Ismail MM, Jayakody RL, Weil GJ, et al. Efficacy of single dose combinations of albendazole, ivermectin and diethylcarbamazine for the treatment of bancroftian filariasis. Transactions of the Royal Society of Tropical Medicine and Hygiene. 1998;92:94-97

[10] Hussain MA, Sitha AK, Swain S, Kadam S, Pati S. Mass drug administration for lymphatic filariasis elimination in a coastal state of India: A study on barriers to coverage and compliance. Infectious Diseases of Poverty. 2014;3:31

[11] Jambulingam P, Subramanian S, de Vlas SJ, Vinubala C, Stolk WA. Mathematical modelling of lymphatic filariasis elimination programmes in India: Required duration of mass drug administration and post-treatment level of infection indicators. Parasites & Vectors. 2016;9:501

[12] Michael E, Bundy DA, Grenfell BT. Re-assessing the global prevalence and distribution of lymphatic filariasis. Parasitology. 1996;112:409-428

[13] Smith ME, Singh BK, Michael E. Assessing endgame strategies for the elimination of lymphatic filariasis: A model-based evaluation of the impact of DEC-medicated salt. Scientific Reports;7:7386. DOI: 10.1038/s41598-017-07782-9

[14] Shriram AN, Premkumar A, Krishnamoorthy K, et al. Elimination of diurnally sub-periodic *Wuchereria bancrofti* in Andaman and Nicobar Islands, India, using mass DEC-fortified salt as a supplementary intervention to MDA. Parasitology Research. 26 March 2020. PMID: 32219550. DOI: 10.1007/s00436-020-06659-7

[15] Lammie P, Milner T, Houston R. Unfulfilled potential: Using diethylcarbamazine-fortified salt to eliminate lymphatic filariasis. Bulletin of the World Health Organization. 2007;85:545-549

[16] Sebasan S, Palaniyandi M, Das PK, Michael E. Mapping of lymphatic filariasis in India. Annals of Tropical Medicine and Parasitology. 2000; 94: 591-606

[17] Laboratory Diagnosis of Lymphatic Filariasis. 2013. Available from: https://microbeonline.com/laboratory-diagnosis-lymphatic-filariasis/

[18] WHO. Lymphatic Filariasis: Diagnosis. 2020. Available from: https://www.who.int/lymphatic_filariasis/epidemiology/epidemiology_diagnosis/en/

[19] Srivastava PK, Dhillon GP, editors. Elimination of lymphatic filariasis in India—A successful endeavour. Journal of the Indian Medical Association. 2008;**106**:673-677

[20] WHO. Global Programme to Eliminate Lymphatic Filariasis—Annual Report on Lymphatic Filariasis. Geneva: WHO; 2002. WHO/CDS/CPE/CEE/2002.28

[21] Srivastava PK, Dhariwal AC. Progress towards morbidity management under elimination of lymphatic filariasis programme in India. Journal of the Indian Medical Association. 2010;**108**:854-862

[22] Srivastava PK, Dhariwal AC, Bhattacharjee J. Status of lymphatic filariasis in India. Health Action. 2013:19

[23] Srivastava PK, Bhattacharjee J, Dhariwal AC, Krishnamoorthy K, Dash AP. Elimination of lymphatic filariasis—Current status and way ahead. Journal of Communicable Diseases. 2014;**46**:85-94

[24] Dhariwal AC, Srivastava PK, Bhattacharjee J. Elimination of lymphatic filariasis in India: An update. Journal of the Indian Medical Association. 2015;**113**:189-190

[25] India Adopts New Strategy to Accelerate Lymphatic Filariasis Elimination. 2018. Available from: https://health.economictimes.indiatimes.com/news/diagnostics/india-adopts-new-strategy-to-accelerate-lymphatic-filariasis-elimination/64574044

[26] WHO. Global Programme to Eliminate Lymphatic Filariasis: Progress Report, 2018. Weekly Epidemiological Record, No. 41. Geneva: WHO; 11 October 2019. Available from: https://www.who.int/publications-detail/who-wer9441-457-472

[27] Ghosh SK, Rahi M. Malaria elimination in India—The way forward. Journal of Vector Borne Diseases. 2019;**56**:32-40

[28] Harsh Vardhan. Scale-Up of Triple-Drug Therapy to Achieve the Elimination of Lymphatic Filariasis by 2021. 2019. Available from: https://pib.gov.in/PressReleasePage.aspx?PRID=1589596

[29] Weil GJ, Bogus J, Christian M, Dubray C, Djuardi Y, Fischer PU, et al. The safety of double- and triple-drug community mass drug administration for lymphatic filariasis: A multicenter, open-label, cluster-randomized study. PLoS Medicine. 2019;**16**(6):e1002839. DOI: 10.1371/journal.pmed.1002839

[30] Addiss DG, Beach MJ, Streit TG, et al. Randomised placebo-controlled comparison of ivermectin and albendazole alone and in combination for *Wuchereria bancrofti* microfilaremia in Haitian children. Lancet. 1997;**350**(9076):480-484

[31] Shenoy RK, Suma TK, Kumaraswami V, et al. Preliminary findings from a cross-sectional study on lymphatic filariasis in children in an area endemic for *Brugia malayi* infection. Annals of Tropical Medicine and Parasitology. 2007;**101**:205-213

[32] Ghosh SK. Human dirofilariasis: A fast emerging zoonosis in India. Indian Journal of Medical Microbiology. 2015;**33**:595-596

[33] Khatri V, Amdare N, Chauhan N, Togre R, Reddy MV, Hoti SL, et al. Epidemiological screening and xenomonitoring for human Lymphatic Filariasis infection in select districts in the states of Maharashtra and Karnataka, India. Parasitology Research. 2019;**118**:1045-1050

[34] Peter B, Fred B, Carlos C, et al. A Roadmap for the development of ivermectin as a complementary malaria vector control tool: The ivermectin roadmappers. American Journal of Tropical Medicine and Hygiene. 2020; **102**:3-24. DOI: 10.4269/ajtmh.19-0620

[35] Ghosh SK, Yadav RS. Naturally acquired concomitant infections of bancroftian filariasis and human plasmodia in Orissa. Indian Journal of Malariology. 1995; 32, 32-36

[36] Ramaiah KD, Das PK, Michael E, et al. Economic burden of lymphatic filariasis in India. Parasitology Today. 2000;**16**:251-255

[37] Ghosh SK, Ghosh C. New ways of tackling malaria. In: Claborn D, Bhattacharya S, Roy S, editors. Current Topics in the Epidemiology of Vector-Borne Diseases. 2019. ISBN: 978-1-83880-022-2. Available from: https://www.intechopen.com/online-first/new-ways-to-tackle-malaria

Chapter 18

State of the Art and Future Directions of *Cryptosporidium* spp.

Helena Lúcia Carneiro Santos, Karina Mastropasqua Rebello and Teresa Cristina Bergamo Bomfim

Abstract

Cryptosporidium species are protozoan parasites that infect epithelium surfaces in gastrointestinal and respiratory tracts of humans and a range of animals worldwide. Cryptosporidiosis has been associated with considerable morbidity and, under certain circumstances, mortality. Humans can acquire it by consuming food and drink containing oocysts, which have been recognised as a major cause for diarrhoeal disease. The ubiquitousness of the infective oocyst, its resilience to environmental pressures, and the low dose of oocyst exposure needed for infection amplify to outbreaks of *Cryptosporidium* traced to drinking and recreational water. Unlike in developing countries where lack of sustained access to safe water creates tremendous burdens of *Cryptosporidium* diarrhoea, this scenario is aggravated due to limited diagnosis and therapeutics. However, over the past few decades, growing information on *Cryptosporidium* genomes have allowed novel insight into the host-parasite relationship. Future field research on potential tools will focus on biology-derived parasite products applicable to drugs and diagnosis. This chapter reviews available data on biology, transmission, life cycle, diagnosis, genome, and a few but important progresses in the field of cryptosporidiosis.

Keywords: cryptosporidiosis, diagnosis, transmission, infectious disease, genome

1. Introduction

Cryptosporidium species are protozoan parasites that infect the epithelial cells of the gastrointestinal and respiratory tracts of humans and a wide range of animals, with a global distribution [1–3]. *Cryptosporidium* represents a major public health concern for waterborne disease and daycare outbreaks of diarrhoeal disease worldwide [2, 4–8]. Human cryptosporidiosis is usually a self-limiting infection in immunocompetent individuals. However, cases of severe diarrhoea and dissemination to extra-intestinal sites can occur in children, the elderly, and individuals with impairment of T-cell functions, mainly those with HIV infection [9–12]. In children, although diarrhoea is a key feature of malabsorption, it may not be apparent at presentation; when the infection becomes chronic, the only symptom may be limited growth. Consequently, chronic infections can culminate in poor growth [5, 13–16]. The epidemiology of infections is complex and involves transmission by a faecal-oral route, either by ingestion of contaminated water or food or by human-to-human or animal-to-human transmission [17, 18]. The oocyst, the environmental stage of *Cryptosporidium,* is incredibly hardy, easily spread through water, and resistant

IntechOpen

to inactivation by chlorine; and without the use of filtration, it is challenging to remove it from drinking water [19–21]. *Cryptosporidium* prevalence is higher in areas lacking a sanitation infrastructure, mainly drinking water and sewage, which led the World Health Organization (WHO) to include it in the water sanitation and health programme [22]. The scarcity of sustained access to safe water creates tremendous burdens of *Cryptosporidium* diarrhoea in developing countries [23]. Treatment and diagnosis options are still not totally effective [2, 24–26]. No fully effective drug therapy or vaccine is available for *Cryptosporidium*, and the diagnosis of cryptosporidiosis has been based on the demonstration of oocysts in faeces, which present low sensibility [25]. However, the ability to culture relevant *Cryptosporidium* isolates in vitro, the development of novel gene-editing tools (knockout genes, CRISPR/Cas9, and RNAi) [26–30], and 'omic' research (genomics, transcriptomics, and proteomics) represent essential paths towards significant advancements in the control of cryptosporidiosis [30–38]. In the future, those approaches will show a holistic view of the biology of *Cryptosporidium*. In this chapter, we present recent advances and remaining challenges regarding human cryptosporidiosis under a public health perspective.

2. Clinical perspective, diagnosis, and treatment

Despite *Cryptosporidium* species infecting the epithelial cells of the gastrointestinal and respiratory epithelium tracts, human cryptosporidiosis is a usually self-limiting infection in immunocompetent individuals with a low fatality rate [39–41]. In general, onset of the symptoms occurs 5–7 days following exposure and resolves in 2–3 weeks [42]. Clinical manifestations vary from subclinical infection to watery diarrhoea, sometimes profuse. Other common symptoms include abdominal cramps, fever, flatulence, nausea, vomiting, and low-grade fever [43–45]. Clinical presentation of cryptosporidiosis in individuals with impairment of T-cell functions, mainly those with HIV infection, varies according to the level of immunosuppression, from asymptomatic disease, to transient disease, to relapsing chronic diarrhoea or even cholera-like diarrhoea that is debilitating and potentially life-threatening [46]. Spreading of infection beyond the extra-intestinal site (in the biliary or respiratory tract) has been documented in children and immunocompromised people, resulting in a potentially life-threatening disease [47, 48]. Sclerosing cholangitis and other biliary involvements are common in AIDS patients with cryptosporidiosis. Both innate and adaptive immunity of the host have major impacts on the severity of cryptosporidiosis and its prognosis.

Cryptosporidium has been diagnosed using a variety of approaches, such as microscopy, immunofluorescent antibody (IFA), enzyme-linked immunosorbent assay (ELISA), and DNA-based detection methods [18]. However, identification of the parasite's morphologic features through examination of stool smears is widely employed in diagnostic laboratories, particularly in resource-limited health systems. The oocysts are shed intermittently [49]; therefore, three faecal samples collected on alternate days are recommended. To maximise the recovery of oocysts, Sheather's sucrose flotation, saturated salt flotation, and Allen and Ridley's formol-ether method are the stool concentration techniques most frequently used prior to the use of the microscopy staining technique [50, 51]. Stain differential is required due to the small size of the specimen (ranging from 4 to 6 μm), similar in shape to yeasts and faecal debris [52]. Safranin-methylene blue, Kinyoun Ziehl-Neelsen, and dimethyl sulfoxide-carbol fuchsin are the most commonly used stain methods [11, 53–55]. However, in the absence of staining solution, phase contrast microscopy has proven to be highly specific for the detection of *Cryptosporidium* oocysts in human stool samples [56]. In general, conventional microscopy lacks sensitivity, is time-consuming, and requires a skilled and well-experienced microscopist [57–59].

Direct fluorescent antibody tests (DFAs), enzyme-immunoassays (EIAs), and rapid immunochromatographic assays (dipsticks) are commercially available [60–63]. The EIA kits have been evaluated with human stool specimens only, presumably from patients infected with *C. hominis* or *C. parvum*. The direct fluorescent antibody tests have been widely used for the detection of *Cryptosporidium* in faecal smears, water, and food [60, 62–66]. However, the antigenic variability of oocyst wall epitopes contributes to reducing specificity, and the sensibility of all immunological-based methods is low. High specificity (99–100%) has been generally reported for EIA kits. Sensitivities, however, have been reported to range from 70 to 100% [62–65]. Dipsticks and EIAs are available for individual and for all-in-one tests for *Giardia*, *Cryptosporidium*, and *Entamoeba histolytica* [66–69]. The tests are fast and easy to perform. However, EIA kits and rapid format assays present a potential problem with false positives, so results need to be interpreted and evaluated with caution [70]. To overcome these barriers, one of the most notable advances in public health in recent decades has been the development of tools based on molecular biology for the diagnosis of infectious diseases. These polymerase chain reaction (PCR) techniques have enabled specific sensitive detection of oocysts (a single oocyst) in clinical and environmental samples [71–77]. Examples of such techniques include conventional PCR, quantitative PCR real time, and high-resolution melt. A wide variety of PCR methods targeting different genes have been developed for the detection of *Cryptosporidium* at the species/genotype/subtype levels. However, no targeted tests have been patterned for the detection of *Cryptosporidium* in clinical laboratories. Recently, the simultaneous qualitative detection and identification of multiple viral, parasitic (including *C. parvum* and *C. hominis*), and bacterial nucleic acids in human stool specimens were approved by the Food and Drug Administration (FDA) [78]. In general, PCR tools solely amplify the DNA of *C. parvum*, *C. hominis*, *C. meleagridis*, and species/genotypes closely related to *C. parvum* [18]. For genotyping, nested PCR-RFLP was the most commonly used method in the past. Nowadays, DNA sequencing of 18S has been required to reliably detect all *Cryptosporidium* spp. The HSP70 and COWP targets fail to detect the DNA of *C. felis*, *C. canis*, and *C. muris* [79]. Subtyping tools are indispensable from the epidemiological point of view and are helpful in knowing the possible transmission routes of *Cryptosporidium* species and zoonotic potential of the parasite. Several subtyping tools have been developed to evaluate the diversity within *C. parvum* or *C. hominis*, including analysis of the microsatellite, GP-60 gene, HSP70 gene, 47-kDa protein, small double-stranded (ds) RNA virus, serine repeat antigen, and T-rich gene fragment [73, 80–85]. The 18S ribosomal RNA (rRNA) gene and the hypervariable 60-kDa glycoprotein (gp60) gene have been widely used as targets to identify species and track transmission [18, 86, 87]. The 60-kDa glycoprotein (gp60, also known as gp40/gp15) gene presents a wide genetic heterogeneity in the number of trinucleotide repeats (TCA, TCG, or TCT). This gene encodes a precursor protein that is cleaved to produce mature cell surface glycoproteins (gp45/gp40 and gp15) implicated in the attachment to, and invasion of, enterocytes [18, 87]. Identification of subtypes using GP60 subtype families has revealed the subtype families (Ia-Ik) in *C. hominis* [87–91] and two zoonotic subtypes (IIa, IId), subtypes (IIb, IIc, IIe, IIf, IIi, IIj-IIt) in *C. parvum* [4, 87, 92–94], and subtype families (IIIa to IIIg) in *C. meleagridis* have been acknowledged [87, 95, 96]. Subtyping tools targeting the gp60 gene have been developed recently for several other human-pathogenic *Cryptosporidium* species [87]. Species and subtype identification are not necessary for clinical care and therapeutic options but are important for epidemiological surveillance and for drug investigations and clinical trials. Novel diagnostic tools and biomarkers for cryptosporidiosis, which could also be used for therapeutic or vaccine trials, are necessary for accurate identification.

Current treatment options for cryptosporidiosis are limited. So far, there is no vaccine against *Cryptosporidium* [97], and nitazoxanide (NTZ) is the only drug approved by the FDA for treatment of cryptosporidiosis in children and immuno-competent adults [98]. However, it is not effective without an appropriate immune status and, consequently, is ineffectual for the treatment of immune-compromised patients, particularly those with AIDS [25, 99]. NTZ is a nitrothiazole benzamide compound with a broad spectrum of activity against a wide range of parasites, bacteria, and viruses. In protozoa, NTZ inhibits the enzyme pyruvate ferredoxin oxidoreductase, which is essential to anaerobic energy metabolism [100]. Due to the prevalence of cryptosporidiosis, the development of novel therapeutic targets and vaccines against *Cryptosporidium* spp. is a public health priority. The ongoing need to develop new anti-cryptosporidial drugs has spurred the process of finding new uses for existing drugs. Repurposing drug provides an attractive alternative to drug development [101]. Two compounds, 3-hydroxy-3-methyl-glutaryl-coenzyme A (HMG-CoA) reductase inhibitor, pitavastatin and auranofin (approved for the treatment of rheumatoid arthritis), have been shown to be effective against *Cryptosporidium* in vitro [102]. Auranofin has been shown to be 10 times more potent than metronidazole against *Entamoeba histolytica*, the protozoan agent of human amoebiasis [103]. HMG-CoA and auranofin have particular promise in fast-tracking for further in vivo testing in animals and humans.

3. Life cycle and classification

The parasite has a complex monoxenous life cycle with both asexual (merogony) and sexual (gametogony) stages. Ingestion of an infective oocyst (containing four sporozoites) by a susceptible host initiates the excystation process in the gastroin-testinal tract. The sporulated oocyst ruptures, releasing sporozoites that invade the enterocytes, inducing the cell membrane to enclose the parasite in the parasitopho-rous vacuole, which then differentiates into a trophozoite. Trophozoites undergo merogony and form either a further type I meront or a type II meront, which con-tains four merozoites that are destined for gametogony. Merozoites can differentiate into sexually distinct stages called macro- and microgametocytes in a process called gametogony. New oocysts are formed in the epithelial cells from the fusion of a macro- and a microgametocyte to form a diploid zygote. The new fused cell evolves and sporulates in situ in a process called sporogony, becoming oocysts containing four sporozoites. Type II meronts attach to the epithelial cell and differentiate into either macrogamonts or microgamonts. The microgametes from the microgamont are released, and each can fertilised a macrogamont to form a diploid zygote. This cell undergoes a process like meiosis (sporogony) to produce an oocyst, either thin- or thick-walled, containing four sporozoites (sporulated oocysts). The thin-walled oocysts are involved in autoinfection, and thick-walled oocysts are released within the faeces to infect new hosts [104–107] (**Figure 1**).

Until relatively recently, *Cryptosporidium* was classified as a coccidian parasite. However, the taxonomic placement of *Cryptosporidium* was altered after revisions to higher-order classifications due to recent particularities observed in *Cryptosporidium*. The parasite can develop in a cell-free culture, while extracellular stages have been observed in both cell-free and cell cultures, in biofilms, and in vivo [108–111]. It pres-ents the ability to grow and amplify without host cell attachment and encapsulation, as well as the insensitivity of all anticoccidial agents [26]. Moreover, the parasite lacks a micropyle, sporocyst, and polar granular [111–113]. Although initially considered

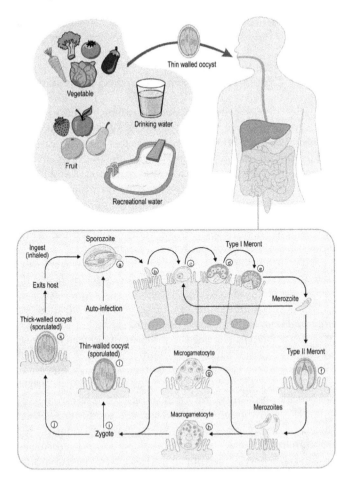

Figure 1.
A schematic diagram of Cryptosporidium *life cycle. After ingestion of contaminated water and/or food, the oocyst wall opens (excystation) triggered by temperature, stomach acid, and bile salts. Then, sporulated oocyst ruptures releasing (a) sporozoites that (b) invade the host cell (c) inducing the cell membrane to enclose the parasite in the parasitophorous vacuole, (d) which then differentiates into a trophozoite that undergoes an asexual reproduction, (e) forming a type I meront that contains 6–8 merozoites. These merozoites can reinfect the epithelial cell, where they undergo merogony and form type I meront or (f) type II meront. (g) Merozoites can differentiate into sexually distinct stages called (g) micro- and (h) macrogametocytes. (i) Zygote is formed after the fertilisation of macrogametocyte by the microgametocyte, (j) and this cell undergoes sporogony and produces a thin-walled oocyst. (k) These thin-walled oocysts are released within faeces to infect new hosts, as well as (l) involved in autoinfection process (adapted from Ref. [104]).*

to be a coccidian, *Cryptosporidium* spp. share features of both the coccidia and gregarines, confirmed by morphological and molecular data. Major similarities between *Cryptosporidium* and gregarine parasites are as follows: (1) the ability to complete its life cycle in the absence of host cells, (2) extracellular gamont-like stages, (3) the process in which two mature trophozoites pair up before the formation of gametocyst (szygy), and (4) changing cell architecture to adapt to diverse environments (biofilms, coelom, intestines, soil, and water) [107, 108, 111, 114]. The most recent classification considers *Cryptosporidium* as a separate group within the Apicomplexa. Analyses of comparative genomics and of phylogenetic inference and the ability of *Cryptosporidium* to complete its life cycle extracellularly confirm its close relationship with gregarines and corroborate the transference of *Cryptosporidium* to the Gregarinomorphea class as a new subclass of Cryptogregaria [111, 115]. Early taxonomy at species level was based originally on morphology and host specificity. Nowadays, the description of species takes molecular analyses, mainly DNA sequencing and PCR-related methods, into account for the detection and differentiation of *Cryptosporidium* spp.

4. Maintenance of *Cryptosporidium* in nature and transmission

Once excreted into the environment, oocysts can be dispersed from the faecal matrix into the terrestrial environment (**Figure 2**). When present on the soil surface, oocysts may be exposed to high temperatures and desiccation, causing their inactivation. Oocysts are sensitive to desiccation and UV-C irradiation [116]. Reports show that desiccation is lethal to oocysts with only 3 and 5% remaining viable after being air-dried at room temperature for 2 and 4 h, respectively [117, 118]. However, when within the soil column, the oocysts were maintained, protected, and viable [119, 120]. Studies have indicated that oocysts at 4°C recovered from soil column may remain infectious for long periods [119, 121]. These findings suggest that the soil column is a sanctuary for *Cryptosporidium*, protecting it until rainfall events scatter them [120]. Oocysts were able to remain viable and infectious after being frozen at –10°C for up to 168 h, at –15°C for up to 24 h, and at –20°C for up to 8 h [122]. Moreover, *Cryptosporidium* oocysts can be carried in the environment due to interactions with biofilms (surface-attached microbial communities). They readily attach to biofilms and persist and subsequently separate from it. High concentrations of oocysts in water biofilms that were maintained over several months maintained viable sporozoites [123]. *Cryptosporidium* oocysts in fresh water and marine water can survive at a range of temperatures. Fayer et al. reported that oocysts maintained at 20°C remain infectious for 12 weeks at salinities of 0 and 10 ppt, for 4 weeks at 20 ppt, and for 2 weeks at 30 ppt [124]. Although salinity can have a pronounced effect on oocyst infectivity, they can survive long enough in marine waters to justify their presence in marine animals.

Cryptosporidium spp. have a huge impact on both human and veterinary health worldwide, aggravated by the limited diagnosis and current therapeutics. *Cryptosporidium* spp. have a worldwide distribution and the ability to infect a wide range of hosts, including humans, and a broad variety of vertebrate [1, 3]. Humans can acquire cryptosporidiosis through several transmission routes, such as direct contact with infected persons or animals and consumption of contaminated water (drinking or recreational) or food (**Figure 3**).

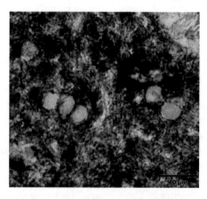

Figure 2.
Cryptosporidium *sp. oocysts in safranin-methylene blue staining method.*

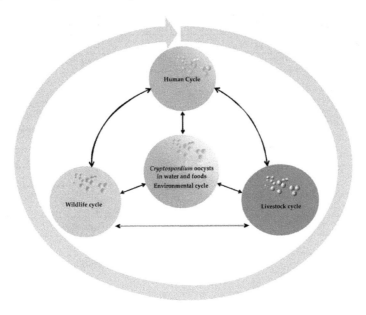

Figure 3.
Transmission cycles of Cryptosporidium *infections.*

The WHO has categorised *Cryptosporidium* as a reference pathogen for the assessment of drinking water quality [125]. Susceptibility to cryptosporidiosis depends on several factors, including environmental conditions, host immune status, age, geographic location, and contact with infected humans/animals [126]. Animals play an important role in the maintenance, amplification, and transmission of *Cryptosporidium* [127]. In fact, a large range of animals are reservoirs for some species, genotypes, and subtypes, which may infect humans [128–130]. The lack of adequate instruments to continuously monitor animal mobility makes it difficult to study the dynamics of transmission [131, 132]. Also, oocysts are ubiquitous in the environment and easily spread via drinking water, recreational water, and food [3, 133, 134]. The ubiquitousness of the infective oocyst, its resilience to environmental pressures [135], and the low-dose oocyst exposure (ingestion of fewer than 10 oocysts can lead to infection) [136, 137] amplify to outbreaks of *Cryptosporidium* traced to drinking and recreational water. In 1993, the largest *Cryptosporidium* waterborne outbreak was recorded in the United States in Milwaukee, where more than 400,000 people were infected by the drinking water supply [138]. The epidemiology of infection is complex and involves transmission by the faecal-oral route, either by indirect transmission through ingestion of contaminated water or food or by direct human-to-human or animal-to-human transmission [3]. The genus *Cryptosporidium* has about 30 species formally described, as well as various genotypes and subtypes. Some species are relatively promiscuous in terms of host specificity, some of which also infected humans. Currently, a wide range of *Cryptosporidium* species and various genotypes have been recognised as responsible for human cryptosporidiosis (**Table 1**).

Human infections predominantly are caused by *C. hominis*, which are considered restricted to humans (anthroponotic transmission), and by *C. parvum*, some of which isolate genotypes and infect ruminants (zoonotic transmission) [18]. However, in recent years, *C. meleagridis*, *C. cuniculus*, and *C. ubiquitum* have also emerged as species relevant to public health, while the other species tend to be associated only with sporadic and rare cases of human infection. Approximately 155

Cryptosporidium spp.	Major host	References
C. andersoni	Cattle	[139–144]
C. baileyi	Chickens and turkeys	[145]
C. bovis	Cattle	[146, 147]
C. canis	Dogs	[148–150]
C. cuniculus	Rabbits	[151–155]
C. fayeri	Marsupials	[141, 156]
C. felis	Cats	[93, 157, 158]
*C. hominis**	Humans	[18]
*C. meleagridis**	Turkeys, chickens, humans	[18, 93, 153, 159, 160]
C. muris	Rodents	[161–163]
*C. parvum**	ruminants, especially calves	[18]
C. scrofarum	Pigs	[164]
C. suis	Pigs	[139, 160, 165–167]
C. tyzzeri	Rodents, snake	[168]
C. ubiquitum	Sheep and cervids	[152, 154, 157, 158, 169]
C. viatorum	Humans	[93, 170]
C. erinacei	Hedgehogs and horses	[171, 172]
C. wrairi	Guinea pigs	[173, 174]
C. xiaoi	Sheep and goat	[174]
Cryptosporidium Chipmunk genotype	Rodents	[93]
Cryptosporidium Horse genotype	Horses	[152, 153]
Cryptosporidium Mink genotype	Minks	[175]
Cryptosporidium Monkey genotype	Monkey	[152]
Cryptosporidium Skunk genotype	Skunk	[152, 153]

*The most prevalent species.

Table 1.
Currently recognised species of Cryptosporidium *spp. associated with human infections.*

species of mammals have been reported as non-human hosts of *C. parvum*, indicating that the parasite is adapting and developing in many hosts [176].

The human-to-human spread is particularly well described within families (often secondary cases after a primary outbreak infection) in childcare nurseries, nursing homes, and hospitals [42, 177, 178]. In addition, contact with production animals, mainly cattle, that are the main hosts of *C. parvum* can potentially infect humans [40, 178, 179]. To date, studies in developing countries have shown a predominance of *C. hominis* in HIV-positive children and adults. These findings are also valid in the United States, Canada, Australia, and Japan. In Europe and New Zealand, several studies have shown a similar prevalence of *C. parvum* and *C. hominis* in immunocompetent and immunocompromised individuals. Thus, in most developing countries, the anthroponotic transmission of *Cryptosporidium* plays an important role in human cryptosporidiosis [18, 180], while in Europe, New Zealand, and rural areas of the United States, there are both anthroponotic and zoonotic transmissions. In Middle Eastern countries, children are mainly infected with *C. parvum*, but the significance of this occurrence is not clear [181]. An exception is *Cryptosporidium* infections in HIV-positive patients in Ababa, Ethiopia, where *C. parvum* is highly endemic and where contact with calves is an important risk factor for cryptosporidiosis [174].

In developing countries, most *C. parvum* infections in HIV-positive children and adults are caused by subtype IIc, with IIa largely absent, indicating that anthroponotic transmission of *C. parvum* is common in these areas. Conversely, families of subtype IIa are commonly diagnosed in humans in industrialised regions, where their occurrence is often associated with contact with calves. Another family of *C. parvum* subtypes commonly found in sheep and goats, IId, is dominant in humans in Middle Eastern countries and is occasionally found in humans in some European countries, such as Sweden, where it is commonly diagnosed in dairy calves. A systematic review of the anthroponotic transmission of *Cryptosporidium* concluded that subtype IIc predominates in low-income countries with poor sanitation and in HIV-positive individuals, unlike in higher-income countries, where it is rarely evident. Lacking effective treatment or vaccine, intervention to improve basic sanitation in these regions is the best option. This prophylactic action certainly may reduce the anthropogenic and zoonotic transmission of cryptosporidiosis, reducing the damage to human health. It is important to emphasise the importance of personal hygiene practices to minimise cryptosporidiosis, in addition to other pathogens transmitted by water and food.

5. Genome of *Cryptosporidium*: new insight and future challenges

Recent years have seen impressive progress of next-generation sequencing technologies in genome assembly and annotation methodologies, mainly by advancements in the fields of molecular biology and technical engineering and by reducing cost. *Cryptosporidium* has been the subject of genome sequencing projects, which have provided valuable insights into the species, biology, and host-parasite relationships. The genomic data of multiple *Cryptosporidium* species are available and accessible in a *Cryptosporidium*-dedicated database, CryptoDB (http://cryptodb.org/cryptodb/) [182], and in the GenBank database (www.ncbi.nlm.nih.gov). Comparative analyses have shown that *Cryptosporidium* genomes are highly compact, containing 8.50–9.50 megabase pairs (Mbp), a total gene count ranging from 3769 to 7610, and coding sequence composition (75–77.6%). Moreover, in general, they share a comparable GC percentage (**Table 2**).

Overall, gene content and genomic organisation among intestinal occurrences of the species are well conserved, with *Cryptosporidium* gene clusters encoding putative secreted proteins. Comparison of the *Cryptosporidium* genomes has identified a core set of proteins commonly studied, as well as major differences in particular gene families, which could be involved in biological differences between species and genotypes [114, 183–185]. Gene encoding proteins that are associated with invasion processes, e.g. protein kinases and thrombospondin-related adhesive proteins (TRAPs), insulinase-like peptidases, MEDLE secretory proteins, and mucin glycoproteins, are observed in genome *Cryptosporidium* spp. [32]. However, some of them differ in copy number variations of genes. Comparative genomic analysis revealed that one of the primary features differentiating *Cryptosporidium* species is the sequence diversity present in major secreted protein families, MEDLE, and insulinase-like proteases [184]. This is consistent with transcriptomic studies

Organism/name	Strain	Bio-sample	Bio-project	Size (Mb)	GC %	Gene	Protein
C. hominis	—	SAMEA 3496639	PRJEB 10000	9.10	30.1	3818	3817
C. hominis	TU502	—	PRJNA 13200	8.74	30.9	3949	3885
C. hominis	TU502_2012	SAMN 02382005	PRJNA 222836	9.10	30.1	3796	3745
C. hominis	UKH1	SAMN 02382004	PRJNA 222837	9.15	30.1	3769	3718
C. hominis	30,976	SAMN 02862040	PRJNA 252787	9.06	30.1	3995	3959
C. parvum	Iowa type II	SAMN 02952908	PRJNA 144	9.10	30.2	7774	7610
C. andersoni	30,847	SAMN 04417240	PRJNA 354069	9.09	28.5	3897	3876
C. meleagridis	UKMEL1	SAMN 02666797	PRJNA 222838	8.97	31.0	3806	3753
C. meleagridis	UKMEL4	SAMN 08383028	PRJNA 315503	8.79	30.9	—	—
C. meleagridis	UKMEL3	SAMN 08383027	PRJNA 315502	8.70	31.0	—	—
C. ubiquitum	39,726	SAMN 02768023	PRJNA 534291	8.97	30.8	3766	3766
Cryptosporidium sp.	Chipmunk LX-2015	SAMN 03281121	PRJNA 272389	9.51	31.9	—	—
Cryptosporidium sp.	37,763	SAMN 10623052	PRJNA 511361	9.05	32.0	—	—
*C. baileyi**	TAMU 09Q1	SAMN 02382006	PRJNA 222835	8.50	24.2	—	—
C. cuniculus	UKCU2	SAMN 08383019	PRJNA 3154496	9.18	25.8	—	—
C. muris	RN66	SAMN 02953683	PRJA 19553	9.25	28.5	—	3934
C. viatorum	UKUIA1	SAMN 10107889	PRJA 492837	9.26	31.1	—	—

Draft genome.

Table 2.
Genomic features of Cryptosporidium *spp.*

of *C. parvum*, which have demonstrated MEDLE proteins in different subcellular locations that may perform their functions in distinct stages of the invasion and development process [33]. Moreover, a reduction in the number of genes encoding secreted MEDLE and insulinase-like proteins was observed in *C. ubiquitum* and *C. andersoni*, whereas the mucin-type glycoproteins are highly divergent between the gastric *C. andersoni* and intestinal *Cryptosporidium* species [184]. Unlike most other apicomplexans, *Cryptosporidium* spp. have no apicoplast or mitochondrial genomes but have remnant ones, the so-called mitosomes. However, *Cryptosporidium* species disagree from each other mostly in mitosome metabolic pathways. *C. parvum, C. hominis*, and *C. andersoni* present more aerobic metabolism and a conventional electron transport chain [114], whereas *C. ubiquitum* has further reductions in ubiquinone and polyisoprenoid biosynthesis and has lost both the conventional and alternative electron transport systems, unlike *C. muris* genome encoding core enzymes for the Krebs cycle and a functional ATP synthase. Thus, the mitosome of *C. muris* functions essentially as a peculiar mitochondrion [186]. However, the loss of biosynthetic pathways is a common feature observed in *Cryptosporidium* spp. genomes, e.g. the cytochrome-based respiratory chain and main de novo synthetic pathways for amino acids, nucleotides, fatty acids, and the Krebs cycle [32, 183]. Conversely, families of transporters to acquire nutrients from the host were expanded, including transporters for amino acids, sugars, and ATP-binding cassettes (ABCs) that drive the transport of various metabolites, lipids/sterols, and drugs [32]. Although these genomic sequences provide valuable data, the genome analyses have revealed contradictory data and inconsistencies between the annotated gene models and transcriptome evidence [31, 36]. Notoriously, those findings are related to sequencing platforms, which have been applied to having different strengths and weaknesses and the use of different strategies and stringencies in gene prediction.

Notwithstanding its novelty, the major challenges for the generation of whole genomes of *Cryptosporidium* are the quality and the yielding of limited DNA. Indeed, this is a critical step, as it is hard to recover enough quantity of DNA (2.5×10^{-5} highly purified oocysts correspondent approximately 10 µg) from faeces from natural infections. A theoretical estimate of the DNA content of one oocyst is of 40 fg [187]; therefore, it is tricky and arduous to recover enough quantity of DNA (2.5×10^{-5} highly purified oocysts correspondent approximately 10 µg) from unculturable samples with the quality necessary for high-throughput sequencing. Non-cultured samples may introduce a level of uncertainty and possess limited metadata. The lower the quality of the initial genome sequence, the higher the likelihood of yielding a missing or misassembled genome. A recent study evaluated an alternative method of preparing faecal samples using the combination of salt flotation, immunomagnetic separation (IMS), and surface sterilisation of oocysts prior to DNA extraction. The method has shown promise when used for the genome sequencing of samples of *C. parvum* and *C. hominis* [36]. This challenging issue can be resolved using a novel approach of *Cryptosporidium* cell-free culture and new long-read sequencing techniques, which will likely be beneficial for improving data. Increases in the quality of the target DNA boost the depth of coverage of the genome in higher levels, so base calls can be made with a higher degree of confidence. Also, the ability to culture relevant *Cryptosporidium* isolates in vitro, the development of novel gene-editing tools (knockout genes, CRISPR/Cas9, and RNAi), and 'omic' research (genomics, transcriptomics, and proteomics) represent essential paths towards significant advancements in the control of cryptosporidiosis.

6. Conclusions and future perspectives

Cryptosporidium is a major cause of diarrhoeal disease in humans worldwide, yet an effective therapy to eradicate the parasite is not available. Also, the diagnosis options remain limited in developing countries, which harm the surveillance and understanding of the epidemiology in resource-poor settings. In developed countries, large waterborne outbreaks in drinking and recreational water continue to occur, emphasising the need for better regulation and for improvements of drinking water treatment processes and control guidelines. However, in recent years, significant improvements have been achieved in understanding the key concepts of the organism, mainly by increasing the use of molecular methods and genome sequences. Recent advancements in knowledge of *Cryptosporidium* provide the basis for the development of effective and practical strategies for the future prevention and control of cryptosporidiosis. The data from *Cryptosporidium* genome sequences have already improved our understanding of the metabolism and cellular processes. In fact, mining the genome and proteome data of *Cryptosporidium* will allow the development of new classes of compounds and molecular targets. However, it is worth underscoring the need for community-wide efforts to generate and integrate high-quality functional datasets that span the full spectrum of biology and life cycles in order to improve the predictive nature of models generated from large-scale system-based resources. Transcriptomes and proteomics from different growth stages are starting to be generated and promise to provide further insight into the biology of *Cryptosporidium*. Also, future studies will require careful validation and follow-up of each finding using in vitro and animal model studies.

Acknowledgements

I would like to thank Victor Ricardo Azevedo for the assistance with **Figure 3**.

Conflict of interest

The authors declare that there is no conflict of interest.

Author details

Helena Lúcia Carneiro Santos[1*], Karina Mastropasqua Rebello[1]
and Teresa Cristina Bergamo Bomfim[2]

1 Oswaldo Cruz Institute/Oswaldo Cruz Foundation, Rio de Janeiro, Brazil

2 Federal Rural University of Rio de Janeiro, Rio de Janeiro, Brazil

*Address all correspondence to: helenalucias@ioc.fiocruz.br

IntechOpen

© 2019 The Author(s). Licensee IntechOpen. This chapter is distributed under the terms of the Creative Commons Attribution License (http://creativecommons.org/licenses/by/3.0), which permits unrestricted use, distribution, and reproduction in any medium, provided the original work is properly cited. (cc) BY

References

[1] Feng Y, Ryan UM, Xiao L. Genetic diversity and population structure of *Cryptosporidium*. Trends in Parasitology. 2018;**34**(11):997-1011. DOI: 10.1016/j.pt.2018.07.009. PubMed PMID: 30108020

[2] Checkley W, White AC Jr, Jaganath D, Arrowood MJ, Chalmers RM, Chen XM, et al. A review of the global burden, novel diagnostics, therapeutics, and vaccine targets for *Cryptosporidium*. The Lancet Infectious Diseases. 2015;**15**(1):85-94. DOI: 10.1016/S1473-3099(14)70772-8. PubMed PMID: 25278220

[3] Ryan U, Fayer R, Xiao L. *Cryptosporidium* species in humans and animals: Current understanding and research needs. Parasitology. 2014;**141**(13):1667-1685. DOI: 10.1017/S0031182014001085. PubMed PMID: 25111501

[4] Ajjampur SS, Liakath FB, Kannan A, Rajendran P, Sarkar R, Moses PD, et al. Multisite study of cryptosporidiosis in children with diarrhea in India. Journal of Clinical Microbiology. 2010;**48**(6):2075-2081. DOI: 10.1128/JCM.02509-09. PubMed PMID: 20392919

[5] Kotloff KL, Blackwelder WC, Nasrin D, Nataro JP, Farag TH, van Eijk A, et al. The global enteric multicenter study (GEMS) of diarrheal disease in infants and young children in developing countries: Epidemiologic and clinical methods of the case/control study. Clinical Infectious Diseases. 2012;**55**(Suppl 4):S232-S245. DOI: 10.1093/cid/cis753. PubMed PMID: 23169936

[6] Shirley DA, Moonah SN, Kotloff KL. Burden of disease from cryptosporidiosis. Current Opinion in Infectious Diseases. 2012;**25**(5):555-563. DOI: 10.1097/QCO.0b013e328357e569. PubMed PMID: 22907279

[7] Korpe PS, Valencia C, Haque R, Mahfuz M, McGrath M, Houpt E, et al. Epidemiology and risk factors for cryptosporidiosis in children from 8 low-income sites: Results from the MAL-ED study. Clinical Infectious Diseases. 2018;**67**(11):1660-1669. DOI: 10.1093/cid/ciy355. PubMed PMID: 29701852

[8] Wheeler C, Vugia DJ, Thomas G, Beach MJ, Carnes S, Maier T, et al. Outbreak of cryptosporidiosis at a California waterpark: Employee and patron roles and the long road towards prevention. Epidemiology and Infection. 2007;**135**(2):302-310. DOI: 10.1017/S0950268806006777. PubMed PMID: 17291365

[9] Baldursson S, Karanis P. Waterborne transmission of protozoan parasites: Review of worldwide outbreaks-An update 2004-2010. Water Research. 2011;**45**(20):6603-6614. DOI: 10.1016/j.watres.2011.10.013. PubMed PMID: 22048017

[10] Navin TR, Juranek DD. Cryptosporidiosis: Clinical, epidemiologic, and parasitologic review. Reviews of Infectious Diseases. 1984;**6**(3):313-327. PubMed PMID: 6377439

[11] Ma P, Soave R. Three-step stool examination for cryptosporidiosis in 10 homosexual men with protracted watery diarrhea. The Journal of Infectious Diseases. 1983;**147**(5):824-828. DOI: 10.1093/infdis/147.5.824. PubMed PMID: 6842020

[12] Guerrant DI, Moore SR, Lima AA, Patrick PD, Schorling JB, Guerrant RL. Association of early childhood diarrhea and cryptosporidiosis with impaired physical fitness and cognitive function four-seven years later in a poor urban community in Northeast Brazil. The

American Journal of Tropical Medicine and Hygiene. 1999;**61**(5):707-713. DOI: 10.4269/ajtmh.1999.61.707. PubMed PMID: 10586898

[13] Operario DJ, Platts-Mills JA, Nadan S, Page N, Seheri M, Mphahlele J, et al. Etiology of severe acute watery diarrhea in children in the global rotavirus surveillance network using quantitative polymerase chain reaction. The Journal of Infectious Diseases. 2017;**216**(2):220-227. DOI: 10.1093/infdis/jix294. PubMed PMID: 28838152

[14] Krause I, Amir J, Cleper R, Dagan A, Behor J, Samra Z, et al. Cryptosporidiosis in children following solid organ transplantation. The Pediatric Infectious Disease Journal. 2012;**31**(11):1135-1138. DOI: 10.1097/INF.0b013e31826780f7. PubMed PMID: 22810017

[15] Wang RJ, Li JQ, Chen YC, Zhang LX, Xiao LH. Widespread occurrence of *Cryptosporidium* infections in patients with HIV/AIDS: Epidemiology, clinical feature, diagnosis, and therapy. Acta Tropica. 2018;**187**:257-263. DOI: 10.1016/j.actatropica.2018.08.018. PubMed PMID: 30118699

[16] Liu L, Johnson HL, Cousens S, Perin J, Scott S, Lawn JE, et al. Global, regional, and national causes of child mortality: An updated systematic analysis for 2010 with time trends since 2000. Lancet. 2012;**379**(9832):2151-2161. DOI: 10.1016/S0140-6736(12)60560-1. PubMed PMID: 22579125

[17] Caccio SM, Chalmers RM. Human cryptosporidiosis in Europe. Clinical Microbiology and Infection. 2016;**22**(6):471-480. DOI: 10.1016/j.cmi.2016.04.021. PubMed PMID: 27172805

[18] Xiao L. Molecular epidemiology of cryptosporidiosis: An update. Experimental Parasitology.

2010;**124**(1):80-89. DOI: 10.1016/j.exppara.2009.03.018. PubMed PMID: 19358845

[19] Carpenter C, Fayer R, Trout J, Beach MJ. Chlorine disinfection of recreational water for *Cryptosporidium parvum*. Emerging Infectious Diseases. 1999;**5**(4):579-584. DOI: 10.3201/eid0504.990425. PubMed PMID: 10458969

[20] Water Safety Plans: Managing Drinking Water Quality from Catchment to Consumer [Internet]. Geneva: World Health Organization; 2005

[21] Pollock KG, Young D, Robertson C, Ahmed S, Ramsay CN. Reduction in cryptosporidiosis associated with introduction of enhanced filtration of drinking water at loch Katrine. Scotland. Epidemiol Infect. 2014;**142**(1):56-62. DOI: 10.1017/S0950268813000678. PubMed PMID: 23591075

[22] WHO. Risk Assessment of *Cryptosporidium* in Drinking-Water Guidelines for Drinking-Water Quality. Geneva: WHO; 2011. pp. 303-304

[23] Manjunatha UH, Chao AT, Leong FJ, Diagana TT. Cryptosporidiosis drug discovery: Opportunities and challenges. ACS Infectious Diseases. 2016;**2**(8):530-537. DOI: 10.1021/acsinfecdis.6b00094. PubMed PMID: 27626293

[24] Ryan U, Paparini A, Oskam C. New technologies for detection of enteric parasites. Trends in Parasitology. 2017;**33**(7):532-546. DOI: 10.1016/j.pt.2017.03.005. PubMed PMID: 28385423

[25] Amadi B, Mwiya M, Sianongo S, Payne L, Watuka A, Katubulushi M, et al. High dose prolonged treatment with nitazoxanide is not effective for cryptosporidiosis in HIV positive Zambian children: A randomised

controlled trial. BMC Infectious Diseases. 2009;**9**:195. DOI: 10.1186/1471-2334-9-195. PubMed PMID: 19954529

[26] Cabada MM, White AC Jr. Treatment of cryptosporidiosis: Do we know what we think we know? Current Opinion in Infectious Diseases. 2010;**23**(5):494-499. DOI: 10.1097/QCO.0b013e32833de052. PubMed PMID: 20689422

[27] Vinayak S, Pawlowic MC, Sateriale A, Brooks CF, Studstill CJ, Bar-Peled Y, et al. Genetic modification of the diarrhoeal pathogen *Cryptosporidium parvum*. Nature. 2015;**523**(7561):477-480. DOI: 10.1038/nature14651. PubMed PMID: 26176919

[28] Beverley SM. Parasitology: CRISPR for *Cryptosporidium*. Nature. 2015;**523**(7561):413-414. DOI: 10.1038/nature14636. PubMed PMID: 26176915

[29] Witola WH, Zhang X, Kim CY. Targeted gene knockdown validates the essential role of lactate dehydrogenase in *Cryptosporidium parvum*. International Journal for Parasitology. 2017;**47**(13):867-874. DOI: 10.1016/j.ijpara.2017.05.002. PubMed PMID: 28606696

[30] Castellanos-Gonzalez A, Perry N, Nava S, White AC. Preassembled single-stranded RNA-Argonaute complexes: A novel method to silence genes in *Cryptosporidium*. The Journal of Infectious Diseases. 2016;**213**(8): 1307-1314. DOI: 10.1093/infdis/jiv588. PubMed PMID: 26656125

[31] Ifeonu OO, Chibucos MC, Orvis J, Su Q, Elwin K, Guo F, et al. Annotated draft genome sequences of three species of *Cryptosporidium*: *Cryptosporidium meleagridis* isolate UKMEL1, *C. baileyi* isolate TAMU-09Q1 and *C. hominis* isolates TU502_2012 and UKH1. Pathogens and Disease. 2016;**74**(7):1-5. DOI: 10.1093/femspd/ftw080. PubMed PMID: 27519257

[32] Xu Z, Guo Y, Roellig DM, Feng Y, Xiao L. Comparative analysis reveals conservation in genome organization among intestinal *Cryptosporidium* species and sequence divergence in potential secreted pathogenesis determinants among major human-infecting species. BMC Genomics. 2019;**20**(1):406. DOI: 10.1186/s12864-019-5788-9. PubMed PMID: 31117941

[33] Su J, Jin C, Wu H, Fei J, Li N, Guo Y, et al. Differential expression of three *Cryptosporidium* species-specific MEDLE proteins. Frontiers in Microbiology. 2019;**10**:1177. DOI: 10.3389/fmicb.2019.01177. PubMed PMID: 31191495

[34] Widmer G. Diverse single-amino-acid repeat profiles in the genus *Cryptosporidium*. Parasitology. 2018;**145**(9):1151-1160. DOI: 10.1017/S0031182018000112. PubMed PMID: 29429420

[35] Nader JL, Mathers TC, Ward BJ, Pachebat JA, Swain MT, Robinson G, et al. Evolutionary genomics of anthroponosis in *Cryptosporidium*. Nature Microbiology. 2019;**4**(5):826-836. DOI: 10.1038/s41564-019-0377-x. PubMed PMID: 30833731

[36] Hadfield SJ, Pachebat JA, Swain MT, Robinson G, Cameron SJ, Alexander J, et al. Generation of whole genome sequences of new *Cryptosporidium hominis* and *Cryptosporidium parvum* isolates directly from stool samples. BMC Genomics. 2015;**16**:650. DOI: 10.1186/s12864-015-1805-9. PubMed PMID: 26318339

[37] Zhang H, Guo F, Zhou H, Zhu G. Transcriptome analysis reveals unique metabolic features in the *Cryptosporidium parvum* oocysts associated with environmental survival and stresses. BMC Genomics. 2012;**13**:647. DOI: 10.1186/1471-2164-13-647. PubMed PMID: 23171372

[38] Xu P, Widmer G, Wang Y, Ozaki LS, Alves JM, Serrano MG, et al. The genome of *Cryptosporidium hominis*. Nature. 2004;**431**(7012):1107-1112. DOI: 10.1038/nature02977. PubMed PMID: 15510150

[39] Clark DP. New insights into human cryptosporidiosis. Clinical Microbiology Reviews. 1999;**12**(4):554-563. PubMed PMID: 10515902

[40] Hunter PR, Hughes S, Woodhouse S, Syed Q, Verlander NQ, Chalmers RM, et al. Sporadic cryptosporidiosis case-control study with genotyping. Emerging Infectious Diseases. 2004;**10**(7):1241-1249. DOI: 10.3201/eid1007.030582. PubMed PMID: 15324544

[41] Chalmers RM, Davies AP. Minireview: Clinical cryptosporidiosis. Experimental Parasitology. 2010;**124**(1):138-146. DOI: 10.1016/j.exppara.2009.02.003. PubMed PMID: 19545516

[42] Hunter PR, Hadfield SJ, Wilkinson D, Lake IR, Harrison FC, Chalmers RM. Subtypes of *Cryptosporidium parvum* in humans and disease risk. Emerging Infectious Diseases. 2007;**13**(1):82-88. DOI: 10.3201/eid1301.060481. PubMed PMID: 17370519

[43] Fayer R. Ungar BL, *Cryptosporidium* spp. and cryptosporidiosis. Microbiology Reviews. 1986;**50**(4):458-483. PubMed PMID: 3540573

[44] Casemore DP. Epidemiological aspects of human cryptosporidiosis. Epidemiology and Infection. 1990;**104**(1):1-28. DOI: 10.1017/s0950268800054480. PubMed PMID: 2407541

[45] Chappell CL, Okhuysen PC, Langer-Curry R, Widmer G, Akiyoshi DE, Tanriverdi S, et al. *Cryptosporidium hominis*: Experimental challenge of healthy adults. American Journal of Tropical Medicine and Hygiene. 2006;**75**(5):851-857. PubMed PMID: 17123976

[46] Ryan U, Zahedi A, Paparini A. *Cryptosporidium* in humans and animals-a one health approach to prophylaxis. Parasite Immunology. 2006;**38**(9):535-547. DOI: 10.1111/pim.12350. PubMed PMID: 27454991

[47] Mercado R, Buck GA, Manque PA, Ozaki LS. *Cryptosporidium hominis* infection of the human respiratory tract. Emerging Infectious Diseases. 2007;**13**(3):462-464. DOI: 10.3201/eid1303.060394. PubMed PMID: 17552101

[48] Xiao L, Feng Y. Zoonotic cryptosporidiosis. FEMS Immunology and Medical Microbiology. 2008;**52**(3):309-323. DOI: 10.1111/j.1574-695X.2008.00377.x. PubMed PMID: 18205803

[49] Vanathy K, Parija SC, Mandal J, Hamide A, Krishnamurthy S. Cryptosporidiosis: A mini review. Tropical Parasitology. 2017;**7**(2):72-80. DOI: 10.4103/tp.TP_25_17. PubMed PMID: 29114483

[50] McNabb SJ, Hensel DM, Welch DF, Heijbel H, McKee GL, Istre GR. Comparison of sedimentation and flotation techniques for identification of *Cryptosporidium* sp. oocysts in a large outbreak of human diarrhea. Journal of Clinical Microbiology. 1985;**22**(4):587-589. PubMed PMID: 2416771

[51] Alles AJ, Waldron MA, Sierra LS, Mattia AR. Prospective comparison of direct immunofluorescence and conventional staining methods for detection of *Giardia* and *Cryptosporidium* spp. in human fecal specimens. Journal of Clinical Microbiology. 1995;**33**(6):1632-1634. PubMed PMID: 7544365

[52] O'Donoghue PJ. *Cryptosporidium* and cryptosporidiosis in man and

animals. International Journal for Parasitology. 1995;**25**(2):139-195. PubMed PMID: 7622324

[53] Baxby D, Blundell N, Hart CA. The development and performance of a simple, sensitive method for the detection of *Cryptosporidium* oocysts in faeces. The Journal of Hygiene. 1984;**93**(2):317-323. DOI: 10.1017/s0022172400064858. PubMed PMID: 6209333

[54] Pohjola S, Jokipii L, Jokipii AM. Dimethylsulphoxide-Ziehl-Neelsen staining technique for detection of cryptosporidial oocysts. The Veterinary Record. 1985;**116**(16):442-443. PubMed PMID: 2408372

[55] Henriksen SA, Pohlenz JF. Staining of cryptosporidia by a modified Ziehl-Neelsen technique. Acta Veterinaria Scandinavica. 1981;**22**(3-4):594-596. PubMed PMID: 6178277

[56] Ignatius R, Klemm T, Zander S, Gahutu JB, Kimmig P, Mockenhaupt FP, et al. Highly specific detection of *Cryptosporidium* spp. oocysts in human stool samples by undemanding and inexpensive phase contrast microscopy. Parasitology Research. 2016;**115**(3):1229-1234. DOI: 10.1007/s00436-015-4859-3. PubMed PMID: 26646397

[57] Smith HV, McDiarmid A, Smith AL, Hinson AR, Gilmour RA. An analysis of staining methods for the detection of *Cryptosporidium* spp. oocysts in water-related samples. Parasitology. 1989;**99**(Pt 3):323-327. PubMed PMID: 2481834

[58] Moodley D, Jackson TF, Gathiram V, van den Ende J. *Cryptosporidium* infections in children in Durban. Seasonal variation, age distribution and disease status. South African Medical Journal. 1991;**79**(6):295-297. PubMed PMID: 2017736

[59] Fall A, Thompson RC, Hobbs RP, Morgan-Ryan U. Morphology is not a reliable tool for delineating species within *Cryptosporidium*. The Journal of Parasitology. 2003;**89**(2):399-402. DOI: 10.1645/0022-3395(2003)089[0399:MINART]2.0.CO;2. PubMed PMID: 12760666

[60] Garcia LS, Bruckner DA, Brewer TC, Shimizu RY. Techniques for the recovery and identification of *Cryptosporidium* oocysts from stool specimens. Journal of Clinical Microbiology. 1983;**18**(1):185-190. PubMed PMID: 6193138

[61] Geurden T, Thomas P, Casaert S, Vercruysse J, Claerebout E. Prevalence and molecular characterisation of *Cryptosporidium* and *Giardia* in lambs and goat kids in Belgium. Veterinary Parasitology. 2008;**155**(1-2):142-145. DOI: 10.1016/j.vetpar.2008.05.002. PubMed PMID: 18565678

[62] Robinson TJ, Cebelinski EA, Taylor C, Smith KE. Evaluation of the positive predictive value of rapid assays used by clinical laboratories in Minnesota for the diagnosis of cryptosporidiosis. Clinical Infectious Diseases. 2010;**50**(8):e53-e55. DOI: 10.1086/651423. PubMed PMID: 20218890

[63] Agnamey P, Sarfati C, Pinel C, Rabodoniriina M, Kapel N, Dutoit E, et al. Evaluation of four commercial rapid immunochromatographic assays for detection of *Cryptosporidium* antigens in stool samples: A blind multicenter trial. Journal of Clinical Microbiology. 2011;**49**(4):1605-1607. DOI: 10.1128/JCM.02074-10. PubMed PMID: 21289154

[64] Garcia LS, Shimizu RY. Evaluation of nine immunoassay kits (enzyme immunoassay and direct fluorescence) for detection of Giardia lamblia and *Cryptosporidium parvum* in human fecal specimens. Journal of Clinical

Microbiology. 1997;**35**(6):1526-1529. PubMed PMID: 9163474

[65] Bialek R, Binder N, Dietz K, Joachim A, Knobloch J, Zelck UE. Comparison of fluorescence, antigen and PCR assays to detect *Cryptosporidium parvum* in fecal specimens. Diagnostic Microbiology and Infectious Disease. 2002;**43**(4):283-288. PubMed PMID: 12151188

[66] Srijan A, Wongstitwilairoong B, Pitarangsi C, Serichantalergs O, Fukuda CD, Bodhidatta L, et al. Re-evaluation of commercially available enzyme-linked immunosorbent assay for the detection of *Giardia lamblia* and *Cryptosporidium* spp. from stool specimens. The Southeast Asian Journal of Tropical Medicine and Public Health. 2005;**36**(Suppl 4):26-29. PubMed PMID: 16438175

[67] Chalmers RL, Wagner H, Mitchell GL, Lam DY, Kinoshita BT, Jansen ME, et al. Age and other risk factors for corneal infiltrative and inflammatory events in young soft contact lens wearers from the Contact Lens Assessment in Youth (CLAY) study. Investigative Ophthalmology & Visual Science. 2011;**52**(9):6690-6696. DOI: 10.1167/iovs.10-7018. PubMed PMID: 21527379

[68] Llorente MT, Clavel A, Varea M, Olivera S, Castillo FJ, Sahagun J, et al. Evaluation of an immunochromatographic dip-strip test for the detection of *Cryptosporidium* oocysts in stool specimens. European Journal of Clinical Microbiology & Infectious Diseases. 2002;**21**(8):624-625. DOI: 10.1007/s10096-002-0778-1. PubMed PMID: 12226697

[69] Weitzel T, Dittrich S, Mohl I, Adusu E, Jelinek T. Evaluation of seven commercial antigen detection tests for *Giardia* and *Cryptosporidium* in stool samples. Clinical Microbiology and Infection. 2006;**12**(7):656-659. DOI: 10.1111/j.1469-0691.2006.01457.x. PubMed PMID: 16774562

[70] Chalmers RM, Campbell BM, Crouch N, Charlett A, Davies AP. Comparison of diagnostic sensitivity and specificity of seven *Cryptosporidium* assays used in the UK. Journal of Medical Microbiology. 2011;**60**(Pt 11):1598-1604. DOI: 10.1099/jmm.0.034181-0. PubMed PMID: 21757501

[71] Soliman RH, Othman AA. Evaluation of DNA melting curve analysis real-time PCR for detection and differentiation of *Cryptosporidium* species. Parasitologists United Journal (PUJ). 2009;**2**(1):47-54

[72] Mary C, Chapey E, Dutoit E, Guyot K, Hasseine L, Jeddi F, et al. Multicentric evaluation of a new real-time PCR assay for quantification of *Cryptosporidium* spp. and identification of *Cryptosporidium parvum* and *Cryptosporidium hominis*. Journal of Clinical Microbiology. 2013;**51**(8):2556-2563. DOI: 10.1128/JCM.03458-12. PubMed PMID: 23720792

[73] Spano F, Putignani L, McLauchlin J, Casemore DP, Crisanti A. PCR-RFLP analysis of the *Cryptosporidium* oocyst wall protein (COWP) gene discriminates between *C. wrairi* and *C. parvum*, and between *C. parvum* isolates of human and animal origin. FEMS Microbiology Letters. 1997;**150**(2):209-217. DOI: 10.1016/s0378-1097(97)00115-8. PubMed PMID: 9170264

[74] Abe N, Matsubayashi M, Kimata I, Iseki M. Subgenotype analysis of *Cryptosporidium parvum* isolates from humans and animals in Japan using the 60-kDa glycoprotein gene sequences. Parasitology Research. 2006;**99**(3):303-305. DOI: 10.1007/s00436-006-0140-0. PubMed PMID: 16565816

[75] Jothikumar N, da Silva AJ, Moura I, Qvarnstrom Y, Hill VR. Detection and differentiation of *Cryptosporidium hominis* and *Cryptosporidium parvum* by dual TaqMan assays. Journal of Medical Microbiology. 2008;**57**(Pt 9):1099-1105. DOI: 10.1099/jmm.0.2008/001461-0. PubMed PMID: 18719179

[76] Sturbaum GD, Reed C, Hoover PJ, Jost BH, Marshall MM, Sterling CR. Species-specific, nested PCR-restriction fragment length polymorphism detection of single *Cryptosporidium parvum* oocysts. Applied and Environmental Microbiology. 2001;**67**(6):2665-2668. DOI: 10.1128/AEM.67.6.2665-2668.2001. PubMed PMID: 11375178

[77] Hadfield SJ, Robinson G, Elwin K, Chalmers RM. Detection and differentiation of *Cryptosporidium* spp. in human clinical samples by use of real-time PCR. Journal of Clinical Microbiology. 2011;**49**(3):918-924. DOI: 10.1128/JCM.01733-10. PubMed PMID: 21177904

[78] Navidad JF, Griswold DJ, Gradus MS, Bhattacharyya S. Evaluation of Luminex xTAG gastrointestinal pathogen analyte-specific reagents for high-throughput, simultaneous detection of bacteria, viruses, and parasites of clinical and public health importance. Journal of Clinical Microbiology. 2013;**51**(9):3018-3024. DOI: 10.1128/JCM.00896-13. PubMed PMID: 23850948

[79] Jiang J, Xiao L. An evaluation of molecular diagnostic tools for the detection and differentiation of human-pathogenic *Cryptosporidium* spp. The Journal of Eukaryotic Microbiology. 2003;**50**:542-547. PubMed PMID: 14736156

[80] Robinson G, Chalmers RM. Assessment of polymorphic genetic markers for multi-locus typing of *Cryptosporidium parvum* and

Cryptosporidium hominis. Experimental Parasitology. 2012;**132**(2):200-215. DOI: 10.1016/j.exppara.2012.06.016. PubMed PMID: 22781277

[81] Sulaiman IM, Lal AA, Xiao L. Molecular phylogeny and evolutionary relationships of *Cryptosporidium* parasites at the actin locus. The Journal of Parasitology. 2002;**88**(2):388-394. DOI: 10.1645/0022-3395(2002)088[0388:MPAERO]2.0.CO;2. PubMed PMID: 12054017

[82] Spano F, Putignani L, Crisanti A, Sallicandro P, Morgan UM, Le Blancq SM, et al. Multilocus genotypic analysis of *Cryptosporidium parvum* isolates from different hosts and geographical origins. Journal of Clinical Microbiology. 1998;**36**(11):3255-3259. PubMed PMID: 9774575

[83] Pedraza-Diaz S, Amar C, McLauchlin J. The identification and characterisation of an unusual genotype of *Cryptosporidium* from human faeces as *Cryptosporidium meleagridis*. FEMS Microbiology Letters. 2000;**189**(2):189-194. DOI: 10.1111/j.1574-6968.2000.tb09228.x. PubMed PMID: 10930736

[84] Feng Y, Yang W, Ryan U, Zhang L, Kvac M, Koudela B, et al. Development of a multilocus sequence tool for typing *Cryptosporidium muris* and *Cryptosporidium andersoni*. Journal of Clinical Microbiology. 2011;**49**(1):34-41. DOI: 10.1128/JCM.01329-10. PubMed PMID: 20980577

[85] Yadav P, Mirdha BR, Makharia GK, Chaudhry R. Multilocus sequence typing of *Cryptosporidium hominis* from northern India. The Indian Journal of Medical Research. 2017;**145**(1):102-111. DOI: 10.4103/ijmr.IJMR_1064_14. PubMed PMID: 28574022

[86] Plutzer J, Karanis P. Genetic polymorphism in *Cryptosporidium* species: An update. Veterinary Parasitology. 2009;**165**(3-4):187-199.

DOI: 10.1016/j.vetpar.2009.07.003.
PubMed PMID: 19660869

[87] Xiao L, Feng Y. Molecular
epidemiologic tools for waterborne
pathogens *Cryptosporidium* spp.
and *Giardia duodenalis*. Food and
Waterborne Parasitology. 2017;**8-9**:14-32

[88] Molloy SF, Smith HV, Kirwan P,
Nichols RA, Asaolu SO, Connelly L,
et al. Identification of a high diversity
of *Cryptosporidium* species genotypes
and subtypes in a pediatric population
in Nigeria. The American Journal
of Tropical Medicine and Hygiene.
2010;**82**(4):608-613. DOI: 10.4269/
ajtmh.2010.09-0624. PubMed PMID:
20348508

[89] Feng Y, Lal AA, Li N, Xiao L.
Subtypes of *Cryptosporidium* spp. in mice
and other small mammals. Experimental
Parasitology. 2011;**127**(1):238-242. DOI:
10.1016/j.exppara.2010.08.002. PubMed
PMID: 20692256

[90] Li W, Kiulia NM, Mwenda JM,
Nyachieo A, Taylor MB, Zhang X, et al.
*Cyclospora papionis, Cryptosporidium
hominis*, and human-pathogenic
Enterocytozoon bieneusi in captive
baboons in Kenya. Journal of Clinical
Microbiology. 2011;**49**(12):4326-4329.
DOI: 10.1128/JCM.05051-11. PubMed
PMID: 21956988

[91] Laatamna AE, Wagnerova P, Sak B,
Kvetonova D, Xiao L, Rost M, et al.
Microsporidia and *Cryptosporidium* in
horses and donkeys in Algeria: Detection
of a novel *Cryptosporidium hominis*
subtype family (Ik) in a horse. Veterinary
Parasitology. 2015;**208**(3-4):135-142.
DOI: 10.1016/j.vetpar.2015.01.007.
PubMed PMID: 25638716

[92] Hira KG, Mackay MR,
Hempstead AD, Ahmed S, Karim MM,
O'Connor RM, et al. Genetic diversity
of *Cryptosporidium* spp. from
Bangladeshi children. Journal of Clinical

Microbiology. 2011;**49**(6):2307-2310.
DOI: 10.1128/JCM.00164-11. PubMed
PMID: 21471344

[93] Insulander M, Silverlas C,
Lebbad M, Karlsson L, Mattsson JG,
Svenungsson B. Molecular epidemiology
and clinical manifestations of
human cryptosporidiosis in Sweden.
Epidemiology and Infection.
2013;**141**(5):1009-1020. DOI: 10.1017/
S0950268812001665. PubMed PMID:
22877562

[94] Liu X, Zhou X, Zhong Z, Zuo Z,
Shi J, Wang Y, et al. Occurrence of
novel and rare subtype families of
Cryptosporidium in bamboo rats
(*Rhizomys sinensis*) in China. Veterinary
Parasitology. 2015;**207**(1-2):144-148.
DOI: 10.1016/j.vetpar.2014.11.009.
PubMed PMID: 25499825

[95] Vermeulen ET, Ashworth DL,
Eldridge MD, Power ML. Diversity
of *Cryptosporidium* in brush-tailed
rock-wallabies (*Petrogale penicillata*)
managed within a species recovery
programme. The International Journal
for Parasitology: Parasites and Wildlife.
2015;**4**(2):190-196. DOI: 10.1016/j.
ijppaw.2015.02.005. PubMed PMID:
25834789

[96] Stensvold CR, Beser J, Axen C,
Lebbad M. High applicability of a novel
method for gp60-based subtyping
of *Cryptosporidium meleagridis*.
Journal of Clinical Microbiology.
2014;**52**(7):2311-2319. DOI: 10.1128/
JCM.00598-14. PubMed PMID:
24740082

[97] Haserick JR, Klein JA, Costello CE,
Samuelson J. *Cryptosporidium parvum*
vaccine candidates are incompletely
modified with O-linked-N-
acetylgalactosamine or contain
N-terminal N-myristate and S-palmitate.
PLoS One. 2017;**12**(8):e0182395. DOI:
10.1371/journal.pone.0182395. PubMed
PMID: 28792526

[98] FDA. New drug for parasitic infections in children. FDA Consumer. 2003;**37**(3):4. PubMed PMID: 12793375.

[99] Gargala G. Drug treatment and novel drug target against *Cryptosporidium*. Parasite. 2008;**15**(3):275-281. DOI: 10.1051/parasite/2008153275. PubMed PMID: 18814694

[100] Singh N, Narayan S. Nitazoxanide: A broad spectrum antimicrobial. Medical Journal, Armed Forces India. 2011;**67**(1):67-68. DOI: 10.1016/S0377-1237(11)80020- 1S0377-1237(11)80020-1. PubMed PMID: 27365765

[101] Debnath A, Ndao M, Reed SL. Reprofiled drug targets ancient protozoans: Drug discovery for parasitic diarrheal diseases. Gut Microbes. 2013;**4**(1):66-71. DOI: 10.4161/gmic.22596. PubMed PMID: 23137963

[102] Bessoff K, Sateriale A, Lee KK, Huston CD. Drug repurposing screen reveals FDA-approved inhibitors of human HMG-CoA reductase and isoprenoid synthesis that block *Cryptosporidium parvum* growth. Antimicrobial Agents and Chemotherapy. 2013;**57**(4):1804-1814. DOI: 10.1128/AAC.02460-12. PubMed PMID: 23380723

[103] Debnath A, Parsonage D, Andrade RM, He C, Cobo ER, Hirata K, et al. A high-throughput drug screen for *Entamoeba histolytica* identifies a new lead and target. Nature Medicine. 2012;**18**(6):956-960. DOI: 10.1038/nm.2758. PubMed PMID: 22610278

[104] Bouzid M, Hunter PR, Chalmers RM, Tyler KM. *Cryptosporidium* pathogenicity and virulence. Clinical Microbiology Reviews. 2013;**26**(1):115-134. DOI: 10.1128/CMR.00076-12. PubMed PMID: 23297262

[105] Tzipori S, Griffiths JK. Natural history and biology of *Cryptosporidium parvum*. Advances in Parasitology. 1998;**40**:5-36. PubMed PMID: 9554069

[106] Leitch GJ, He Q. Cryptosporidiosis—An overview. Journal of Biomedical Research. 2011;**25**(1):1-16. DOI: 10.1016/S1674-8301(11)60001-8. PubMed PMID: 22685452

[107] O'Hara SP, Chen XM. The cell biology of *Cryptosporidium* infection. Microbes and Infection. 2011;**13**(8-9):721-730. DOI: 10.1016/j.micinf.2011.03.008. PubMed PMID: 21458585

[108] Koh W, Thompson A, Edwards H, Monis P, Clode PL. Extracellular excystation and development of *Cryptosporidium*: Tracing the fate of oocysts within Pseudomonas aquatic biofilm systems. BMC Microbiology. 2014;**14**:281. DOI: 10.1186/s12866-014-0281-8. PubMed PMID: 25403949

[109] Aldeyarbi HM, Karanis P. Electron microscopic observation of the early stages of *Cryptosporidium parvum* asexual multiplication and development in in vitro axenic culture. European Journal of Protistology. 2016;**52**:36-44. DOI: 10.1016/j.ejop.2015.07.002. PubMed PMID: 26587578

[110] Karanis P, Aldeyarbi HM. Evolution of *Cryptosporidium* in vitro culture. International Journal for Parasitology. 2011;**41**(12):1231-1242. DOI: 10.1016/j.ijpara.2011.08.001. PubMed PMID: 21889507

[111] Ryan U, Paparini A, Monis P, Hijjawi N. It's official-*Cryptosporidium* is a gregarine: What are the implications for the water industry? Water Research. 2016;**105**:305-313. DOI: 10.1016/j.watres.2016.09.013. PubMed PMID: 27639055

[112] Tzipori S, Widmer G. A hundred-year retrospective on cryptosporidiosis. Trends in

Parasitology. 2008;**24**(4):184-189. DOI: 10.1016/j.pt.2008.01.002. PubMed PMID: 18329342

[113] Petry F. Structural analysis of *Cryptosporidium parvum*. Microscopy and Microanalysis. 2004;**10**(5):586-601. DOI: 10.1017/S1431927604040929. PubMed PMID: 15525433

[114] Liu S, Roellig DM, Guo Y, Li N, Frace MA, Tang K, et al. Evolution of mitosome metabolism and invasion-related proteins in *Cryptosporidium*. BMC Genomics. 2016;**17**(1):1006. DOI: 10.1186/s12864-016-3343-5. PubMed PMID: 27931183

[115] Cavalier-Smith T. Gregarine site-heterogeneous 18S rDNA trees, revision of gregarine higher classification, and the evolutionary diversification of Sporozoa. European Journal of Protistology. 2014;**50**(5):472-495. DOI: 10.1016/j.ejop.2014.07.002. PubMed PMID: 25238406

[116] Johnson AM, Linden K, Ciociola KM, De Leon R, Widmer G, Rochelle PA. UV inactivation of *Cryptosporidium hominis* as measured in cell culture. Applied and Environmental Microbiology. 2005;**71**(5):2800-2802. DOI: 10.1128/AEM.71.5.2800-2802.2005. PubMed PMID: 15870378

[117] Robertson LJ, Campbell AT, Smith HV. Survival of *Cryptosporidium parvum* oocysts under various environmental pressures. Applied and Environmental Microbiology. 1992;**58**(11):3494-3500. PubMed PMID: 1482175

[118] Deng MQ, Cliver DO. *Cryptosporidium parvum* studies with dairy products. International Journal of Food Microbiology. 1999;**46**(2):113-121. PubMed PMID: 10728612

[119] Davies CM, Altavilla N, Krogh M, Ferguson CM, Deere DA, Ashbolt NJ. Environmental inactivation of *Cryptosporidium* oocysts in catchment soils. Journal of Applied Microbiology. 2005;**98**(2):308-317. DOI: 10.1111/j.1365-2672.2004.02459.x. PubMed PMID: 15659185

[120] King BJ, Monis PT. Critical processes affecting *Cryptosporidium* oocyst survival in the environment. Parasitology. 2007;**134**(Pt 3):309-323. DOI: 10.1017/S0031182006001491. PubMed PMID: 17096874

[121] Jenkins MB, Bowman DD, Fogarty EA, Ghiorse WC. *Cryptosporidium parvum* oocyst inactivation in three soil types at various temperatures and water potentials. Soil Biology and Biochemistry. 2002;**34**:1101-1109

[122] Fayer R, Nerad T. Effects of low temperatures on viability of *Cryptosporidium parvum* oocysts. Applied and Environmental Microbiology. 1996;**62**(4):1431-1433. PubMed PMID: 8919806

[123] Keevil CW. Rapid detection of biofilms and adherent pathogens using scanning confocal laser microscopy and episcopic differential interference contrast microscopy. Water Science and Technology. 2003;**47**(5):105-116. PubMed PMID: 12701914

[124] Fayer R, Graczyk TK, Lewis EJ, Trout JM, Farley CA. Survival of infectious *Cryptosporidium parvum* oocysts in seawater and eastern oysters (*Crassostrea virginica*) in the Chesapeake Bay. Applied and Environmental Microbiology. 1998;**64**(3):1070-1074. PubMed PMID: 9501446

[125] World Health Organization. Water, Sanitation and Health Team. Risk Assessment of *Cryptosporidium* in Drinking Water. Geneva: World Health Organization; 2009

[126] Putignani L, Menichella D. Global distribution, public health and clinical

impact of the protozoan pathogen
Cryptosporidium. Interdisciplinary
Perspectives on Infectious
Diseases. 2010;**2010**:1-39. DOI:
10.1155/2010/753512. PubMed PMID:
20706669

[127] Parsons MB, Travis D,
Lonsdorf EV, Lipende I, Roellig DM,
Collins A, et al. Epidemiology and
molecular characterization of
Cryptosporidium spp. in humans, wild
primates, and domesticated animals in
the greater Gombe ecosystem, Tanzania.
PLoS Neglected Tropical Diseases.
2015;**9**(2):e0003529. DOI: 10.1371/
journal.pntd.0003529. PubMed PMID:
25700265

[128] Caccio SM, Sannella AR, Mariano V,
Valentini S, Berti F, Tosini F, et al. A
rare *Cryptosporidium parvum* genotype
associated with infection of lambs and
zoonotic transmission in Italy. Veterinary
Parasitology. 2013;**191**(1-2):128-131.
DOI: 10.1016/j.vetpar.2012.08.010.
PubMed PMID: 22954678

[129] Casemore DP. Sheep as a source of
human cryptosporidiosis. The Journal of
Infection. 1989;**19**(2):101-104. PubMed
PMID: 2809233

[130] Current WL, Reese NC,
Ernst JV, Bailey WS, Heyman MB,
Weinstein WM. Human
cryptosporidiosis in immunocompetent
and immunodeficient persons. Studies
of an outbreak and experimental
transmission. The New England Journal
of Medicine. 1983;**308**(21):1252-1257.
DOI: 10.1056/NEJM198305263082102.
PubMed PMID: 6843609

[131] Efstratiou A, Ongerth JE,
Karanis P. Waterborne transmission
of protozoan parasites: Review of
worldwide outbreaks—An update 2011-
2016. Water Research. 2017;**114**:14-22

[132] Ryan U, Hijjawi N, Xiao L.
Foodborne cryptosporidiosis.
International Journal for Parasitology.

2018;**48**(1):1-12. DOI: 10.1016/j.
ijpara.2017.09.004. PubMed PMID:
29122606

[133] Hlavsa MC, Roberts VA,
Anderson AR, Hill VR, Kahler AM,
Orr M, et al. Surveillance for waterborne
disease outbreaks and other health
events associated with recreational
water—United States, 2007-2008.
MMWR Surveillance Summaries.
2011;**60**(12):1-32. PubMed PMID:
21937976

[134] Hunter PR, Zmirou-Navier D,
Hartemann P. Estimating the impact on
health of poor reliability of drinking
water interventions in developing
countries. Science of the Total
Environment. 2009;**407**(8):2621-2624.
DOI: 10.1016/j.scitotenv.2009.01.018.
PubMed PMID: 19193396

[135] Reinoso R, Becares E, Smith HV.
Effect of various environmental factors
on the viability of *Cryptosporidium
parvum* oocysts. Journal of Applied
Microbiology. 2008;**104**(4):980-986.
DOI: 10.1111/j.1365-2672.2007.03620.x.
PubMed PMID: 17973913

[136] Chappell CL, Okhuysen PC,
Sterling CR, DuPont HL.
Cryptosporidium parvum: Intensity of
infection and oocyst excretion patterns
in healthy volunteers. The Journal of
Infectious Diseases. 1996;**173**(1):232-236.
DOI: 10.1093/infdis/173.1.232. PubMed
PMID: 8537664

[137] Chappell CL, Okhuysen PC,
Sterling CR, Wang C,
Jakubowski W, Dupont HL. Infectivity
of *Cryptosporidium parvum* in healthy
adults with pre-existing anti-*C.
parvum* serum immunoglobulin G. The
American Journal of Tropical Medicine
and Hygiene. 1999;**60**(1):157-164. DOI:
10.4269/ajtmh.1999.60.157. PubMed
PMID: 9988341

[138] MacKenzie WR, Schell WL,
Blair KA, Addiss DG, Peterson DE,

Hoxie NJ, et al. Massive outbreak of waterborne *Cryptosporidium* infection in Milwaukee, Wisconsin: Recurrence of illness and risk of secondary transmission. Clinical Infectious Diseases. 1995;**21**(1):57-62. DOI: 10.1093/clinids/21.1.57. PubMed PMID: 7578760

[139] Leoni F, Amar C, Nichols G, Pedraza-Diaz S, McLauchlin J. Genetic analysis of *Cryptosporidium* from 2414 humans with diarrhoea in England between 1985 and 2000. Journal of Medical Microbiology. 2006;**55**(Pt 6):703-707. DOI: 10.1099/jmm.0.46251-0. PubMed PMID: 16687587

[140] Morse TD, Nichols RA, Grimason AM, Campbell BM, Tembo KC, Smith HV. Incidence of cryptosporidiosis species in paediatric patients in Malawi. Epidemiology and Infection. 2007;**135**(8):1307-1315. DOI: 10.1017/S0950268806007758. PubMed PMID: 17224087

[141] Waldron LS, Cheung-Kwok-Sang C, Power ML. Wildlife-associated *Cryptosporidium fayeri* in human, Australia. Emerging Infectious Diseases. 2010;**16**(12):2006-2007. DOI: 10.3201/eid1612.100715. PubMed PMID: 21122247

[142] Agholi M, Hatam GR, Motazedian MH. HIV/AIDS-associated opportunistic protozoal diarrhea. AIDS Research and Human Retroviruses. 2013;**29**(1):35-41. DOI: 10.1089/AID.2012.0119. PubMed PMID: 22873400

[143] Jiang Y, Ren J, Yuan Z, Liu A, Zhao H, Liu H, et al. *Cryptosporidium andersoni* as a novel predominant *Cryptosporidium* species in outpatients with diarrhea in Jiangsu Province, China. BMC Infectious Diseases. 2014;**14**:555. DOI: 10.1186/s12879-014-0555-7. PubMed PMID: 25344387

[144] Liu H, Shen Y, Yin J, Yuan Z, Jiang Y, Xu Y, et al. Prevalence and genetic characterization of *Cryptosporidium*, *Enterocytozoon*, *Giardia* and *Cyclospora* in diarrheal outpatients in China. BMC Infectious Diseases. 2014;**14**:25. DOI: 10.1186/1471-2334-14-25. PubMed PMID: 24410985

[145] Ditrich O, Palkovic L, Sterba J, Prokopic J, Loudova J, Giboda M. The first finding of *Cryptosporidium baileyi* in man. Parasitology Research. 1991;**77**(1):44-47. PubMed PMID: 1825238

[146] Khan SM, Debnath C, Pramanik AK, Xiao L, Nozaki T, Ganguly S. Molecular characterization and assessment of zoonotic transmission of *Cryptosporidium* from dairy cattle in West Bengal, India. Veterinary Parasitology. 2010;**171**(1-2):41-47. DOI: 10.1016/j.vetpar.2010.03.008. PubMed PMID: 20356678

[147] Helmy YA, Krucken J, Nockler K, von Samson-Himmelstjerna G, Zessin KH. Molecular epidemiology of *Cryptosporidium* in livestock animals and humans in the Ismailia province of Egypt. Veterinary Parasitology. 2013;**193**(1-3):15-24. DOI: 10.1016/j.vetpar.2012.12.015. PubMed PMID: 23305974

[148] Gatei W, Barrett D, Lindo JF, Eldemire-Shearer D, Cama V, Xiao L. Unique *Cryptosporidium* population in HIV-infected persons, Jamaica. Emerging Infectious Diseases. 2008;**14**(5):841-843. DOI: 10.3201/eid1405.071277. PubMed PMID: 18439378

[149] Gatei W, Suputtamongkol Y, Waywa D, Ashford RW, Bailey JW, Greensill J, et al. Zoonotic species of *Cryptosporidium* are as prevalent as the anthroponotic in HIV-infected patients in Thailand. Annals of Tropical Medicine and Parasitology. 2002;**96**(8):797-802. DOI: 10.1179/000349802125002202. PubMed PMID: 12625934

[150] Lucio-Forster A, Griffiths JK, Cama VA, Xiao L, Bowman DD. Minimal zoonotic risk of cryptosporidiosis from pet dogs and cats. Trends in Parasitology. 2010;**26**(4):174-179. DOI: 10.1016/j.pt.2010.01.004. PubMed PMID: 20176507

[151] Robinson G, Chalmers RM. The European rabbit (*Oryctolagus cuniculus*), a source of zoonotic cryptosporidiosis. Zoonoses and Public Health. 2010;**57**(7-8):e1-e13. DOI: 10.1111/j.1863-2378.2009.01308.x. PubMed PMID: 20042061

[152] Elwin K, Hadfield SJ, Robinson G, Chalmers RM. The epidemiology of sporadic human infections with unusual cryptosporidia detected during routine typing in England and Wales, 2000-2008. Epidemiology and Infection. 2012;**140**(4):673-683. DOI: 10.1017/S0950268811000860. PubMed PMID: 21733255

[153] Chalmers RM, Robinson G, Elwin K, Hadfield SJ, Xiao L, Ryan U, et al. *Cryptosporidium* sp. rabbit genotype, a newly identified human pathogen. Emerging Infectious Diseases. 2009;**15**(5):829-830. DOI: 10.3201/eid1505.081419. PubMed PMID: 19402985

[154] Chalmers RM, Elwin K, Hadfield SJ, Robinson G. Sporadic human cryptosporidiosis caused by *Cryptosporidium cuniculus*, United Kingdom, 2007-2008. Emerging Infectious Diseases. 2011;**17**(3):536-538. DOI: 10.3201/eid1703.100410. PubMed PMID: 21392453

[155] Koehler AV, Whipp MJ, Haydon SR, Gasser RB. *Cryptosporidium cuniculus*— New records in human and kangaroo in Australia. Parasites & Vectors. 2014;**7**:492. DOI: 10.1186/s13071-014-0492-8. PubMed PMID: 25359081

[156] Ryan U, Power M. *Cryptosporidium* species in Australian wildlife and domestic animals. Parasitology. 2012;**139**(13):1673-1688. DOI: 10.1017/S0031182012001151. PubMed PMID: 22906836

[157] Raccurt CP. Worldwide human zoonotic cryptosporidiosis caused by *Cryptosporidium* felis. Parasite. 2007;**14**(1):15-20. DOI: 10.1051/parasite/2007141015. PubMed PMID: 17432054

[158] Cieloszyk J, Goni P, Garcia A, Remacha MA, Sanchez E, Clavel A. Two cases of zoonotic cryptosporidiosis in Spain by the unusual species *Cryptosporidium ubiquitum* and *Cryptosporidium felis*. Enfermedades Infecciosas y Microbiología Clínica. 2012;**30**(9):549-551. DOI: 10.1016/j.eimc.2012.04.011. PubMed PMID: 22728073

[159] Silverlas C, Mattsson JG, Insulander M, Lebbad M. Zoonotic transmission of *Cryptosporidium meleagridis* on an organic Swedish farm. International Journal for Parasitology. 2012;**42**(11):963-967. DOI: 10.1016/j.ijpara.2012.08.008. PubMed PMID: 23022616

[160] Cama VA, Ross JM, Crawford S, Kawai V, Chavez-Valdez R, Vargas D, et al. Differences in clinical manifestations among *Cryptosporidium* species and subtypes in HIV-infected persons. The Journal of Infectious Diseases. 2007;**196**(5):684-691. DOI: 10.1086/519842. PubMed PMID: 17674309

[161] Palmer CJ, Xiao L, Terashima A, Guerra H, Gotuzzo E, Saldias G, et al. *Cryptosporidium muris*, a rodent pathogen, recovered from a human in Peru. Emerging Infectious Diseases. 2003;**9**(9):1174-1176. DOI: 10.3201/eid0909.030047. PubMed PMID: 14519260

[162] Al-Brikan FA, Salem HS, Beeching N, Hilal N. Multilocus genetic

analysis of *Cryptosporidium* isolates from Saudi Arabia. Journal of the Egyptian Society of Parasitology. 2008;**38**(2):645-658. PubMed PMID: 18853635

[163] Muthusamy D, Rao SS, Ramani S, Monica B, Banerjee I, Abraham OC, et al. Multilocus genotyping of *Cryptosporidium* sp. isolates from human immunodeficiency virus-infected individuals in South India. Journal of Clinical Microbiology. 2006;**44**(2):632-634. DOI: 10.1128/JCM.44.2.632-634.2006. PubMed PMID: 16455931

[164] Kvac M, Kvetonova D, Sak B, Ditrich O. *Cryptosporidium* pig genotype II in immunocompetent man. Emerging Infectious Diseases. 2009;**15**(6):982-983. DOI: 10.3201/eid1506.071621. PubMed PMID: 19523313

[165] Wang L, Zhang H, Zhao X, Zhang L, Zhang G, Guo M, et al. Zoonotic *Cryptosporidium* species and *Enterocytozoon bieneusi* genotypes in HIV-positive patients on antiretroviral therapy. Journal of Clinical Microbiology. 2013;**51**(2):557-563. DOI: 10.1128/JCM.02758-12. PubMed PMID: 23224097

[166] Xiao L, Bern C, Arrowood M, Sulaiman I, Zhou L, Kawai V, et al. Identification of the *Cryptosporidium* pig genotype in a human patient. The Journal of Infectious Diseases. 2002;**185**(12):1846-1848. DOI: 10.1086/340841. PubMed PMID: 12085341

[167] Bodager JR, Parsons MB, Wright PC, Rasambainarivo F, Roellig D, Xiao L, et al. Complex epidemiology and zoonotic potential for *Cryptosporidium suis* in rural Madagascar. Veterinary Parasitology. 2015;**207**(1-2):140-143. DOI: 10.1016/j.vetpar.2014.11.013. PubMed PMID: 25481280

[168] Raskova V, Kvetonova D, Sak B, McEvoy J, Edwinson A, Stenger B,

et al. Human cryptosporidiosis caused by *Cryptosporidium tyzzeri* and *C. parvum* isolates presumably transmitted from wild mice. Journal of Clinical Microbiology. 2013;**51**(1):360-362. DOI: 10.1128/JCM.02346-12. PubMed PMID: 23100342

[169] Li N, Xiao L, Alderisio K, Elwin K, Cebelinski E, Chalmers R, et al. Subtyping *Cryptosporidium ubiquitum*, a zoonotic pathogen emerging in humans. Emerging Infectious Diseases. 2014;**20**(2):217-224. DOI: 10.3201/eid2002.121797. PubMed PMID: 24447504

[170] Elwin K, Hadfield SJ, Robinson G, Crouch ND, Chalmers RM. *Cryptosporidium viatorum* n. sp. (Apicomplexa: Cryptosporidiidae) among travellers returning to Great Britain from the Indian subcontinent, 2007-2011. International Journal for Parasitology. 2012;**42**(7):675-682. DOI: 10.1016/j.ijpara.2012.04.016. PubMed PMID: 22633952

[171] Garcia RJ, French N, Pita A, Velathanthiri N, Shrestha R, Hayman D. Local and global genetic diversity of protozoan parasites: Spatial distribution of *Cryptosporidium* and *Giardia* genotypes. PLoS Neglected Tropical Diseases. 2017;**11**(7):e0005736. DOI: 10.1371/journal.pntd.0005736. PubMed PMID: 28704362

[172] Kvac M, Hofmannova L, Hlaskova L, Kvetonova D, Vitovec J, McEvoy J, et al. *Cryptosporidium erinacei* n. sp. (Apicomplexa: Cryptosporidiidae) in hedgehogs. Veterinary Parasitology. 2014;**201**(1-2):9-17. DOI: 10.1016/j.vetpar.2014.01.014. PubMed PMID: 24529828

[173] Azami M, Moghaddam DD, Salehi R, Salehi M. The identification of *Cryptosporidium* species (protozoa) in Ifsahan, Iran by PCR-RFLP analysis of the 18S rRNA gene. Molekuliarnaia

Biologiia. 2007;**41**(5):934-939. PubMed PMID: 18240576

[174] Adamu H, Petros B, Zhang G, Kassa H, Amer S, Ye J, et al. Distribution and clinical manifestations of *Cryptosporidium* species and subtypes in HIV/AIDS patients in Ethiopia. PLoS Neglected Tropical Diseases. 2014;**8**(4):e2831. DOI: 10.1371/journal. pntd.0002831. PubMed PMID: 24743521

[175] Ng-Hublin JS, Combs B, Mackenzie B, Ryan U. Human cryptosporidiosis diagnosed in Western Australia: A mixed infection with *Cryptosporidium meleagridis*, the *Cryptosporidium mink* genotype, and an unknown *Cryptosporidium* species. Journal of Clinical Microbiology. 2013;**51**(7):2463-2465. DOI: 10.1128/ JCM.00424-13. PubMed PMID: 23637295

[176] Slapeta J. Cryptosporidiosis and *Cryptosporidium* species in animals and humans: A thirty colour rainbow? International Journal for Parasitology. 2013;**43**(12-13):957-970. DOI: 10.1016/j. ijpara.2013.07.005. PubMed PMID: 23973380

[177] Pintar KD, Pollari F, Waltner-Toews D, Charron DF, McEwen SA, Fazil A, et al. A modified case-control study of cryptosporidiosis (using non-*Cryptosporidium*-infected enteric cases as controls) in a community setting. Epidemiology and Infection. 2009;**137**(12):1789-1799. DOI: 10.1017/S0950268809990197. PubMed PMID: 19527550

[178] Roy SL, DeLong SM, Stenzel SA, Shiferaw B, Roberts JM, Khalakdina A, et al. Risk factors for sporadic cryptosporidiosis among immunocompetent persons in the United States from 1999 to 2001. Journal of Clinical Microbiology. 2004;**42**(7):2944-2951. DOI: 10.1128/ JCM.42.7.2944-2951.2004. PubMed PMID: 15243043

[179] Yoder JS, Beach MJ. *Cryptosporidium* surveillance and risk factors in the United States. Experimental Parasitology. 2010;**124**(1):31-39. DOI: 10.1016/j.exppara.2009.09.020. PubMed PMID: 19786022

[180] King P, Tyler KM, Hunter PR. Anthroponotic transmission of *Cryptosporidium parvum* predominates in countries with poorer sanitation: A systematic review and meta-analysis. Parasites & Vectors. 2019;**12**(1):16. DOI: 10.1186/s13071-018-3263-0. PubMed PMID: 30621759

[181] Nazemalhosseini-Mojarad E, Feng Y, Xiao L. The importance of subtype analysis of *Cryptosporidium* spp. in epidemiological investigations of human cryptosporidiosis in Iran and other mideast countries. Gastroenterology and Hepatology from Bed to Bench. 2012;**5**(2):67-70. PubMed PMID: 24834202

[182] Heiges M, Wang H, Robinson E, Aurrecoechea C, Gao X, Kaluskar N, et al. CryptoDB: A *Cryptosporidium* bioinformatics resource update. Nucleic Acids Research. 2006;**34**:D419-D422. DOI: 10.1093/nar/gkj078. PubMed PMID: 16381902

[183] Abrahamsen MS, Templeton TJ, Enomoto S, Abrahante JE, Zhu G, Lancto CA, et al. Complete genome sequence of the apicomplexan, *Cryptosporidium parvum*. Science. 2004;**304**(5669):441-445. DOI: 10.1126/ science.1094786. PubMed PMID: 15044751

[184] Guo Y, Tang K, Rowe LA, Li N, Roellig DM, Knipe K, et al. Comparative genomic analysis reveals occurrence of genetic recombination in virulent *Cryptosporidium hominis* subtypes and telomeric gene duplications in *Cryptosporidium parvum*. BMC Genomics. 2015;**16**:320. DOI: 10.1186/ s12864-015-1517-1. PubMed PMID: 25903370

[185] Feng Y, Li N, Roellig DM, Kelley A, Liu G, Amer S, et al. Comparative genomic analysis of the IId subtype family of *Cryptosporidium parvum*. International Journal for Parasitology. 2017;**47**(5):281-290. DOI: 10.1016/j.ijpara.2016.12.002. PubMed PMID: 28192123

[186] Mogi T, Kita K. Diversity in mitochondrial metabolic pathways in parasitic protists *Plasmodium* and *Cryptosporidium*. Parasitology International. 2010;**59**(3):305-312. DOI: 10.1016/j.parint.2010.04.005. PubMed PMID: 20433942

[187] Guy RA, Payment P, Krull UJ, Horgen PA. Real-time PCR for quantification of *Giardia* and *Cryptosporidium* in environmental water samples and sewage. Applied and Environmental Microbiology. 2003;**69**(9):5178-5185. DOI: 10.1128/aem.69.9.5178-5185.2003. PubMed PMID: 12957899

Printed in the USA
CPSIA information can be obtained
at www.ICGtesting.com
LVHW051341011023
759814LV00010B/1185